BIOMEDICAL ENGINEERING

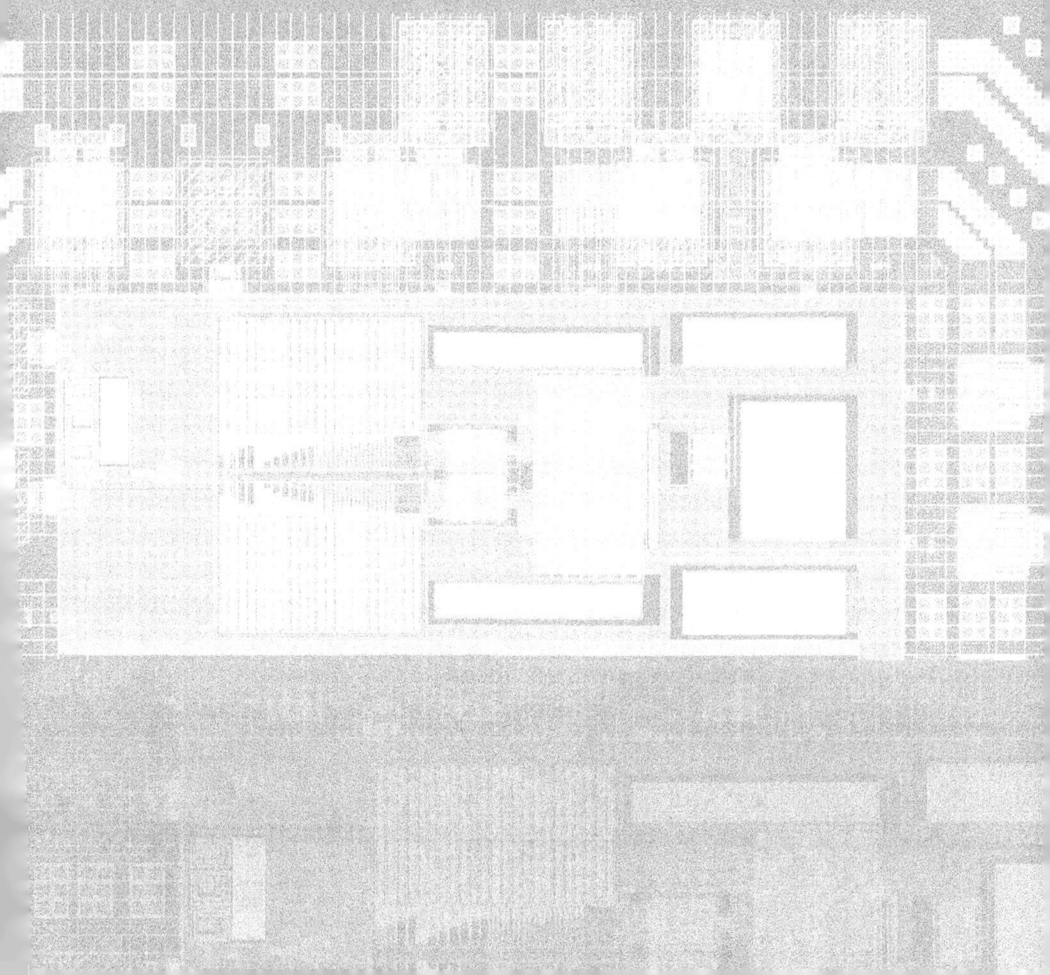

Jenny Stanford Series on Biomedical Engineering *Vol. I*

BIOMEDICAL ENGINEERING

Imaging Systems, Electric Devices, and Medical Materials

edited by

Akihiro Miyauchi

Hiroyuki Kagechika

JENNY STANFORD
PUBLISHING

Published by

Jenny Stanford Publishing Pte. Ltd.
101 Thomson Road
#06-01, United Square
Singapore 307591

Email: editorial@jennystanford.com
Web: www.jennystanford.com

British Library Cataloguing-in-Publication Data
A catalogue record for this book is available from the British Library.

Biomedical Engineering: Imaging Systems, Electric Devices, and Medical Materials

ISBN 978-981-5129-16-8 (Hardcover)
ISBN 978-1-003-46404-4 (eBook)

Contents

Preface

With the coming of an aging society, how to ensure a healthy life expectancy has become a social issue. In addition, the global epidemic of infectious diseases such as COVID-19 has caused confusion in the medical field, and we have witnessed the collapse of medical care in the world. Various issues such as early diagnosis and prevention, minimally invasive treatment, and countermeasures against infectious diseases were reconfirmed in future medical care. Currently, health care workers are demanding the practical realization of new drugs, medical devices, and medical systems that will help solve these problems. Therefore, engineering researchers must translate their advanced technologies into medical applications rapidly.

Against this backdrop, the Research Center of Biomedical Engineering (RCBE) was established in April 2016 through collaboration among four distinguished Japanese institutes: the Institute of Biomaterials and Bioengineering, Tokyo Medical and Dental University; Laboratory for Future Interdisciplinary Research of Science and Technology, Tokyo Institute of Technology; Research Institute for Nanodevices, Hiroshima University; and the Research Institute of Electronics, Shizuoka University. Endorsed by the Japan Ministry of Education, Culture, Sports, Science and Technology, the RCBE aims to promote interaction and collaboration between engineers and medical researchers to revolutionize future medicine and healthcare through the development of innovative technologies. These four research institutes have their own core competencies in different areas of science and technology and the RCBE strengthens their potentials and enhances the collaborations through collaboration with advanced research institutes around the world. The center also fosters young researchers in this interdisciplinary field between medicine and engineering.

This book presents real medical problems and their solutions by leading-edge researchers in engineering. If the readers in this growing research field can get hints or new ideas from this book, it is a pleasure for us.

Akihiro Miyauchi and
Hiroyuki Kagechika
2023

Chapter 1

Manipulation of Mechanical and Functional Properties of the Ti-Au-Based Shape Memory Alloys by Transition Metal Introduction

Wan-Ting Chiu, Masaki Tahara, and Hideki Hosoda

Institute of Innovative Research (IIR), Tokyo Institute of Technology, 4259 Nagatsuta-cho, Midori-ku, Yokohama 226-8501, Japan

chiu.w.aa@m.titech.ac.jp

Shape memory alloys (SMAs) and superelastic (SE) alloys are critical materials among the issues of the urgently demanded biomedical applications and biomaterials. In this chapter, a series of highly potential near-eutectoid Ti-4Au-5M (mol%) (M = transition metals of V, Cr, Mn, Fe, Co, Ni, Cu, and Mo) specimens were systematically explored. Specimens were prepared by physical metallurgy procedures and were evaluated by XRD measurements, microstructure observations, chemical composition analysis, bending examinations, tensile examinations, and so on. Outstanding shape memory effect (SME) exhibiting around 94% shape recovery rate (SR%) was discerned in the Cr element

Biomedical Engineering: Imaging Systems, Electric Devices, and Medical Materials
Edited by Akihiro Miyauchi and Hiroyuki Kagechika

ISBN 978-981-5129-16-8 (Hardcover), 978-1-003-46404-4 (eBook)
www.jennystanford.com

introduced Ti-4Au-based alloy. Furthermore, as the introduced third elements V, Cr, Mn, and Mo, the Ti-4Au-based ternary specimens exhibit slight pseudoelastic (PE) behavior. While no PE is found when the introduced third metals are Fe and Co elements, respectively. Based on the investigations of mechanical behavior, the introduced third metals Cr, Mn, and Mo could be categorized as the optimized group. Judging from the evaluations of their mechanical behavior, SME, and SE effect, respectively, these alloys clearly surpass others. In brief, first, this study systematically investigated the effects of transition metals on the mechanical and functional behaviors of the near-eutectoid Ti-4Au-5M (mol%) SMAs. Second, the Cr-introduced alloy, which is sorted as the optimized group, was further subjected to the manipulation of its chemical composition. Last, fine tailoring of the Ti-4Au-5Cr-based ternary alloy was done by an introduction of the Ta element, which possesses high X-ray contrast and is suitable for biomedical applications. Through step-by-step optimizations, the mechanical behaviors and functionalities of these SMAs have been greatly enhanced. These findings could be guidelines for further investigations of the Ti-4Au-based alloys.

1.1 Introduction

Due to the rapidly growing aging population [1], biomedical applications and biomaterials, such as stents, implant materials, and other surgery materials, are now urgently required [2]. Among the candidates, shape memory alloys (SMAs) and superelastic (SE) alloys, performing a manipulatable shape deformation via controlling the applied stress and/or temperature [3, 4], are considered promising materials for the usages of biomaterials. There are a few essential prerequisites for SMAs toward the aforementioned applications, such as non-toxicity and non-hypersensitivity to the human body, high interfacial adaptableness, high corrosion resistance, and appropriate mechanical behaviors [5]. Among the SMAs, the β-type Ti SMAs have attracted much interest for their outstanding properties, which fulfill the abovementioned critical demands [6]. This work; thus, systematically worked on the β-Ti SMAs for the crucial issues of the urgently required materials for these biomedical applications.

To tune the essential properties and impose functionalities on the β-Ti SMAs, some additional elements have been introduced. Due to a requirement of high biocompatibility to the human body [7], gold (Au) element was chosen for tailoring the β-Ti-based SMAs in view of its non-toxic and non-allergic characteristics. Furthermore, in consideration of long-term usage (i.e., implantation materials) in the human body, Au possesses excellent resistance to corrosion [8], which is a crucial issue for long-term usage in aqueous solutions, such as implant materials. Besides the abovementioned requirements of biocompatibility and corrosion resistance in aqueous solutions, it is also essential to fine-tune the martensitic transformation start temperature (M_s) to around the human body temperature to meet the prerequisites of operation temperature of biomedical materials in the human body. It has been reported that introducing a third element to the aforementioned Ti-Au-based binary SMAs for regulating M_s could be both effective and facile [9, 10]. Elements in the transition metals, such as 3d, 4d, and 5d transition metals, were selected for the reasons of their low-cost, comparatively low melting temperature, comparatively low density, and being earth-abundant metals [11]. Additionally, it has also been claimed that there is a good relationship between the behaviors of phase transformation of the Ti-based alloys and the electron configurations of transition metals [9, 12]. Accordingly, following the Au addition, a screening of the Ti-Au-M ternary SMAs via the introduction of different transition metals (M = V, Cr, Mn, Fe, Co, Ni, Cu, and Mo) into the Ti-Au-based SMAs as third metals were carried out.

Some reports have proven that the chosen transition metals are considered to be biocompatible as merely a small additional amount is introduced into the Ti alloys. Moreover, most of the selected elements have been claimed as essential metals for the human body [13–15]. It, therefore, could consider that, overall, the chosen alloys are basically biocompatible. Nevertheless, Sc and Zn were not preferred for the 3d transition metal elements. The reason to exclude the Sc element is because of its low biocompatibility, relatively high price, and great inclination to be oxidized [16]. In the case of Zn, the relatively low boiling temperature could result in problematic procedures in the alloying procedure [17] (i.e., the comparatively non-manipulatable chemical composition of specimens); therefore, as an additional element, Zn was also ruled out.

Despite the potential candidates of the binary Ti-Au-based SMAs and their corresponding ternary and quaternary alloy systems for the communities of biomedical applications and biomaterials, the binary Ti-Au correlated literature is relatively inadequate compared to the Ti-Ni, Ti-Nb, Ti-Zr, and their higher order system alloys [18–22]. Concerning the Ti-Au binary alloy systems, the phase transformation of $\beta \rightarrow \alpha_m$ was reported by Plichta and the collaborators. Here, the α-massive (α_m) martensite is generated from the massive transformation of the binary Ti-Au alloy system and other Ti-based systems [23, 24]. To screen a wide range of the Ti-Au alloys, Xin et al. investigated hardness and observed microstructures of six different $Ti_{1-x}Au_x$ alloys by a casting method (Au molar fraction = 0.220–0.800, respectively), which were broadly distributed in this binary Ti-Au phase diagram [25].

In addition to the abovementioned binary Ti-Au alloy system, a few of its ternary and quaternary systems were also carried out. Regarding the near-equivalent $Ti_{50}Au_{50}$ intermetallic compound, Kawamura et al. studied the influences of the third addition element on the M_s and further investigated the factors for manipulating their M_s in the $Ti_{50}Au_{50}$-based alloys [9]. Wadood et al. studied the phase constituents, phase transformation, oxidation behaviors, and SME of the Ti-Au-Ag-Zr quaternary alloys [26] and ternary Ti-50Au-10Zr alloys [10]. Shinohara et al. investigated the effects of various temperatures for annealing treatments on the development of alloy microstructures and variations of the SE behaviors of the Ti-Au-Cr-Zr quaternary alloys; in addition, their deformation behaviors were also studied [27, 28]. Zadorozhnyy et al. worked on the analysis of micro-structures, mechanical behaviors, and biocompatible characteristics of the Ti-Fe-Au-Nb alloy system [29]. The abovementioned articles revealed various influences of the third and the fourth introduced elements on the performances of the binary Ti-Au-based alloy systems.

However, no report concerning the influences of the addition of transition metals on the features of the promising near-eutectoid Ti-4Au (mol%) specimen has been studied. Additionally, given that the phase transformation behavior is strongly affected by electron configurations as mentioned above, this chapter; therefore, systematically studied the influences of the transition metal additions on the phase constituents, mechanical behaviors, SME, and SE effect of the near-eutectoid Ti-4Au-5M (mol%) (M = V, Cr, Mn, Fe, Co, Ni, Cu, and Mo transition metals) systems. A succession of basic evaluations was provided and the high-potential specimens were pointed out. This chapter could be an imperative database and a guideline for the research of this promising near-eutectoid Ti-4Au-5M (mol%) alloy. Please note that due to both the considerations of the alloy design and heat treatments, the Au element with 4 mol% was selected for the eutectoid phase transformation in this binary Ti-Au alloy system and also for the relatively low temperature for the heat-treatment process [25]. Likewise, the cause for the introduction of the transition metals of 5 mol% was also by reason of their eutectoid transformation at approximately 5 mol% in most of the introduced metals, which have been selected. Moreover, based on some preliminary findings, good mechanical behaviors via the 5 mol% addition concentration have been observed in some of the ternary systems [30–33].

A research flow chart, which demonstrates the development history of the Ti-Au-based SMAs, is summarized in Figure 1.1. Some results are extracted and shown in this chapter. First, part (A), which corresponds to the aforementioned screening of the transition metals, is discussed in Section 1.3. Second, based on the results of the screening of the transition elements, it was found that the Cr-introduced specimens performed high shape recovery strain (SRS), proper mechanical behaviors, and good cold workability (CW). The Ti-Au-Cr alloys, which have been discussed in our publication [34], were subjected to further optimization via the manipulation of their chemical composition.

Besides the aforesaid elements, tantalum (Ta), which is a β-stabilizer, was designated for further fine-modification of the functionalities (i.e., SME and SE) of the Ti-4Au-5Cr-based

SMAs [8]. Judging from the phase diagram of the Ti-Ta binary alloy, a solid-solution phase region (i.e., isomorphous) exists throughout the entire Ta concentration range [17]. The abovementioned α-massive martensite, which performs neither SME nor SE, could also be constrained by the introduction of Ta element and could be transformed into the functional α″-martensite phase by undergoing the martensitic transformation (MT) [18–20]. Besides the purpose of imposing functionalities on the alloys, Ta, as a heavy element, performs high X-ray contrast for the uses of biomedical materials (i.e., guidewires) [21, 22]. Moreover, regarding the biocompatible issues to the human body, Ta also performs high biocompatibility [23–25]. In consideration of the aforementioned merits of the Ta element, it thus was selected as the fourth element for the operation of the Ti-Au-Cr-based SMAs toward biomedical applications. The Ta-introduced Ti-Au-Cr-based SMAs are discussed in Section 1.4 and are symbolized as part (B) in Figure 1.1.

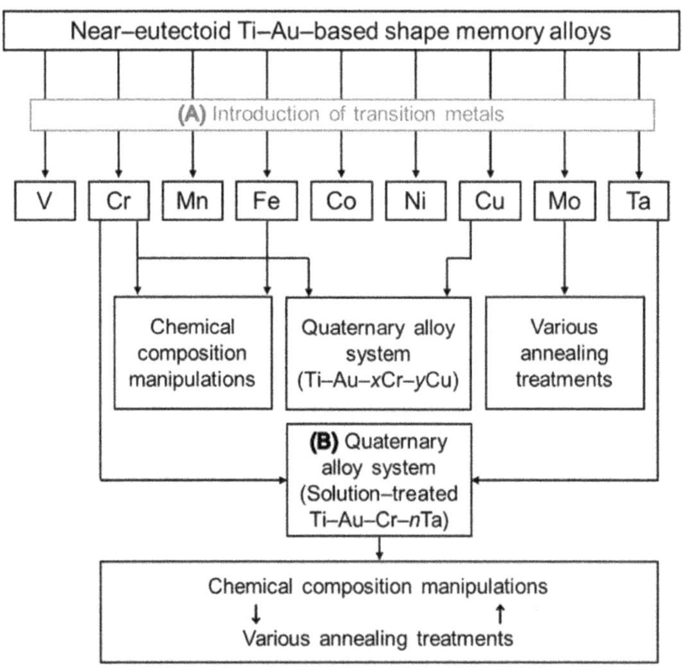

Figure 1.1 Research flow chart of the Ti-Au-based SMAs.

1.2 Experimental

1.2.1 Chemicals

Titanium (Ti), gold (Au), vanadium (V), chromium (Cr), magnesium (Mn), iron (Fe), cobalt (Co), nickel (Ni), copper (Cu), molybdenum (Mo), and tantalum (Ta) are high purity (purity ≥ 99.9%) raw metals, which were utilized to fabricate the specimens. Each raw metal was obtained from Kojundo Chemical Lab. Co., Ltd. Among all metals, Ti sponge and Fe powder were re-melted followed by a cold-rolling (CR) to obtain Ti and Fe sheets. The edges of sheet metals were excluded to heighten their purity. The purified sheets were then used as starting materials to manufacture the designated specimens with a particular composition. The Ar-1H_2 (vol.%) atmosphere was applied during this high-temperature procedure for reducing oxidation reactions of the specimens while they were applied in the high-temperature molten process. As-received chemicals of perchloric acid ($HClO_4$; 60–62%, Kanto Chemical Co. Inc.), butanol (C_4H_9OH; 99.0%, Kanto Chemical Co. Inc.), and methanol (CH_3OH, 99.8%, Kishida Chemical Co. Ltd.) were utilized for conducting an electropolishing.

1.2.2 Alloy Fabrication

In this chapter, two different groups of alloys were fabricated, respectively. The (A) ternary Ti-4Au-5M (mol%) (M = V, Cr, Mn, Fe, Co, Ni, Cu, and Mo) alloys and the (B) Ti-4Au-5Cr-*n*Ta (mol%) (n = 1, 2, 3, 4, 5, 6, 7, and 9) alloys (Figure 1.1) were fabricated by using an arc-melting system equipped with a non-consumable tungsten electrode under the Ar-1H_2 (vol.%) atmosphere, respectively. The specimens of the Ti-4Au-5M (mol%) alloys of the group (A) are abbreviated as "Ti-4Au-5M" by excluding the unit of mol% in the entire article unless otherwise mentioned. The group (B) is also abbreviated as "Ti-4Au-5Cr-*n*Ta" alloys.

The aforementioned alloyed ingots were subsequently sealed into quartz tubes and homogenized at 1273 K for 7.2 ks under high purity Ar atmosphere. The homogenization treatment was followed by a water-quenching (W.Q.) of the specimens by immersing the specimens rapidly into iced water. The homogenized ingots are abbreviated as "HT ingots" unless otherwise mentioned. The surface of HT ingots was then mechanically ground for removing surface contaminations. Cleaned HT ingots were thereafter cold-worked until a 98% reduction of specimen thickness. The cold-worked specimens show a thickness of about 0.2 mm, respectively. For those ingots, which were not able to be cold-worked up to 98% reduction of thickness, they were subjected to an annealing process and were cold-worked again until the 98% reduction in thickness was achieved.

These cold-worked alloys were shaped into particular structures and dimensions, wrapped by Ti-foil, vacuum-sealed into quartz tubes, immersed into a high-purity Ar atmosphere, and solution-treated (ST) at 1173 K for 0.9 ks. Please note that the temperature of 1173 K indicates the region of the single β-phase in the phase diagram of the binary Ti-Au alloy system [35]. The ST specimens were eventually immersed in iced water for conducting a quenching process. An illustration to show the overall thermal-mechanical procedures is revealed in Figure 1.2. Please note that the alloys in two different groups (i.e., group (A) and (B)) were fabricated by exactly identical procedures except for the alloy compositions.

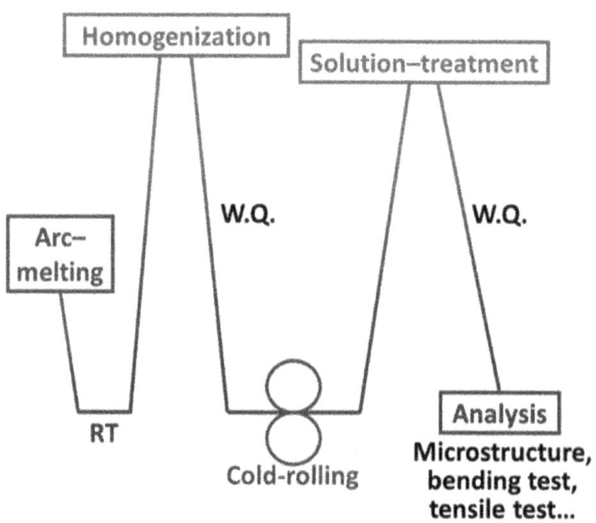

Figure 1.2 Illustration of overall thermal-mechanical processes.

1.2.3 Phase Identification and Lattice Parameter Analysis

An X-ray diffractometer (XRD; X'Pert PRO MPD, PANalytical) was carried out to characterize the phase constituents and crystal structures of the alloys. Before these XRD measurements, ST alloys were ground by SiC papers (from #800 to #4000) and also polished by diamond pastes (from 5 μm to 1 μm), followed by an electro-polishing method in an electrolyte of 6% $HClO_4$: 35% C_4H_9OH : 59% CH_3OH at the temperature range of 213–223 K for 0.6 ks. The XRD examination was conducted at room temperature (RT; i.e., 296±3 K) with radiation of CuK_α by utilizing a Philips X'Pert-Pro Galaxy system. A silicon plate was used as a standard material for the correction of system errors. Concerning the calculation of lattice parameters, a unit cell parameter refinement program on a Windows computer was utilized to precisely determine their lattice parameters [36]. Here, the CellCalc is based on the method of least-square by using the reciprocal lattice parameters. The lattice parameters of the orthorhombic α''-martensite phase are labeled as $a_{\alpha''}$, $b_{\alpha''}$, and $c_{\alpha''}$ and are defined as $b_{\alpha''} > c_{\alpha''} > a_{\alpha''}$.

1.2.4 Microstructure Observation and Composition Analysis

Microstructure observations were carried out by using a scanning electron microscopy (SEM) and the chemical compositions were also examined by an energy-dispersive spectroscopy (EDS), which was attached to the SEM. The elemental mapping of chemical compositions of different elements was further carried out for the observations of the distribution of each element. Besides the elemental mapping, a point analysis was also carried out at least 10 times at random positions for precise detection and also for building error bars. Prior to the microstructure observations and chemical composition analysis, specimens are subjected to the identical pre-treatments that were carried out before the X-ray diffraction measurements were conducted. The chemical composition of each phase was eventually determined by averaging the point analysis results, whose top 2 and bottom 2 data were ruled out.

1.2.5 Mechanical Property Evaluations

1.2.5.1 Bending examinations

Bending examinations were conducted to estimate the SME of the specimens. The alloys were bent up to a 5% surface strain first, followed by a heating-up process via a lighter or a furnace secondly to determine their strain recovery behaviors. The heating-up temperature for activating their shape recovery behaviors was approximately 900–1300 K.

1.2.5.2 Tensile examinations

Mechanical behaviors of the alloys were exanimated by utilizing an Instron-type universal testing machine (AG1kNI Autograph, Shimadzu). Two different tensile examinations were conducted at RT under ambient. They are (1) continuous tensile examinations until the fracture of the alloys and (2) cyclic loading-unloading tensile examinations. The "cyclic loading-unloading tensile examination" is abbreviated as "cyclic examination" unless otherwise mentioned. A strain rate of ~8×10^{-4} s^{-1} was imposed on the alloys in both the abovementioned tensile examinations. The gauge length, width, and thickness of the alloys were approximately 10 mm, 2 mm, and 0.2 mm, respectively. External stress loading direction to the alloys was along with the rolling direction (RD). The (2) cyclic examinations were carried out with a 1% constant strain increase each cycle and the cycle was repeated up to the overall strain of 10% or a fracture of the testing alloys.

1.3 Ti-4Au-5M Alloy Systems

1.3.1 Cold Workability

CW of the Ti-4Au-5M specimens is revealed in Figure 1.3. Among all the specimens, essentially, there are three different outcomes in the results of the CW.

Firstly, the group (I) of the Cr, Fe, Co, and Mo introduced alloys, which were capable to be cold-rolled up to 98% reduction of thickness without any annealing procedure, perform an excellent CW. Second, the group (II) of the V- and Mn-introduced alloys were merely capable to be cold-worked up to around 50% thickness reduction in the first CR procedure. As expressed in the experimental section, a specific annealing treatment was carried out after the first CR procedure. The group (II) specimens of the V and Mn were then capable to be cold-worked up to the 98% reduction of thickness after performing an annealing process. Lastly, the group (III) of the Ni- and Cu-introduced alloys were not capable to be cold-worked even an annealing procedure was carried out, implying their inferior CW. The group (I), (II), and (III) are symbolized as solid red circles, green solid and networked circles, and blue open circles in Figure 1.3. The specimens, which are not subjected to any annealing treatment, are denoted by solid circle symbols, while the specimens, which experienced a specific annealing process, are symbolized as network-structured circles. The specimens, which show deteriorated CW, are indicated by open-circle symbols.

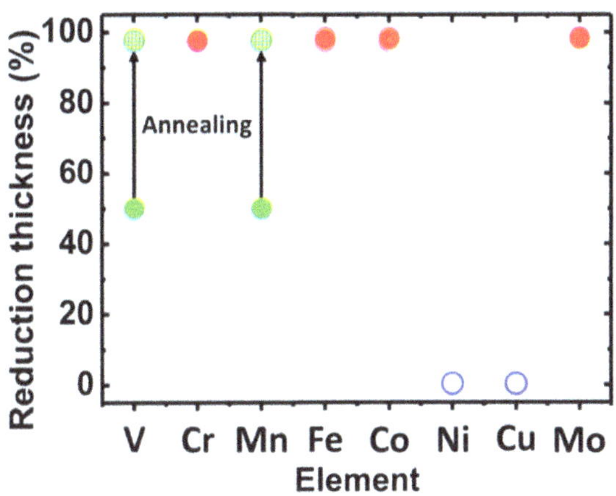

Figure 1.3 CW of all specimens with transition metal introduced.

1.3.2 Phase Identification

The XRD patterns of the Ti-4Au-5M specimens at RT under ambient are shown in Figure 1.4. The phase constituents in nine different specimens, which were with different introductions of transition metals, are distributed into four different categories: (i) the single α′-martensite phase, (ii) the dual α′+β-phase, (iii) the parent β-phase + limited precipitates with an A15 crystal structure, and (iv) the single parent β-phase.

First, the apparent phase of the (a) Ti-4Au binary alloy as well as the (b) V-, (c) Cr-, and (h) Cu-introduced ternary alloys, which was the single α′-phase with an hcp crystal structure, are classified into the group (I). Whether the phase with an hcp crystal structure in the (a) binary Ti-4Au alloy, (b) V-, (c) Cr-, and (h) Cu-introduced ternary alloys are the martensitic α (α′)-phase or a massive α (α_m)-phase was not recognized. The phase with an hcp crystal structure is simply labeled as α′ in the XRD profiles in Figure 1.4. Judging from the (a) Ti-4Au binary alloy, (b) V-, and (c) Cr-introduced ternary alloys, their diffraction peak intensities in the XRD profiles vary from specimen to specimen. High intensities of the $100_{\alpha'}$ and the $101_{\alpha'}$ diffraction peaks were observed in the (a) Ti-4Au binary specimen; inversely, high intensities of the $002_{\alpha'}$ and the $101_{\alpha'}$ were discerned in the (c) Ti-4Au-5Cr ternary specimen. Additionally, diffraction peaks at a high angle range were not detected in the (c) Ti-4Au-5Cr ternary alloy, while they were obviously detected in the (a) Ti-4Au binary alloy. The XRD pattern of the (b) Ti-4Au-5V ternary alloy was in the middle of the (a) Ti-4Au binary alloy and the (c) Ti-4Au-5Cr ternary alloy. This result indicates that the crystal orientations, which were caused by the introduction of the third metal, follow the inclination of the atomic number of the added transition metals. The differences imply that the alloy texture after recrystallization by the ST process is influenced by the third element introduced.

Second, following the (a) Ti-4Au binary alloy, (b) V-, and (c) Cr-introduced ternary alloys, which show the single α′-phase, the (d) Mn-introduced specimen is composed of a dual phase of α′+β. Third, the phase constituents of the (e) Fe- and (f) Co-introduced alloys are the parent β-phase; in addition, some diffraction peaks of a phase possessing a crystal structure of A15 in low intensity were further discerned in these two alloys. Lastly, the phase constituents in the (g) Ni- and (i) Mo-introduced alloys are the single parent β-phase.

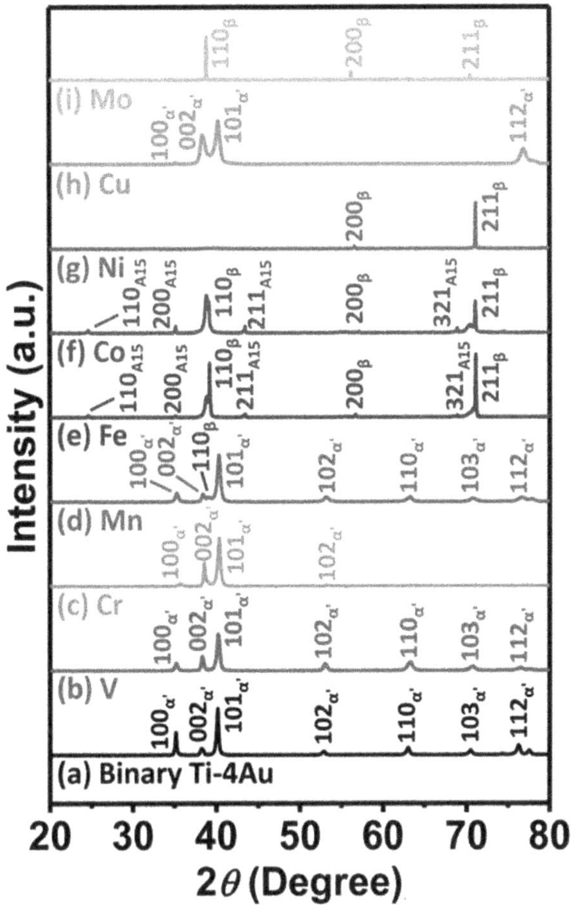

Figure 1.4 The XRD profiles of the (a) binary Ti-4Au specimen and the Ti-4Au-5M (M = V (b); Cr (c); Mn (d); Fe (e); Co (f), Ni (g); Cu (h); Mo (i)) ternary specimens at RT under ambient.

Regarding the XRD profiles, it is obvious that along with the increasing atomic number of the introduced elements, the apparent phases transformed in the sequence of (i) single α′-phase → (ii) α′+β-dual phase → (iii) parent β-phase with a phase possessing a crystal structure of A15 → (iv) single parent β-phase without any other secondary phase. The evolution of the phase transformation essentially follows the atomic number of the transition metals, indicating a reverse relationship of the MT (or massive transformation) temperature to the atomic number of the introduced transition metals as a third element. In brief, the higher the atomic number of the transition metal elements the lower the temperature of MT. It is needed to mention that there is an abrupt variation of the phase constituents of the (h) 5Cu-introduced alloy. It has been revealed that the Cu element in the raw of the 3d transition metal merely stabilizes the β-phase slightly [9], implying that the phase constituent formed could be the single α′-phase rather than the parent β-phase.

In addition to the abovementioned phase transformation from the α′-phase to the β-phase, it is also observed that with the rise in the atomic number (i.e., from Fe element to Ni element), the 110_β intensity at approximately $2\theta = 40^\circ$ decreases. Similar to the (a) Ti-4Au binary alloy, (b) V-, and (c) Cr-introduced ternary alloys, this result indicates that the crystal structure orientations, which were the outcomes of the introduced third elements, follow a good inclination of the atomic number of the introduced transition metals. This evolution tendency of the diffraction peak intensities indicates that the alloy texture after the recrystallization by the ST process is changed by the introduced third elements in a good correlation.

As stated previously, an abrupt alteration of the apparent phase in the (h) Ti-4Au-5Cu specimen was found; therefore, the reasons are explained as follows. First, it is known that the electron configurations of the Cr and Cu elements are $[Ar]3d^54s^1$ and $[Ar]3d^{10}4s^1$, respectively. In contrast, in the raw of the 3d transition metal, electron configurations of the Mn, Fe, Co, and Ni elements, which are composed of the dual α′+β-phase or the single parent β-phase (with or without the phase possessing the A15 crystal structure), are $[Ar]3d^54s^2$, $[Ar]3d^64s^2$, $[Ar]3d^74s^2$, and $[Ar]3d^84s^2$, respectively. The valence shell electron configuration of the 4s-orbital is known to be a primary reason for the resulting apparent phase of the β-Ti-based alloys [9]. Here, please note that the phase possessing the A15 crystal structure is recognized as the Ti_3Au phase in advance. Analysis in detail is discussed in the following chemical composition analysis results.

Second, besides the abovementioned electron configuration of the introduced third elements, it is also well-known that the MT is strongly altered by the electron-to-atom (e/a) ratio [9, 37]. The values of (s + d) are 4 for Ti, 11 for Au, and 11 for Cu. For instance, in Ti-4Au-5Cu alloy, its e/a ratio is 0.91 × 4 of Ti + 0.04 × 11 of Au + 0.05 × 11 of Cu. Because the total number of electrons in the s- and d-orbitals of Au and Cu elements are identical, the e/a values are exactly identical for these two specimens (i.e., with or without Cu replacement). The impact of the Cu introduction into the Ti-4Au binary alloy could merely be minor due to the same e/a ratio of these two elements. From the aforementioned two explanations, it thus could be concluded that the abrupt change of the apparent phase in the ternary (h) 5Cu-introduced specimen to the single α'-phase, which is the same as the (a) Ti-4Au binary alloy, would be also a result of the influence of the e/a ratios.

1.3.3 Mechanical Behavior Evaluations

1.3.3.1 Bending examinations

Figure 1.5 shows the different shapes in the bending examinations. State (i) before bending deformation, state (ii) after bending deformation with a surface strain of 5%, and state (iii) upon heating process are displayed at the top columns, respectively, representing different statuses in the bending examinations. In Figure 1.5, first, the (b) Cr-, (c) Mn-, and (f) Mo-introduced alloys obviously perform SME (i.e., open circle symbols in the righthand-side column). Among them, the recovery strains of the (b) Cr- and (f) Mo-introduced specimens are superior to that of the (c) Mn alloyed specimen. Second, (a) the V-introduced specimen exhibits a slight SRS (i.e., open triangle in the righthand-side column). Lastly, the (d) Fe- and (e) Co-introduced alloys do not perform SME (i.e., cross symbols in the righthand-side column). The shape recovery strain percentage (SRS%) of the Ti-4Au-5M (M = V (a); Cr (b); Mn (c); Mo (f)) specimens, performing SME, are calculated to be 20%, 94%, 59%, and 89%, respectively.

It is supposed that the SME of the (f) Mo-introduced alloy origins from the stress-induced martensitic transformation (SIMT) and its reverse transformation since its phase constituent before bending deformation is the single β-phase (Figure 1.4). While the SME of the (c) Mn-introduced specimen is triggered by both the SIMT and martensite variant reorientations (MVR) and their reverse transformations due to the dual $\alpha'+\beta$-phase before bending deformation (Figure 1.4). On the other hand, it is unexpected that the (a) V- and (b) Cr-introduced alloys possessed SME even though their phase constituents before deformation by bending was the non-thermoelastic α′-martensite phase, which is considered to possess no SME. Here, it is speculated that the α′-phase is at the exact borderline of the α′-phase and the α″-phase. Accordingly, it is inferred that the SME originates from the thermoelastic α″-phase, which is a martensite phase possessing shape memory behavior. Further studies relating to the recognition of the α′-phase and the α″-phase are necessary.

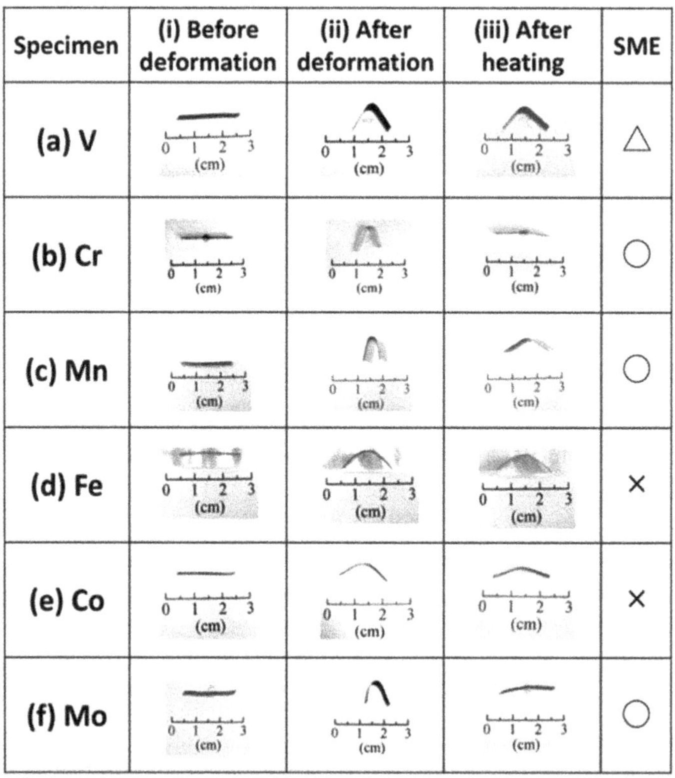

Figure 1.5 Optical images of the Ti-4Au-5M (M = V (a); Cr (b); Mn (c); Fe (d); Co (e); Mo (f)) specimens at the states of (i) before applying bending stress, (ii) after applying bending stress, and (iii) upon a heating process.

Oppositely, no SME is revealed as the introduced third metals were the (d) Fe and (e) Co elements (Figure 1.5). From the XRD patterns in Figure 1.4, it is apparent that the Ti_3Au phase was merely found in the Ti-4Au-5Fe alloy and the Ti-4Au-5Co alloy, respectively. Among all the specimens, those specimens, which do not perform SME, are the Ti-4Au-5Fe and the Ti-4Au-5Co alloys coincidentally. It is, therefore, concluded that the vanishing of the SME was strongly related to the presence of the Ti_3Au phase. It is also worth noticing that the abovementioned phenomenon was exactly the same as those revealed in the earlier reports [29]. For further information, please refer to the literature concerning the Ti-Au-Fe alloy [38].

1.3.3.2 Continuous tensile examinations

Stress-strain (SS) curves of the Ti-4Au-5M specimens are shown in Figure 1.6. Please note that, among the specimens, the Ti-4Au-5Ni and Ti-4Au-5Cu specimens were not examined, owing to their poor workability as shown in Figure 1.3. It was discovered that there are stress plateaus in the (c) Cr-, (d) Mn-, and (g) Mo-introduced alloys. These plateau regimes after the first yielding (marked by dashed lines), which could be caused by the MVR and/or the SIMT, were observed clearly in these three specimens. Based on the XRD profiles (Figure 1.4), the apparent phases of the (c) Cr-, (d), Mn-, and (g) Mo-introduced specimens are the single α'-phase, the dual α'+β-phase, and the single parent β-phase, respectively. Thus, the stress plateaus of these three specimens were deduced to be the commencement of the single MVR, mixed MVR and/or SIMT, and the single SIMT, respectively. In contrast, given that the Ti-4Au-5V alloy shows merely smear SME (Figure 1.5(a)), no obvious stress plateau could be found in its SS curves by the continuous tensile examinations (Figure 1.6(b)).

The ultimate tensile strength (UTS) and the fracture strain (ε_f) of the Ti-4Au-5M ternary specimens were read from Figure 1.6 and then plotted in Figure 1.7. Obviously, the UTS of each ternary specimen is higher than that of the Ti-4Au binary specimen because of the contribution from the strengthening of solid solution and/or precipitation. First, the UTS of the 5V-, 5Mn-, and 5Co-introduced specimens are about double that of the binary alloy Ti-4Au. Second, the 5Cr- and the 5Mo-introduced specimens are about 1.5 times greater than the Ti-4Au binary alloy. Lastly, the 5Fe-introduced specimen is even three times greater than the Ti-4Au binary alloy. On the whole, the UTS increases with the atomic number, reaches the greatest UTS by the Fe introduction, and decreases after the maximum of UTS caused by the Ti-4Au-5Fe sample.

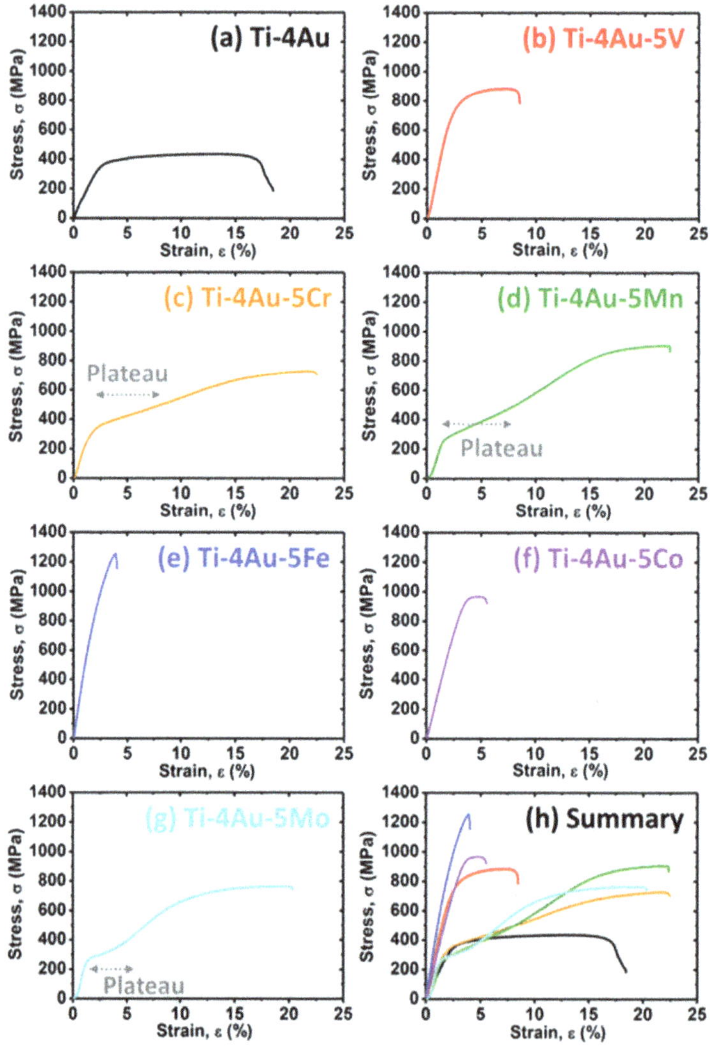

Figure 1.6 SS curves attained from the continuous tensile examinations of the (a) Ti-4Au binary alloy, Ti-4Au-5M (M = V (b); Cr (c); Mn (d); Fe (e); Co (f); Mo (g)) ternary alloys at RT. (h) Summary of all specimens. Both the 5Ni- and 5Cu-introduced samples were not examined because of their poor CW.

However, the ε_f of the ternary specimens are not enhanced in all element introduction circumstances (Figure 1.7(b)). In all alloys, ε_f of V-, Fe-, and Co-introduced specimens are poorer than that of the binary Ti-4Au alloy; inversely, the ε_f of the Cr-, Mn-, and Mo-introduced specimens are enhanced than that of the Ti-4Au binary alloy. The ε_f of the Ti-4Au-5V specimen is half that of the binary one; while the Fe- and Co-introduced alloys are almost 4 times more deteriorated than that of the binary Ti-4Au alloy (Figure 1.7(b)). As expected, the Ti-4Au-5Fe and Ti-4Au-5Co alloys perform the lowest two ε_f since the Ti_3Au intermetallic compound is considered to be brittle and hard, leading to a deteriorated elongation behavior of the specimens [39].

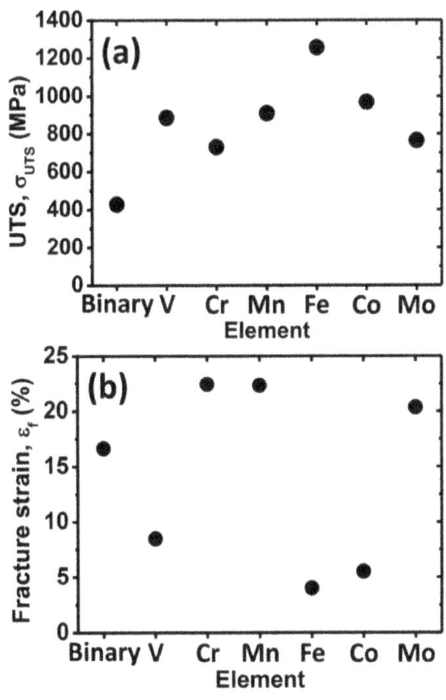

Figure 1.7 (a) UTS and (b) ε_f acquired from the continuous tensile examinations of the binary Ti-4Au specimen and the Ti-4Au-5M (M = V; Cr; Mn; Fe; Co; Mo) ternary specimens. The 5Ni- and 5Cu-introduced specimens were not conducted, owing to their poor CW.

The correlation of the UTS and the ε_f of each specimen is plotted in Figure 1.8. Although the 5V-introduced specimen deviates from the tendency to some extent in UTS and ε_f, it is clear that the UTS of the specimens increases with the atomic number of the third element, reached the utmost UTS by the Ti-4Au-5Fe specimen, and decreases after the maximum UTS. On the other hand, ε_f of the specimens is lowered to its minimum via the Fe-tailoring and is enhanced after the minimum point. These show the nearly reverse tendency between the strength and elongation of the specimens. The strength and elongation of the specimens, which are traded off at the upper-right corner of Figure 1.8, are circled by a gray square with dashed lines. It is noticed that these Ti-4Au-5M ternary specimens with the elements such as Cr, Mn, and Mo metals are the optimized ones in terms of the mechanical behaviors compared to the addition-free one and other ternary ones.

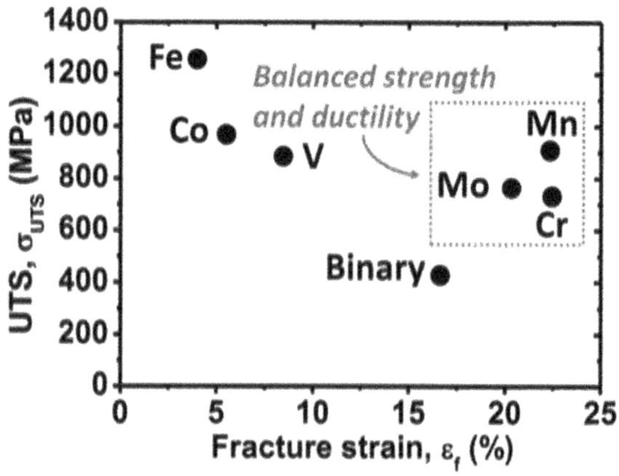

Figure 1.8 The correlation between UTS and ε_f of the Ti-4Au binary specimen and the Ti-4Au-5M (M = V; Cr; Mn; Fe; Co; Mo) ternary alloys. The Ti-4Au-5Ni and Ti-4Au-5Cu alloys were not exanimated owing to their non-workability.

Basically, in Figure 1.8, all the specimens are sorted into three categories. The Ti-4Au-5Fe and Ti-4Au-5Co alloys are in the high-strength classification presenting high strength, low elongation, and no SME. The Ti-4Au-5Cr, Ti-4Au-5Mn, and Ti-4Au-5Mo specimens are the optimized ones, exhibiting proper strength, good elongation, and excellent SME. The Ti-4Au-5V specimen, which is distributed to the medium group, possesses the strength and ductility between the high-strength group and the optimized group. Further explorations of the optimized alloys, such as the management of the microstructures and phase constituents by fine-adjusting the chemical composition, are stated in Section 1.4.

It is worth noting that, in terms of mechanical behaviors, the Ti-4Au-5Mn specimen showed slight improvement as compared to the Ti-4Au-5Mo specimen in the optimized classification. Besides the mechanical behaviors, the Mn element, which is lighter than Mo [40], is thought to be a better candidate for the applications of biomedical materials. Additionally, the Mn ion, which is considered an essential trace element in the human body, indicates better biocompatibility than the Mo-introduced specimen [41]. Moreover, according to Figure 1.8, the Ti-4Au-5Cr alloy is also comparable to the Ti-4Au-5Mo specimen. Cr element further possesses low density, being an essential trace element in the human body, and low price as compared to the Mo metal. In addition, both Cr and Mn elements possess lower melting points than the Mo element [42], suggesting less energy consumption during the manufacture of the specimens. Therefore, based on the aforementioned truths, better applicability of Ti-4Au-5Cr and Ti-4Au-5Mn alloys than that of the Ti-4Au-5Mo alloy was found in this chapter.

1.3.3.3 Cyclic loading-unloading tensile examinations

The SS curves of the cyclic examinations of the Ti-4Au-5M ternary specimens are shown in Figure 1.9. Among all these specimens, the (a) V-, (b) Cr-, (c) Mn-, and (f) Mo-introduced specimens performed slight pseudoelasticity (PE) and/or limited superelasticity (SE) effect. Since the (a) V and (b) Cr alloys are composed of the single α'-martensite phase (Figure 1.4) at RT before loading of tensile stress. The slight PE effect of these two specimens was considered to be due to reversible MVR during the cyclic process. The limited PE of the (c) Ti-4Au-5Mn specimen was caused by the reversible MVR (major) and/or the SIMT (minor). While the limited SE of the (f) Ti-4Au-5Mo alloy could be attributed to the SIMT during first loading and MVR during first unloading due to its single parent β-phase at RT (Figure 1.4(i)). From the second cycle, SIMT and/or MVR took place during loading while MVR commenced during unloading.

On the other hand, no SE nor PE effect is observed in the (d) Fe- and (e) Co-introduced ternary specimens.

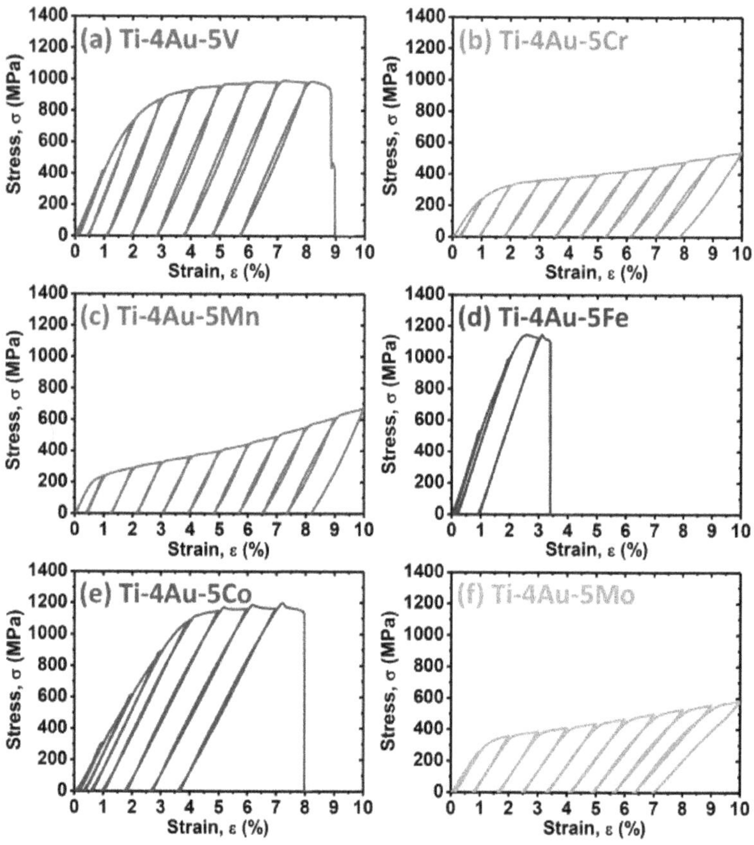

Figure 1.9 SS curves of cyclic examinations of the Ti-4Au-5M (M = V (a); Cr (b); Mn (c); Fe (d); Co (e); Mo (f)) ternary ST specimens. The 5Ni- and 5Cu-introduced alloys were not conducted, owing to their limited workability by a CR process.

This chapter shows a screening of the ternary Ti-4Au-5M specimens (M = numerous transition metals), and the fundamental results acquired could be a database and a useful guideline for future investigations of the highly potential near-eutectoid ternary Ti-4Au-5M-based alloy systems. Judging from the abovementioned results achieved, the thirdly introduced elements of Cr and Mn metals, which were categorized as the optimized classification based on the trade-off between UTS and fracture strain, could be promising candidates for the SMA applications. In addition, it was further found that the Ti-4Au-5Cr specimen possesses a much better SME than that of the Ti-4Au-5Mn alloy (Figure 1.5). Further research concerning these Ti-4Au-5Cr-based specimens was thus conducted and discussed in the following Section 1.4.

1.3.4 Brief Summaries of the Ti-4Au-5M Alloys

The phase constituents and the fundamental mechanical behaviors of the Ti-4Au-5M (M = V; Cr; Mn; Fe; Co; Ni; Cu; Mo) ternary specimens were systematically investigated. The important discoveries of this Ti-4Au-based alloy system are listed as follows:

(1) Among all the tested transition metals, when the thirdly introduced elements are V, Cr, Mn, Fe, Co, and Mo elements, proper CW was found.

(2) The specimens, except for V and Mn elements, were able to be cold-worked with a 98% reduction of thickness without introducing any annealing process.

(3) The parent β-phase remained at RT via the introduction of the third element of Mn, Fe, Co, Ni, and Mo metals to the Ti-4Au binary specimen. The influence of the transition metals on reducing the martensitic transformation start temperature (M_s) of the Ti-4Au-based specimens is consistent with that of the Ti-18Nb-based specimens in the literature.

(4) The alloys, which were alloyed with the third metals of Cr, Mn, and Mo elements, obviously perform the shape memory effect (SME). It was expected that the SME of the Ti-4Au-5Cr alloy was caused by the martensite variant reorientation (MVR) during loading and reverse MT upon heating since its apparent phase at RT was believed to locate at exactly the borderline of the α′-martensite phase and the α″-martensite phase.

(5) Different from the Ti-4Au-5Cr alloy, the reason for the observed shape memory behavior of the Ti-4Au-5Mn could be attributed to its dual α′+β-phase, which could undergo reversible MVR and/or SIMT.

(6) The alloys, which are alloyed with the third element of Cr, Mn, and Mo metals, are categorized as the optimized group

with balanced strength and ductility. These alloys are superior in the mechanical behaviors, such as strength and elongation, to the Ti-Au binary alloy and other transition metal introduced ternary specimens based on the fundamental evaluations of the strength, elongation, and also SME.

(7) As the introduced third elements were V, Cr, Mn, and Mo elements, the specimens exhibit slight pseudoelastic (PE) behavior. While there was no PE that could be observed when the introduced third elements were Fe and Co elements.

(8) The Ti-4Au-5Cr and Ti-4Au-5Mn alloys could be better selections than the Ti-4Au-5Mo alloy, owing to their promoted mechanical behaviors, low price, lightweight, relatively low melting temperature, and being essential trace elements in the human body from the application point of view.

(9) Especially, the Ti-4Au-5Cr alloy even wins over the Ti-4Au-5Mn alloy, due to its high SRS of 94% upon a heating process.

1.4 Ti-4Au-5Cr-*n*Ta Alloy System

In this section, the Ti-4Au-5Cr-*n*Ta solution-treated (ST) alloys were further investigated and discussed due to the following reasons. First, in Section 1.3, it is discovered that the Ti-4Au-5Cr alloy was in the optimized group, showing proper mechanical behaviors, excellent SME, and good workability. Second, the 5 mol% addition of Cr was also confirmed to be the optimized addition concentration to the Ti-4Au alloys by our previous study [34]. Finally, the advantages of the Ta element, such as high biocompatibility and high X-ray contrast, are also mentioned in Section 1.1. Therefore, the quaternary Ti-4Au-5Cr-*n*Ta (n = 1, 2, 3, 4, 5, 6, 7, and 9 mol%) ST alloys were further studied and stated in this section.

1.4.1 Cold Workability

Figure 1.10 reveals the CW of the Ti-4Au-5Cr-*n*Ta (n = 1 mol%-9 mol%) ST specimens. Solid red circles suggest the reduction percentage by the initial CR of these specimens without any annealing treatment, while the open red circles imply the reduction of thickness reached 98% with an annealing procedure for 30 s at 1273 K.

Specimens with comparatively low Ta introduction amount (i.e., n = 1 mol%–3 mol% Ta), which exhibit less CW, show a reduction of thickness at about 60% in the initial CR procedure. After an annealing process for 30 s at 1273 K, a reduction of 98% was obtained in these three alloys by the subsequent CR procedure. In contrast, it is noticed that specimens with comparatively moderate Ta introduction amount (i.e., n = 4–6 mol%) and great Ta introduction amount (i.e., n = 7 mol% and 9 mol%) were thinned down to the 98% decrease of thickness successfully without any annealing treatment. Nevertheless, some small cracks could be observed in the moderate and great Ta amount alloyed specimens after CR processes. It is evident that the CW of these specimens could be enhanced by this Ta introduction because the annealing treatment was not required to be carried out on these specimens with Ta introduction amount from n = 4 mol% to n = 9 mol% (i.e., comparatively moderate and great Ta introduction amounts). These outcomes are also in good agreement with those in the reference representing that the CW of specimens could be promoted by the Ta introduction [43, 44].

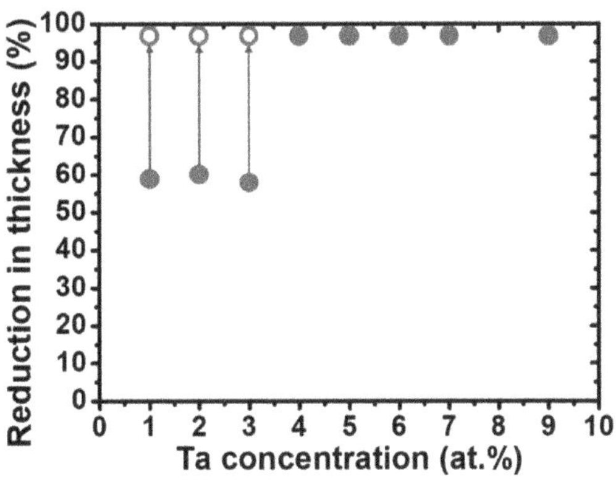

Figure 1.10 The CW of the Ti-4Au-5Cr-*n*Ta (n = 1–9 mol%) ST alloys. Solid red circles imply those specimens are not subjected to any annealing treatment, while open red circles indicate those specimens were subjected to an annealing treatment for 30 s at 1273 K followed by a succeeding CR process.

1.4.2 Phase Identification

Figure 1.11 reveals XRD profiles of the quaternary Ti-4Au-5Cr-*n*Ta (n = (a) 1 mol%–(h) 9 mol%) ST specimens under ambient at RT. It is observed that when the Ta introduction amount is < 3 mol% (Figure 1.11(a) and (b)), the phase constituent was a dual-phase of the α''-martensite with an orthorhombic structure, and the β-phase with a bcc structure. The phase constituent entirely developed into the β-phase while the Ta addition amount is ≥ 3 mol% (Figure 1.11(c–h)). This implies that the β-phase is wholly stabilized when the Ta addition amount > 2 mol% in this Ti-4Au-5Cr-*n*Ta specimens because the Ta element is sorted as a β-stabilizer [45, 46]. Hence, regarding the temperatures of phase transformation in the 1Ta introduced specimen (Figure 1.11(a)) and the 2Ta introduced specimen (Figure 1.11(b)), it is speculated that the M_s is beyond RT, while its A_s is lower than RT. Furthermore, it is also clear that with the addition of third and fourth metals (i.e., Cr and Ta elements in this chapter), the phase transformation reaction evolved successfully into the desired MT rather than the massive transformation, which results in a generation of a functionless α_m-phase from the high-temperature β-phase during cooling [23, 24].

Basically, the 110_β characteristic peaks of (b) n = 2 mol%–(h) n = 9 mol% alloys show high intensity (Figure 1.11). It was claimed that, in the Ti-Mo-Al-Zr specimens, owing to the development of alloy texture after recrystallization, the 110_β characteristic peak was also generated by the CR process followed by a 1273 K ST procedure [47]. Henceforth, it could be speculated that the development of the alloy texture after recrystallization of the Ti-4Au-5Cr-*n*Ta specimens is quite close to those of the quaternary Ti-Mo-Al-Zr specimens showing a well-developed texture of $\{110\}_\beta$ $\langle 100\rangle_\beta$ (i.e., the so-called GOSS orientation) of the β-phase. These results might be explained by the likeness of the crystal structures of the Ti-4Au-5Cr-*n*Ta alloys to the Ti-Mo-Al-Zr specimens and also their inclination to undergo MT in a CR procedure. Contrarily, it was observed that the development of alloy texture varied from the Ti-Nb-based specimens, which possess strong $\{112\}_\beta\langle 110\rangle_\beta$ and $\{001\}_\beta\langle 110\rangle_\beta$ textures after some specific mechanical procedures and certain ST processes [48].

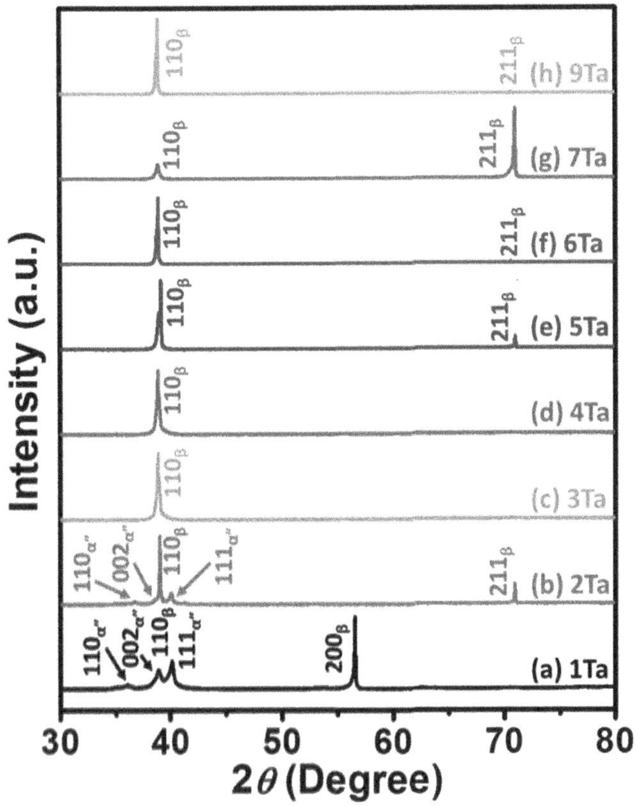

Figure 1.11 XRD profiles of the quaternary Ti-4Au-5Cr-*n*Ta (*n* = 1–9 mol%) ST specimens under ambient at RT. The alloys are shortened as 1Ta (a); 2Ta (b); 3Ta (c); 4Ta (d); 5Ta (e); 6Ta (f); 7Ta (g); 9Ta (h) by ruling out the partition of "Ti-4Au-5Cr".

Please note that a different texture in the 7Ta introduced alloy (Figure 1.11(g)) from other specimens would be due to the comparatively larger grain of the β-Ti-based specimens than other ST processed specimens. It was revealed that grains of β-Ti ST materials would be as large as 500 μm [49, 50]; therefore, in their XRD patterns, it is highly probable that the high intensity of the 211_β characteristic peak located at approximately $2\theta = 72^\circ$ was observed by chance. Further investigations regarding the influences of the CR procedures and ST processes on the evolution of alloy texture must be carried out to figure out the complicated development of alloy texture after recrystallization.

1.4.3 Mechanical Behavior Evaluations

1.4.3.1 Continuous tensile examinations

The SS curves of the Ti-4Au-5Cr-*n*Ta (*n* = (a) 1 mol%–(h) 9 mol%) ST specimens by the continuous tensile examinations under ambient at RT are revealed in Figure 1.12. Apparent two-stage yielding is discerned in the (a) 1Ta, (b) 2Ta, and (c) 3Ta introduced Ti-4Au-5Cr-based specimens. However, no two-stage yielding could be observed in other specimens. This two-stage yielding behavior also has been stated in the earlier reports [38, 51–54], which also worked on the Ti-Au-based and/or the Ti-Cr-based alloy systems. Stress for the first-yielding indicates the SIMT and/or MVR depending on the phase constituents of the alloys. While stress for the second-yielding corresponds to the initiation of plastic deformation (i.e., movement of dislocations) [38, 51–54].

Judging from the phase constituents revealed by the XRD profiles, it is deduced that those stress plateaus in the (a) 1Ta and the (b) 2Ta introduced Ti-4Au-5Cr-based alloys (Figure 1.12(a, b)), suggest SIMT and/or MVR because of the dual-phase of the α''-phase and the β-phase. Similar outcomes have also been stated in the former reports [55, 56]. On the other hand, the observed stress plateau of the 3–9Ta introduced Ti-4Au-5Cr-based alloys (Figure 1.12) suggests the initiation and continuing of SIMT only, since they are composed of the single β-phase revealed in their XRD patterns (Figure 1.11).

It is greatly recognized that the deformation behavior of these β-Ti specimens commences from SIMT followed by a deformation mode of twinning, and eventually shifted into a plastic deformation (i.e., dislocations slip) [57–59] when the parent β-phase is progressively stabilized by introducing β-stabilizers. An obvious serration in the SS curves during the continuous tensile examinations is detected when the deformation behavior is in the transition state of the twinning mode and the plastic deformation mode [60–62] of the β-Ti specimens. Henceforth, it is apparent that obvious serration behaviors in the SS curves are observed in the 7Ta and the 9Ta introduced Ti-4Au-5Cr alloys (Figure 1.12(g, h)). Inversely, merely faint serration behavior could be observed in the 5Ta and the 6Ta introduced alloys (Figure 1.12(e, f)), owing to their comparatively little amount of plastic

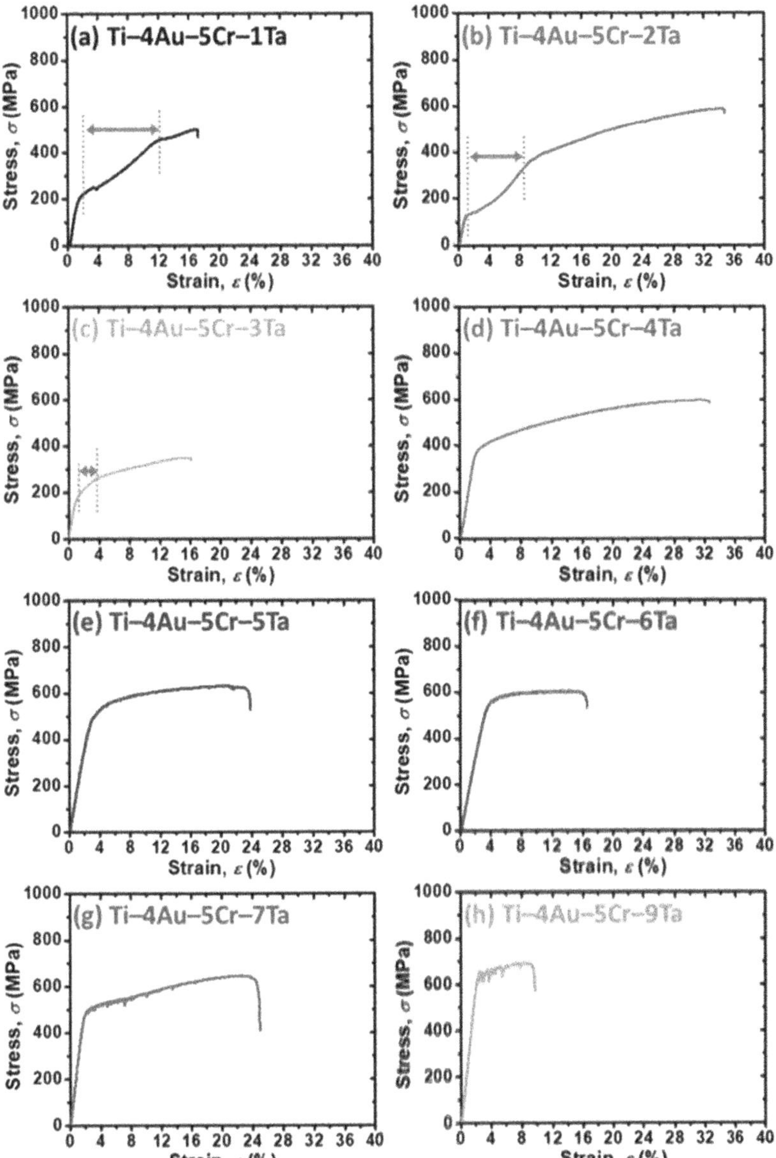

Figure 1.12 SS curves of the Ti-4Au-5Cr-*n*Ta (*n* = (a) 1 mol%–(h) 9 mol%) ST specimens by the continuous tensile examinations under ambient at RT. (Plateaus, which are marked by upright dotted lines and solid horizontal lines with arrows in (a–c) specimens, specify the propagation of MVR and/or SIMT.)

deformation. Nevertheless, relatively obvious serration behaviors are revealed in the tensile examinations of the cyclic examinations, which are stated in the following section. So far, there are different explanations for the appearance of the serration observed in the β-Ti alloys and other alloy systems. However, this is out of the scope of this chapter, to figure out its mechanism, more research is necessitated.

Please also note that it is probable that the brittle ω-phase might be the reason for the low ductility of the 3Ta introduced specimen (Figure 1.12(c)) [52]. This ω-phase is often observed when the dual-phase of the α″(minor)+β(major) alloy transforms into the single meta-stabilized β-phase (i.e., competition between the formation of the α″-phase and the ω-phase in a cooling procedure from a β-phase). Hence, it is reasonable to infer that the abrupt drop of alloy elongation property of the 3Ta introduced alloy (Figure 1.12(c)) might be ascribed to the existence of the undesired ω-phase.

It has been reported that the strength and ductility of the alloys could both be raised when the transformation-induced plasticity (TRIP) and the twinning-induced plasticity (TWIP) are activated simultaneously [62–64]. Hereafter, the 4Ta introduced alloy (Figure 1.12(d)) performs a comparatively superior ductility compared to the other specimens, as shown in Figure 1.12, due to the initiation and propagation of both the deformation modes of TRIP and the TWIP during deformation. Conversely, with the increased introduction of Ta amount from (d) 4 mol% to (g) 7 mol%, the extent of the TRIP deformation mode could be diminished progressively, in the meanwhile, the extent of the TWIP deformation manner could be relatively raised. Consequently, the ductility of the 5–7Ta introduced alloys (Figure 1.12(e–g)) deteriorated to about 20% of the ε_f along with small deviations. Lastly, the most deteriorated ductility is noted in the 9Ta introduced specimen (Figure 1.12(h)) as the deformation manner transforms into a mixture of the twinning (minor) motion and the plastic deformation (major, i.e., motions of dislocation slip).

In general, the results of the specimen strength and ductility by the continuous tensile examinations (Figure 1.12) are well explained by the progress of deformation motions from SIMT to twinning mode, and in the end to slip deformation mode. They are also explained by the discerned deformation behaviors from a plateau to serration and finally to reduced elongation. Further details regarding mechanical behaviors are also stated in the following section.

1.4.3.2 Elongation vs Ta amount

The correlation between the (a) ε_f, (b) σ_y, and (c) σ_{UTS} and the Ta introduction amount are shown in Figure 1.13. In Figure 1.13(a), black circles suggest ε_f, and a dotted line with an arrow indicates the ε_f tendency with Ta introduction concentration. While, in Figure 1.13(b, c), blue triangles represent the σ_y and red squares correspond to the σ_{UTS}, respectively. An upright gray broken line at 2 mol% Ta stands for the boundary of phase stability, while two dotted light-blue lines in reverse tendency suggest the trends of the σ_y more and less than 2 mol% Ta, respectively.

In Figure 1.13, basically, the Ta-tailored specimens show enhanced ductility of more than about 12% compared to the binary Ti-Au-based alloys and/or the Ti-Cr-based specimens [51–53, 63]; in addition, by ruling out the 9Ta introduced specimen (Figure 1.12(h) and Figure 1.13(a)), all specimen ε_f is higher than about 16% (Figure 1.13(a)). Again, as aforesaid, the decreased ductility of the 3Ta introduced specimen (Figure 1.12(c) and Figure 1.13(a)) could be due to the generations of the fine ω-phase, which is undesired. Even though the fine ω-phase is not observed via the XRD measurements, owing to its limited quantity, the influences of the Ta element introduction amount on the β-Ti SMAs have been claimed [65] and the inclination of the formations of the ω-phase in the previous works are in good accordance with the phenomenon revealed in this chapter. Additionally, it is well-known that the β-Ti alloys usually show relatively coarse grain; thus, abrupt alterations of performances, such as mechanical behaviors or alloy textures after recrystallization are frequently observed in these β-Ti-based alloys. Nevertheless, it is apparent that, concerning their overall inclination, the alloy ductility was deteriorated by the addition of Ta element into these Ti-4Au-5Cr-based specimens (Figure 1.12 and Figure 1.13).

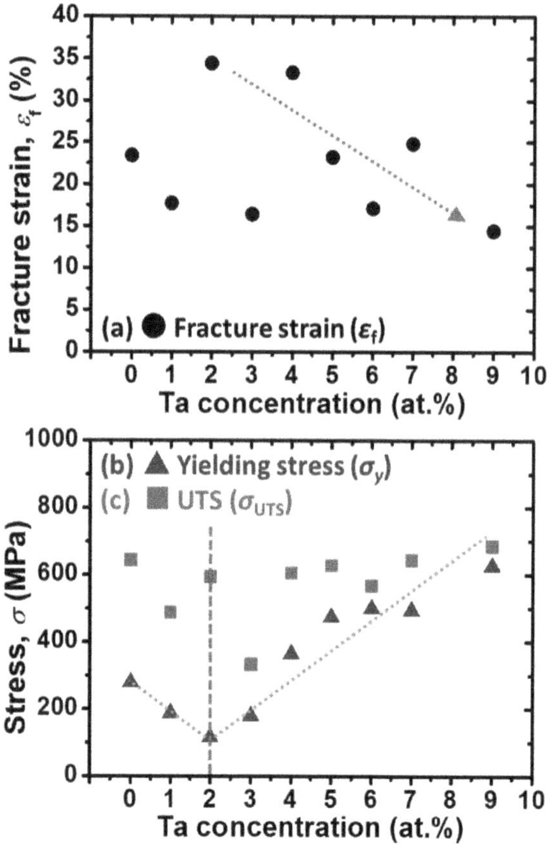

Figure 1.13 (a) ε_f, (b) σ_y, and (c) σ_{UTS} as a function of Ta addition amount. (Black circles: ε_f; Gray dotted line with an arrow: The tendency of ε_f as a function of Ta introduction amount as specimens are the single β-phase; Blue triangles: σ_y; Red squares: σ_{UTS}; Gray broken upright line: Ta at 2 mol%; Light-blue dotted lines: tendencies for σ_y.)

It is necessary to mention that the 2Ta introduced alloy (Figure 1.12(b)) and the 4Ta introduced specimen (Figure 1.12(d)), before fractures, show especially a good ductility of about 35% and 33%, respectively. It was observed that the {332}<113> twinning could be triggered during tensile deformation and result in an enhanced ductility when the β-phase is meta-stabilized [65, 66]. In addition, similar behavior of the {332}<113> twinning was also discerned in the binary Ti-V-based and the binary Ti-Cr-based specimens [67, 68]. Since it is found that the phase constituent developed from the dual α″+β-phase to the single β-phase as the introduction concentration of the Ta element was increased from 2 mol% (Figure 1.11(b)) to 3–4 mol% (Figure 1.11(c, d)), it is thus speculated that the β-phase in the 2–4 mol% Ta introduced specimens stay in its meta-stabilized state. Therefore, based on the determinations of the phase constituents by the XRD patterns and those of the previous studies [64–66], this good ductility of the 4Ta tailored alloy (Figure 1.12(d)) might be ascribed to the twinning of {332}<113> resulting in a promoted ductility before a fracture happens. Different from the aforementioned 3Ta added specimen (Figure 1.12(c)), the ω-phase might be suppressed via further addition of Ta (i.e., 4 mol% Ta introduction) [43]; therefore, an advanced elongation behavior is found in the 4 mol% Ta introduced specimen (Figure 1.12(d)).

In contrast, reverse to the excellent elongation of the 4 mol% Ta introduced specimen (Figure 1.12(d) and Figure 1.13(a)), the 9 mol% Ta introduced specimen (Figure 1.12(h) and Figure 1.13(a)), which was tailored by the maximum Ta addition amount exhibits the most deteriorated elongation behavior before its fracture happens, among all specimens. Judging from the XRD patterns (Figure 1.11), it is apparent that the β-phase, which is completely stabilized from the 3 mol% Ta introduced alloy (Figure 1.11(c)), showed the single β-phase as its apparent phase. With the increment of additional concentration of Ta element, the β-phase was progressively stabilized from the meta-stabilized state to the fully-stabilized state because the fourthly introduced Ta element is sorted as a β-stabilizer, which could stabilize the parent β-phase [43]. Hence, lastly, among all the specimens, the β-phase in this 9 mol% Ta introduced specimen (Figure 1.12(h)) would be the utmost stabilized alloy (i.e., greatly stabilized β-phase) and this specimen probably experienced the plastic deformation mode (i.e., dislocation slip motion) during the loading of an external force before the SIMT takes place in the tensile examinations. Consequently, a deteriorated fracture strain of the 9 mol% Ta introduced alloy (Figure 1.12(h) and Figure 1.13(a)) was discovered.

Furthermore, generally, it is observed that the fracture strain of the samples is reduced with Ta introduction concentration while certain deviations could be found (Figure 1.13(a)). Hence, the ε_f of the specimens, which are composed of the single β-phase, show a good inclination with Ta amount (implied by a gray dotted line with an arrow in Figure 1.13(a)). Basically, the overall ductility of these specimens is in good agreement with the progress of the deformation mode by tensile examinations, such as SIMT → twinning motion → plastic deformation (i.e., slip motion), which is also stated in detail in the former section.

1.4.3.3 Yielding stress vs Ta amount

Correlation of the (b) σ_y-Ta introduction concentration (solid blue triangles), which is obtained from the SS curves (Figure 1.12), is shown in Figure 1.13(b). It is observed that the σ_y decreases progressively from nearly 288 MPa to around 127 MPa when the Ta introduction concentration is raised from 0 mol% to 2 mol%. According to their XRD patterns, the phase constituents of 0–2 mol% Ta introduced specimens are composed of the dual-phase of the α″+β-phase (Figure 1.11(a, b)). Hence, their deformation mechanisms are deduced to be MVR and/or SIMT. As previously stated, as the metastable β-phase is constructed, low σ_y could be expected [65, 66]. This reduced σ_y could therefore be ascribed to the arising amount of the meta-stabilized β-phase, that is to say, decreasing amount of the α″-phase, via the fine-adjustment of Ta addition concentration. Meanwhile, this could also be explicated that because the α″-phase was tuned stably when the Ta introduction amount decreases; accordingly, a relatively high stress to trigger the MVR is required. As a result, an inverse relationship between the σ_y and Ta amount is observed before 2 mol% Ta.

Different from the aforementioned phenomenon, σ_y increases from around 179 MPa to approximately 622 MPa while the Ta introduction amount increases from 3 mol% Ta to 9 mol% Ta. According to their XRD patterns, these specimens consist of a single β-phase (Figure 1.11(c-h)). Therefore, the major deformation mechanism is speculated to gradually progress from SIMT to twinning mode and eventually transform to a plastic deformation mode produced by dislocation slip in these specimens. Once again, as previously stated, the strength of specimens could be advanced as the TWIP and TRIP initiate together [62]. Apparently, with the introduction of the β-stabilizer element of Ta, the β-phase could progressively be stabilized, resulting in a promoted σ_y from the 3 mol% Ta introduced specimen to the 9 mol% Ta introduced specimen in Figure 1.13(b). Briefly, phase stability, which is regulated by adding Ta into the Ti-4Au-5Cr-based alloys for fine-tuning, corresponds well with the σ_y discerned. A gray broken line is exhibited in Figure 1.13(b,c) at the Ta amount of 2 mol% for illustrating the borderline of different phase constituents, phase stability, and altering point of the σ_y.

1.4.3.4 UTS vs Ta amount

Correlation of the (c) UTS-Ta introduction amount (solid red squares), which is also obtained from their SS curves (Figure 1.12), is plotted and revealed in Figure 1.13(c). In general, UTS follows an almost similar inclination with the σ_y (Figure 1.13(b)) with certainly acceptable deviations because UTS is also influenced by multi-factors. Comparatively high UTS of the specimens with the Ta introduction amount less than the 3 mol% Ta introduced alloy could be attributed to the dual-phase of the α″+β-phase, which results in a precipitation-hardening effect. While the UTS of the specimens could be enhanced by the Ta addition amount slightly from 3 mol% Ta to 9 mol% Ta, owing to the truth of the effect of solid-solution hardening.

1.4.3.5 UTS vs yielding stress

The functional mapping of UTS and ε_f of the Ti-4Au-5Cr-*n*Ta (*n* = 1–9 mol%) ST specimens (Figure 1.14) is read from the corresponding SS curves (Figure 1.12). It is discovered that the UTS of the specimens of 2Ta introduced and the 4Ta introduced alloys are quite close to the Ta-free alloy while a great enhancement of the ductility is practiced by the 2 mol% Ta and the 4 mol% Ta introduced alloys. This phenomenon suggests that, from the standpoint of mechanical behaviors, with the addition of certain Ta (i.e., < 4 mol%), strength of the specimen remains unchanged; moreover, enhanced ductility could also be realized. In the meanwhile, from the viewpoint of actual applications, a high X-ray contrast [69] and a high biocompatible behavior [70, 71] are also realized in biomedical applications via the modification of the Ta element.

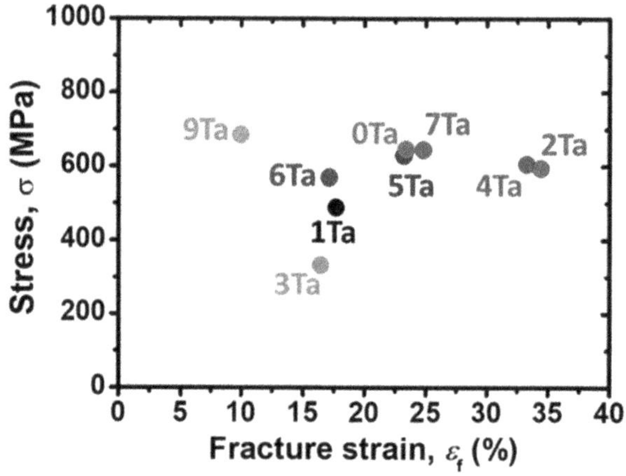

Figure 1.14 Functional mapping of UTS and ε_f of all ST Ti-4Au-5Cr-*n*Ta (n = 0–9 mol%) specimens.

1.4.3.6 Cyclic loading-unloading tensile examinations

Figure 1.15 shows the cyclic examinations of the ST Ti-4Au-5Cr-*n*Ta (n = 1–9 mol%) alloys under ambient at RT. It is observed that a small SRS in the unloading process by not only the recovery brought about by the elastic behavior is discerned in the 1–4Ta introduced alloys (Figure 1.15(a–d)) to a certain extent, revealing a representative non-linear behavior of shape recovery. Different from the aforementioned ones, nearly no SRS could be found from PE behavior in the 5–9Ta introduced alloys (Figure 1.15(e–h)). Here, elastic shape recovery suggests the linear behavior in the unloading process, while a non-linear recovery in the unloading procedure indicates the propagation of the PE behavior (i.e., reverse MVR during unloading). The SS curves of the final cycle have been extracted and revealed in the following section, for analysis in detail.

Both 1Ta and 2Ta introduced specimens are composed of the α''+β dual-phase based on their XRD patterns (Figure 1.11(a, b)); therefore, both MVR and SIMT are triggered in a loading process. In the unloading process, a non-linear behavior of recovery originates from the PE behavior (i.e., reverse MVR). It is thus speculated that the A_s is beyond the operating temperature at RT of the cyclic examinations.

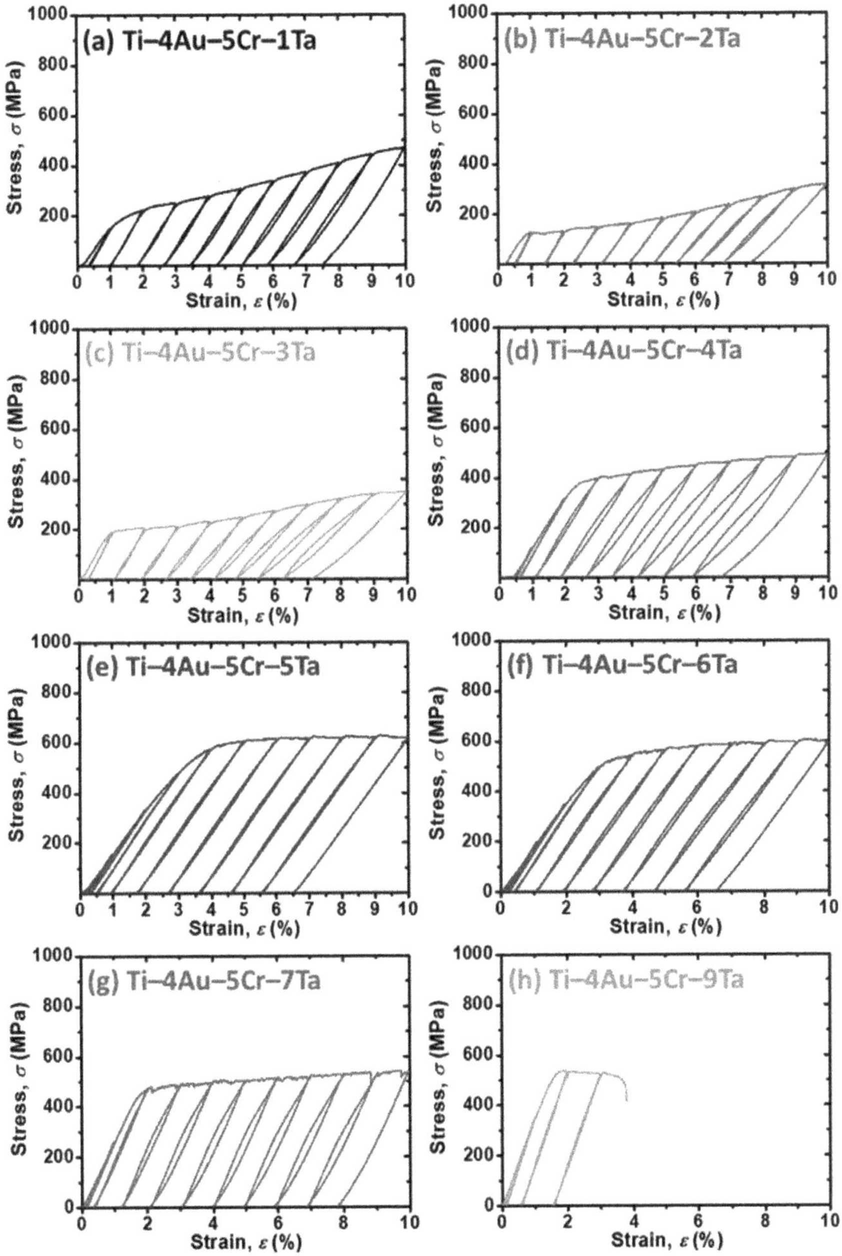

Figure 1.15 The SS curves of the Ti-4Au-5Cr-*n*Ta (*n* = (a) 1 mol%–(h) 9 mol%) ST alloys by cyclic examinations under ambient at RT.

Similar to the Ti-4Au-5Cr-1–2Ta alloys, the 3 mol% Ta and 4 mol% Ta introduced alloys in Figure 1.15(c, d) also perform a slight PE behavior in the unloading process demonstrating a representative non-linear recovery. Because the phase constituents of the 3 mol% Ta and 4 mol% Ta introduced specimens are both the single β-phase (Figure 1.11(c, d)), it is rational to consider that, in the first cycle, these alloys underwent SIMT in a loading process, while they underwent reverse MVR in an unloading process, owing to the remained α″-phase. From the second cycle, due to the remaining α″-phase, the SIMT+MVR took place during loading while reverse MVR commenced during unloading. It is also believed that the A_s, which is beyond the operating temperature (i.e., RT in this case) of the cyclic examinations, is explained below. Additionally, the abovementioned recovery behavior to a comparatively small extent is due to the plastic deformation, which took place along with SIMT in the loading process; accordingly, SRS was suppressed to a certain level in unloading.

Differently, no PE behavior could be observed in the remaining specimens (i.e., the 5–9 mol% Ta introduced specimens) in Figure 1.15(e–h). The recovery behavior, which originates from a non-linear shape recovery almost disappeared in these specimens. The deteriorated recovery behaviors in these specimens are ascribed to the accompanying plastic deformations in the cyclic examinations since plastic deformations (i.e., twinning motion and/or slip of dislocations) were introduced into the alloys before and/or together with when the SIMT took place. That is to say, the stress for initiation of plastic deformation is lower and/or similar to the stress for SIMT in these alloys since the β-phase is greatly stabilized. It was also discovered that the 9Ta-introduced alloy, which possesses the poorest ductility in the continuous tensile examinations (Figure 1.12(h)), fractured before the assigned 10% deformation strain was reached (Figure 1.15(h)). This suggests that the findings in the continuous tensile examinations are in consistent with the observations of these cyclic examinations.

1.4.4 Shape Recovery

For figuring out the recovery behavior in an unloading process, 4Ta and 9Ta introduced alloys, which perform absolutely different recovery behaviors in the cyclic examinations, were chosen and analyzed. The last cycles of these two specimens in the SS curves are revealed in Figure 1.16(a, b), respectively. Definitions of the stress and strains are also illustrated (Figure 1.16(c)).

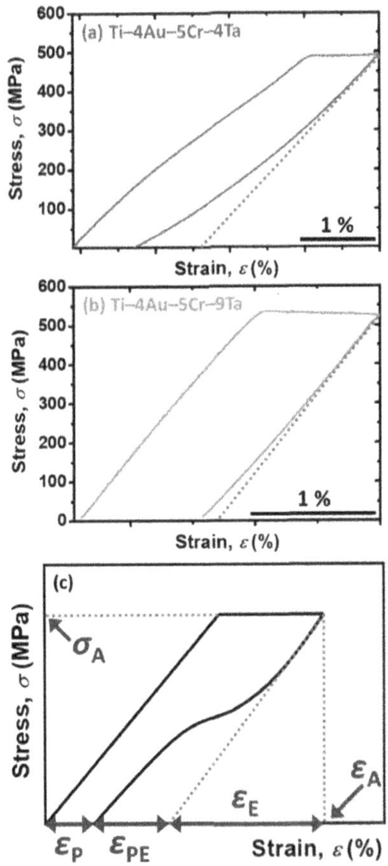

Figure 1.16 The last cycles of the (a) 4Ta and (b) 9Ta introduced alloys read from the cyclic examinations. (c) Definitions in the SS curve. (ε_A: Applied overall strain; ε_E: Recovery strain from elastic behavior; ε_{PE}: Recovery strain from PE; ε_P: Permanent strain; σ_A: Applied overall stress.)

In Figure 1.16(c), ε_A suggests applied strain, ε_E indicates recovery from elastic behavior, ε_{PE} represents recovery strain from a PE behavior, ε_P suggests a permanent strain, and σ_A corresponds to an overall applied stress, respectively.

It is apparent that the 4Ta introduced alloy (Figure 1.16(a)) exhibits particular recovery strain due to a PE behavior, while the 9Ta alloy (Figure 1.16(b)) performed smear recovery strain brought about by this PE behavior, which is almost not detectable. It is recognized that this non-linear recovery behavior originates from a reverse MVR in an unloading process. Since no clear plateau is observed in Figure 1.16(a) during unloading, it is thus deduced that the cause of the SRS was because of the reverse MVR (i.e., a PE behavior) instead of a SE behavior. Different deformation motions between these two specimens are explained in detail in the previous sub-section, the maximum SRS brought about by the PE behavior of the 4Ta introduced specimen (Figure 1.16(a)) is at about 0.84%; in contrast, the smallest recovery strain brought about by the PE behavior of the 9Ta introduced alloy (Figure 1.16(b)) is merely at about 0.1%.

SRS of the ST Ti-4Au-5Cr-nTa (x = 1–9 mol%) alloys due to PE behavior under ambient at RT are read from Figure 1.15 and summarized in Figure 1.17. Please note that, here, the strain is evaluated by ruling out the SRS brought by ε_E during unloading; hence, merely the SRS originating from the ε_{PE} is evaluated. In Figure 1.17, ε_{PE} could be approximately distributed into three different categorizations: the (a) high, (b) medium, and (c) low SRS, respectively, are marked by gray dotted squares. The greatest ε_{PE} could be acquired from the 4Ta introduced specimens, whose shape recovery originates from the reverse MVR in an unloading process for releasing the internal stress. This is a frequently-observed deformation behavior in SMAs.

It is required to declare that the 4Ta introduced specimen with the greatest performance not only exhibits the maximum SRS in an unloading process among all specimens in the cyclic examinations but also performs a good ductility in the continuous tensile examination (Figure 1.12). In addition, its strength remains almost unchanged compared to the Ta-free ternary specimen of the Ti-4Au-5Cr alloy (Figure 1.14). These discoveries indicate that this 4Ta-introduced alloy is a prospective candidate for biomedical applications, owing to its proper strength, good ductility, high X-ray contrast, excellent biocompatibility, and certain SRS in an unloading process. These Ti-Au-based, Ti-Cr-based, and Ti-Au-Cr-based SMAs are still under investigation by our research group, further details concerning these promising materials would be published in the future.

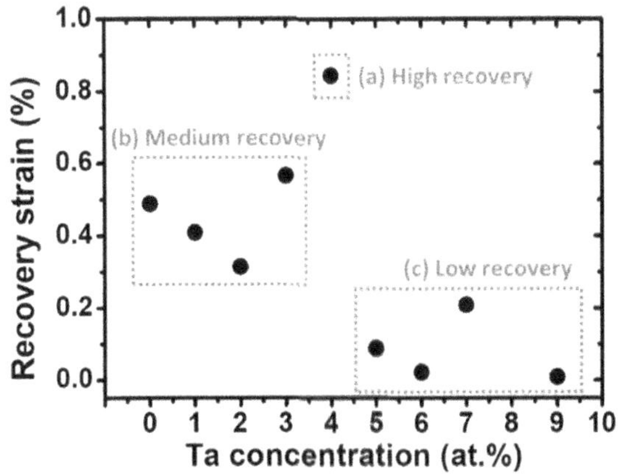

Figure 1.17 SRS of the ST Ti-4Au-5Cr-*n*Ta (*x* = 1–9 mol%) alloys due to the PE behavior under ambient at RT. These values of SRS are generally distributed into three groups of the (a) high, (b) medium, and (c) low sorts, respectively.

1.4.5 Brief Summaries of the Ti-4Au-5Cr-*n*Ta Alloys

The influences of the Ta introduction amount on the CW, phase constituents, mechanical behaviors, and tensile deformation behaviors of the Ti-4Au-5Cr-based SMAs were investigated thoroughly. Critical results are concluded as follows.

(1) Via the addition of Ta metals into the Ti-4Au-5Cr ternary specimens, their CW is significantly advanced. In the CR process, annealing treatment was not required to be carried out to acquire the 98% reduction of specimen thickness when the Ta introduction amount is ≥ 4 mol%.

(2) Apparent phases in the alloys developed progressively from a dual α''+β-phase (i.e., when Ta is < 3 mol%) to a single β-phase (i.e., when Ta is ≥ 3 mol%) with the Ta addition

amount in a good tendency. Specifically, phase stability of the β-phase is elevated with increasing Ta addition amount.

(3) In the continuous tensile examinations, almost all the alloys except for the 9Ta introduced alloy display good ductility higher than 16%.

(4) A representative trend of SMAs in terms of yielding stress is found in the functional mapping of strength vs Ta concentration, which shows an altering point at 2 mol% Ta introduced specimen. This alloy is mostly composed of the β-phase showing the lowest yielding strength among all alloys.

(5) The relationship of the UTS vs Ta addition concentration shows an inclination in a similar way to the yielding stress.

(6) Clear plateaus, corresponding to the MVR and/or SIMT, are observed in the 1Ta and 2Ta introduced specimens. While a relatively faint plateau could be observed in the 3Ta introduced specimen, owing to the probable formation of the ω-phase, which suppresses its SIMT in a loading process.

(7) Functional mappings of the fracture strain, yielding stress, and UTS to the Ta introduction amount were revealed to point out the inclination of various mechanical behaviors and indicate the optimized specimens of 2Ta and 4Ta introduced alloys.

(8) In the cyclic examinations, PE behavior is obviously discerned in the 1–4Ta introduced alloys due to the reverse MVR in an unloading process, showing a slight SRS. The maximum SRS was fulfilled by the 4Ta introduced specimen.

(9) Amongst alloys examined, the 4Ta-introduced alloy shows optimized mechanical behaviors, performing high elongation while its strength remains undamaged. In addition, the maximum SRS in an unloading process is also observed in the cyclic examinations. Therefore, the 4Ta-introduced alloy is considered a potential material for biomedical usage.

Acknowledgments

This work is supported financially by the research grant of the Hitachi Metals and Materials Science Foundation, the Iwatani Naoji Foundation, the Tanaka Kikinzoku Memorial Foundation, the Japan

Society for the Promotion of Science (JSPS) (KAKENHI 22K14491), the Japan Society for the Promotion of Science (JSPS) (KAKENHI 22H05276), the Japan Society for the Promotion of Science (JSPS) (KAKENHI 22K18899), the Japan Society for the Promotion of Science (JSPS) (KAKENHI 20K20544), and the Japan Society for the Promotion of Science (JSPS) (KAKENHI 22H00256). All figures are reproduced with the permission of Elsevier.

References

1. Kong F., (2018). *Aging Trend of the World, the Structure of Healthy Life Determinants*, **18**, Springer, Berlin.
2. Hernlund E., Svedbom A., Ivergård M., Compston J., Cooper C., Stenmark J., McCloskey E.V., Jönsson B., Kanis J., (2013). Osteoporosis in the European Union: Medical management, epidemiology and economic burden, *Arch. Osteoporos.*, **8**, p. 136.
3. Otsuka K., Wayman C.M., (1999). *Shape Memory Materials*, Cambridge University Press, Cambridge.
4. Yamauchi K., Ohkata I., Tsuchiya K., Miyazaki S., (2011). *Shape Memory and Superelastic Alloys*, Woodhead Publishing, Cambridge.
5. Rezaie H.R., Bakhtiari L., Öchsner A., (2015). *Biomaterials and Their Applications*, Springer, Berlin.
6. Gepreel M.A.-H., Niinomi M., (2013). Biocompatibility of Ti-alloys for long-term implantation, *J. Mech. Behav. Biomed. Mater.*, **20**, pp. 407–415.
7. Manam N.S., Harun W.S.W., Shri D.N.A., Ghani S.A.C., Kurniawan T., Ismail M.H., Ibrahim M.H.I., (2017). Study of corrosion in biocompatible metals for implants: A review, *J. Alloys Compd.*, **701**, pp. 698–715.
8. Craig B.D., Anderson D.S., (1994). *Handbook of Corrosion Data*, ASM International, Ohio.
9. Kawamura T., Tachi R., Inamura T., Hosoda H., Wakashima K., Hamada K., Miyazaki S., (2006). Effects of ternary additions on martensitic transformation of TiAu, *Mater. Sci. Eng. A*, **438–440**, pp. 383–386.
10. Wadood A., Hosoda H., Yamabe-Mitarai Y., (2014). Phase transformation, oxidation and shape memory properties of Ti-50Au-10Zr alloy for high temperature applications, *J. Alloys Compd.*, **595**, pp. 200–205.

11. Buschow K.H.J., (2003). *Handbook of Magnetic Materials*, Elsevier, Amsterdam.
12. Horiuchi Y., Inamura T., Kim H.Y., Miyazaki S., Wakashima K., Hosoda H., (2006). X-ray diffraction analysis of Ti-18 mol% Nb based shape memory alloys containing 3d transition metal elements, *Mater. Trans.*, **47**(4), pp. 1209–1213.
13. Biological Response to Metal Implants, (2019). U.S. Food & Drug Administration, September.
14. Liang H., Yang Y., Xie D., Li L., Mao N., Wang C., Tian Z., Jiang Q., Shen L., (2019). Trabecular-like Ti-6Al-4V scaffolds for orthopedic: Fabrication by selective laser melting and in vitro biocompatibility, *J. Mater. Sci. Technol.*, **35**(7), pp. 1284–1297.
15. Trumbo P., Yates A.A., Schlicker S., Poos M., (2001). *Dietary Reference Intakes: Vitamin A, Vitamin K, Arsenic, Boron, Chromium, Copper, Iodine, Iron, Manganese, Molybdenum, Nickel, Silicon, Vanadium, and Zinc*, **101**(3), National Academies Press, Washington (DC).
16. Nikolaychuk P.A., (2016). The revised potential-pH diagram of Sc-H_2O system, *Belgorod State University Scientific Bulletin: Nat. Sci.*, **37**(25), pp. 70–87.
17. Asadian M., (2013). Thermodynamic analysis of ZnO crystal growth from the melt, *J. Cryst. Process Technol.*, **3**(3), p. 33870.
18. Pérez-Sierra A.M., Pons J., Santamarta R., Karaman I., Noebe R.D., (2016). Stability of a Ni-rich Ni-Ti-Zr high temperature shape memory alloy upon low temperature aging and thermal cycling, *Scr. Mater.*, **124**, pp. 47–50.
19. Li S., Kim Y.-W., Choi M.-S., Nam T.-H., (2020). Microstructure, mechanical and superelastic behaviors in Ni-free Ti-Zr-Nb-Sn shape memory alloy fibers prepared by rapid solidification processing, *Mater. Sci. Eng. A*, **782**, p. 139283.
20. Song X., Xiong C., Zhang F., Nie Y., Li Y., (2020). Strain induced martensite stabilization in b Ti-Zr-Nb shape memory alloy, *Mater. Lett.*, **259**, p. 126914.
21. Qu W.-T., Sun X.-G., Yuan B.-F., Li K.-M., Wang Z.-G., Li Y., (2017). Tribological behaviour of biomedical Ti-Zr-based shape memory alloys, *Rare Met.*, **36**, pp. 478–484.
22. Li S., Choi M.-S., Nam T.-H., (2020). Role of fine nano-scaled isothermal omega phase on the mechanical and superelastic properties of a high Zr-containing Ti-Zr-Nb-Sn shape memory alloy, *Mater. Sci. Eng. A*, **782**, p. 139278.
23. Plichta M.R., Williams J.C., Aaronson H.I., (1977). On the existence of

the β/α_m transformation in the alloy systems Ti-Ag, Ti-Au, and Ti-Si, *Metall. Trans. A*, **8**(A), pp. 1885–1892.

24. Plichta M.R., Perepezko J.H., Aaronson H.I., Lange W.F., (1980). Part I Nucleation kinetics of the β/α_m transformation in Ti-Ag and Ti-Au alloys, *Acta Metall.*, **28**(8), pp. 1031–1040.
25. Xin Y., Han K., Svanidze E., Besara T., Siegrist T., Morosan E., (2019). Microstructure of hard biocompatible $Ti_{1-x}Au_x$ alloys, *Mater. Char.*, **149**, pp. 133–142.
26. Wadood A., Yamabe-Mitarai Y., (2015). Silver and Zirconium added ternary and quaternary TiAu based high temperature shape memory alloys, *J. Alloys Compd.*, **646**, pp. 1172–1177.
27. Shinohara Y., Tahara M., Inamura T., Miyazaki S., Hosoda H., (2015). Effect of annealing temperature on microstructure and super elastic properties of Ti-Au-Cr-Zr alloy, *Mater. Trans.*, **56**(3), pp. 404–409.
28. Shinohara Y., Tahara M., Inamura T., Miyazaki S., Hosoda H., (2015). Deformation behavior of Ti-4Au-5Cr-8Zr superelastic alloy with or without containing Ti_3Au precipitates, *Mater. Today Proc.*, **2S**, pp. S821–S824.
29. Zadorozhnyy V. Yu, Shi X., Kopylov A.N., Shchetinin I.V., Wada T., Louzguine-Luzgin D.V., Kato H., (2017). Mechanical properties, structure, and biocompatibility of dual-axially forged $Ti_{94}Fe_3Au_3$, $Ti_{94}Fe_3Nb_3$, and $Ti_{94}Au_3Nb_3$ alloys, *J. Alloys Compd.*, **707**, pp. 269–274.
30. Ishigaki T., Matsuki Y., Inamura T., Wakashima K., Hosoda H., (2007). *Phase Constitution and Mechanical Properties of Near-Eutectoid Ti-Au Alloys Containing Transition Metal Elements*, ASM International, Ohio, pp. 559–564.
31. Kasuya K., Inamura T., Wakashima K., Hosoda H., (2007). *Phase Constitution and Mechanical Properties of Ti-Sn Alloys Containing 3d Transition Metal Elements*, ASM International, Ohio, pp. 553–558.
32. Saito H., Inamura T., Wakashima K., Hosoda H., (2007). *Mechanical Properties of Ti-Mo Alloys Containing 3d Transition Metal Elements*, ASM International, Ohio, pp. 565–570.
33. Okimori Y., Tsugane Y., Inamura T., Wakashima K., Hosoda H., (2007). *Shape Memory Properties of TiAu Base Alloys and Composites*, ASM International, Ohio, pp. 571–576.
34. Chiu W.-T., Wakabayashi K., Umise A., Tahara M., Inamura T., Hosoda H., (2022). Investigations of mechanical properties and deformation behaviors of the Cr modified Ti-Au shape memory alloys, *J. Alloys Compd.*, **897**, p. 163134.

35. Murray J.L., (1983). The Au-Ti (gold-titanium) system, *Bull. Alloy Phase Diagrams*, **4**, pp. 278–283.

36. Miura H., (2003). A unit cell parameter refinement program on windows computer, *J. Crystallogr. Soc. Jpn.*, **45**, p. 145.

37. Hosoda H., Enami K., Kamio A., Inoue K., (1996). Alloys design of PdTi-based shape memory alloys based on defect structures and site preference of ternary elements, *J. Intell. Mater. Syst. Struct.*, **7**, pp. 312–320.

38. Chiu W.-T., Ishigaki T., Nohira N., Umise A., Tahara M., Inamura T., Hosoda H., (2021). Influence of the precipitates on the shape memory effect and superelasticity of the near-eutectoid Ti-Au-Fe alloy towards biomaterial applications, *Intermetallics*, **133**, p. 107180.

39. Shinohara Y., Ishigaki T., Inamura T., Kanetaka H., Miyazaki S., Hosoda H., (2010). Phase constituents of Ti-Cr-Au and Ti-Cr-Au-Zr alloy systems, *Mater. Sci. Forum*, **654–656**, pp. 2122–2125.

40. Kremer G.O., Chiu M.-C., Lin C.-Y., Gupta S., Claudio D., Thevenot H., (2012). Application of axiomatic design, TRIZ, and mixed integer programming to develop innovative designs: A locomotive ballast arrangement case study, *Int. J. Adv. Manuf. Technol.*, **61**, pp. 827–842.

41. Hambidge M., (2003). Biomarkers of trace mineral intake and status, *Nutr. J.*, **133**(3), pp. 948S–955S.

42. Haynes W.M., (2016). *Handbook of Chemistry and Physics*, CRC Press, Ohio.

43. Buenconsejo P.J.S., Kim H.Y., Hosoda H., Miyazaki S., (2009). Shape memory behavior of Ti-Ta and its potential as a high-temperature shape memory alloy, *Acta Mater.*, **57**(4), pp. 1068–1077.

44. Buenconsejo P.J.S., Kim H.Y., Miyazaki S., (2011). Novel β-TiTaAl alloys with excellent cold workability and a stable high-temperature shape memory effect, *Scr. Mater.*, **64**(12), pp. 1114–1117.

45. Gloriant T., Texier G., Prima F., Laillé D., Gordin D.-M., Thibon I., Ansel D., (2006). Synthesis and phase transformations of beta metastable Ti-based alloys containing biocompatible Ta, Mo and Fe beta-stabilizer elements, *Adv. Eng. Mater.*, **8**(10), pp. 961–965.

46. Kim H.Y., Hashimoto S., Kim J.I., Inamura T., Hosoda H., Miyazaki S., (2006). Effect of Ta addition on shape memory behavior of Ti-22Nb alloy, *Mater. Sci. Eng. A*, **417**(1–2), pp. 120–128.

47. Hiramatsu K., Tahara M., Inamura T., Hosoda H., Miyazaki S., (2013). Effect of cold-rolling rate on texture in Ti-Mo-Al-Zr shape memory alloy, *Mater. Sci. Forum*, **738–739**, pp. 262–266.

48. Inamura T., Shimizu R., Hosoda H., Miyazaki S., (2012). Deformation texture of Ti-26mol%Nb-3mol%Al β-titanium alloy, *Mater. Sci. Forum*, **706–709**, pp. 1899–1902.

49. Wadood A., Inamura T., Yamabe-Mitarai Y., Hosoda H., (2013). Strengthening of β Ti-6Cr-3Sn alloy through β grain refinement, α phase precipitation and resulting effects on shape memory properties, *Mater. Sci. Eng. A*, **559**, pp. 829–835.

50. Ma J., Karaman I., Kockar B., Maier H.J., Chumlyakov Y.I., (2011). Severe plastic deformation of Ti74Nb26 shape memory alloys, *Mater. Sci. Eng. A*, **528**(25–26), pp. 7628–7635.

51. Chiu W.-T., Ishigaki T., Nohira N., Umise A., Tahara M., Hosoda H., (2021). Effect of 3d transition metal additions on the phase constituent, mechanical properties, and shape memory effect of near-eutectoid Ti-4Au biomedical alloys, *J. Alloys Compd.*, **857**, p. 157599.

52. Chiu W.-T., Wakabayashi K., Umise A., Tahara M., Inamura T., Hosoda H., (2021). Enhancement of mechanical properties and shape memory effect of Ti-Cr-based alloys via Au and Cu modifications, *J. Mech. Behav. Biomed. Mater.*, **123**, p. 104707.

53. Chiu W.-T., Wakabayashi K., Umise A., Tahara M., Inamura T., Hosoda H., (2021). Enhancement of the shape memory effect by the introductions of Cr and Sn into the β-Ti alloy towards the biomedical applications, *J. Alloys Compd.*, **875**, p. 160088.

54. Chiu W.-T., Ishigaki T., Nohira N., Umise A., Tahara M., Inamura T., Hosoda H., (2021). Evaluations of mechanical properties and shape memory behaviors of the aging-treated Ti-Au-Mo alloys, *Mater. Chem. Phys.*, **269**, p. 124775.

55. Chiu W.-T., Fuchiwaki K., Umise A., Tahara M., Inamura T., Hosoda H., (2022). Enhancement of the superelastic behavior of the Ti-Au-Cr-based shape memory alloys via the manipulations of annealing-treatments and Ta additions, *Mater. Sci. Eng. A*, **847**, p. 143312.

56. Wang L., Fu C., Wu Y., Li R., Wang Y., Hui X., (2019). Ductile Ti-rich high-entropy alloy controlled by stress induced martensitic transformation and mechanical twinning, *Mater. Sci. Eng. A*, **763**, p. 138147.

57. Bortolan C.C., Campanelli L.C., Paternoster C., Giguère N., Brodusch N., Bolfarini C., Gauvin R., Mengucci P., Barucca G., Mantovani D., (2021). Effect of oxygen content on the mechanical properties and plastic deformation mechanisms in the TWIP/TRIP Ti-12Mo alloy, *Mater. Sci. Eng. A*, **817**, p. 141346.

58. Brozek C., Sun F., Vermaut P., Millet Y., Lenain A., Embury D., Jacques P.J., Prima F., (2016). A β-titanium alloy with extra high strain-hardening rate: Design and mechanical properties, *Scr. Mater.*, **114**, pp. 60–64.

59. Abdel-Hady M., Hinoshita K., Morinaga M., (2006). General approach to phase stability and elastic properties of β-type Ti-alloys using electronic parameters, *Scr. Mater.*, **55**(5), pp. 477–480.

60. Zang M.C., Niu H.Z., Zhang H.R., Tan H., Zhang D.L., (2021). Cryogenic tensile properties and deformation behavior of a superhigh strength metastable beta titanium alloy Ti-15Mo-2Al, *Mater. Sci. Eng. A*, **817**, p. 141344.

61. Mantri S.A., Choudhuri D., Alam T., Ageh V., Sun F., Prima F., Banerjee R., (2017). Change in the deformation mode resulting from beta-omega compositional partitioning in a TiMo alloy: Room versus elevated temperature, *Scr. Mater.*, **130**, pp. 69–73.

62. Sun F., Zhang J.Y., Brozek C., Marteleur M., Veron M., Rauch E., Gloriant T., Vermaut P., Curfs C., Jacques P.J., Prima F., (2015). The role of stress induced martensite in ductile metastable beta Ti-alloys showing combined TRIP/TWIP effects, *Mater. Today: Proc.*, **2**(3), pp. S505–S510.

63. Chiu W.-T., Ishigaki T., Nohira N., Umise A., Tahara M., Inamura T., Hosoda H., (2021). Effect of Cr additions on the phase constituent, mechanical properties, and shape memory effect of near-eutectoid Ti-4Au towards the biomaterial applications, *J. Alloys Compd.*, **867**, p. 159037.

64. Hanada S., Yoshio T., Izumi O., (1986). Effect of plastic deformation modes on tensile properties of beta titanium alloys, *Trans. Jan. Inst. Metals*, **27**(7), pp. 496–503.

65. Hanada S., (1986). {332}<113> mechanical twinning in metastable β phase titanium alloys and alloy design, *J. Jpn. Inst. Metals*, **25**, pp. 755–764.

66. Hanada S., T. Yoshio, Izumi O., (1986). Plastic deformation mode of retained β phase in β-eutectoid Ti-Fe alloys, *J. Mater. Sci.*, **21**, pp. 866–870.

67. Hanada S., Izumi O., (1986). Transmission electron microscopic observations of mechanical twinning in metastable beta titanium alloys, *Metall. Trans. A*, **17**, pp. 1409–1420.

68. Hanada S., Izumi O., (1986). Deformation behaviour of retained β phase in β-eutectoid Ti-Cr alloys, *J. Mater. Sci.*, **21**, pp. 4131–4139.

69. Hainfeld J.F., Slatkin D.N., Focella T.M., Smilowitz H.M., (2014). Gold nanoparticles: A new X-ray contrast agent, *Br. J. Radiol.*, **79**(939), pp. 248–253.
70. Biesiekierski A., Wang J., Gepreel M.A.-H., Wen C., (2012). A new look at biomedical Ti-based shape memory alloys, *Acta Biomater.*, **8**(5), pp. 1661–1669.
71. Wataha J.C., (2000). Biocompatibility of dental casting alloys: A review, *J. Prosthet. Dent.*, **83**(2), pp. 223–234.

Chapter 2

Ceramics for Bone Repair and Cancer Therapy

Masaya Shimabukuro, Taishi Yokoi, and Masakazu Kawashita

Institute of Bioengineering and Biomaterials,
Tokyo Medical and Dental University,
2-3-10 Kanda-Surugadai, Chiyoda-ku, Tokyo, 101-0062, Japan

kawashita.bcr@tmd.ac.jp

Ceramics, such as Bioglass®, hydroxyapatite, and glass-ceramic A-W, can bond to living bone. These are known as bioactive ceramics and are used clinically as bone substitutes. Inorganic-organic composite materials such as hydroxyapatite-collagen and octacalcium phosphate-collagen composites, and carbonate apatite are also used clinically. In addition, ceramics are being applied for cancer treatment. Radioactive yttrium aluminosilicate glass microspheres are used for intra-arterial radiotherapy for unresectable hepatocellular carcinoma, and magnetic fluid containing magnetite nanoparticles is used in hyperthermia treatment for brain tumors. Thus, ceramics have great potential as biomaterials for bone repair and cancer treatment. In recent years, ceramics with superior therapeutic effects and novel functions

Biomedical Engineering: Imaging Systems, Electric Devices, and Medical Materials
Edited by Akihiro Miyauchi and Hiroyuki Kagechika

ISBN 978-981-5129-16-8 (Hardcover), 978-1-003-46404-4 (eBook)
www.jennystanford.com

have been proposed, such as yttrium oxide microspheres for intra-arterial radiotherapy, and iron nitride for hyperthermia treatment, as well as bioresponsive and antibacterial materials.

2.1 Introduction

Bones support the human body and protect vital organs such as the brain, lungs, heart, etc. The human skeleton consists of 206 bones, which are connected to one another by joints to allow for a wide range of movement. As such, even a single breakdown in a bone or joint can immediately impact daily life. Osteoarthritis and bone fractures are the second leading cause of elderly people becoming bedridden in Japan. To prevent this, diseased or broken bones are sometimes replaced using artificial joints or bones. Ceramics—which to date have been used mainly as structural and electronic materials—have been used in the field of orthopedics and dentistry since the 1970s.

In 1981, cancer surpassed stroke as the leading cause of death among the Japanese. The primary treatment for cancer is surgical removal; however, the function of the affected organ is often not fully recovered. Therefore, it is desirable to develop therapies that specifically target cancer cells and allow normal tissue to regenerate after treatment. Radiotherapy, chemotherapy, immunotherapy, and hyperthermia have such potential. In chemotherapy, molecular-targeted drugs that suppress cancer growth, by targeting specific molecules involved in cancer cell growth, have attracted attention in recent years. However, complete elimination of the side effects of chemotherapeutics is a challenge. Immunotherapy has been investigated as a treatment method following surgery, radiation therapy, and chemotherapy, but only some drugs, such as immune checkpoint inhibitors, have demonstrated therapeutic efficacy. Meanwhile, ceramics can play a major role in radiotherapy and hyperthermia.

This chapter focuses on ceramics for bone repair and cancer therapy. Ceramics in clinical use are described briefly, and ceramics under research for future applications are introduced.

2.2 Ceramics for Bone Repair

Ceramics for bone repair are classified into three types: bioinert, bioactive, and biodegradable ceramics, according to the responsiveness of the bone tissue. When bioinert ceramics are implanted into bone tissues, they are encapsulated by fibrous tissues. Aluminum oxide (Al_2O_3) and zirconium oxide (ZrO_2) are typical bioinert ceramics and have excellent strength and wear resistance. However, they do not have the property to bond directly to bone tissues. Hence, they are not used for bone repair, even though the thickness of the fibrous tissue formed at the interface between the ceramics and the bone tissue is very thin and the ceramics can be fixed to the bone tissue by mechanical interlocking. However, because of their excellent mechanical properties, these ceramics are used as dental materials today.

Bioactive and biodegradable ceramics are mainly used as bone substitutes. Bioactive ceramics bond directly to bone, and biodegradable ceramics are also capable of such bonding with a few exceptions. The first bioactive ceramics were developed by Hench in the early 1970s [1], who discovered that glasses of specific compositions, later referred to as Bioglass®, bond to the bone as well as soft tissues. Since the discovery of Bioglass®, various bioactive glasses and glass ceramics have been developed. A detailed description of bioactive glasses and glass ceramics can be found in the 1993 book by Hench and Wilson [2]. Calcium phosphate materials are now more common as bone substitutes than glass-based materials. Phosphate ions can exist as mono- to tri-valent anions and thus form compounds with calcium ions in various Ca/P molar ratios. Table 2.1 shows representative calcium phosphate compounds [3].

2.2.1 Bioresponsive Materials

In the above section, traditional ceramic bone substitutes, namely bioinert, bioactive, and biodegradable ceramics, were described. These ceramic biomaterials have been used clinically. In this section, a recently proposed ceramic bone substitute, which is in a new category and is at the research stage, is introduced.

Table 2.1 Representative calcium phosphate compounds [3]

Compound	Abbreviation	Formula	Ca/P molar ratio
Monocalcium phosphate monohydrate	MCPM	$Ca(H_2PO_4)_2 \cdot H_2O$	0.5
Monocalcium phosphate anhydrate	MCPA	$Ca(H_2PO_4)_2$	0.5
Dicalcium phosphate dihydrate	DCPD	$CaHPO_4 \cdot 2H_2O$	1.0
Dicalcium phosphate anhydrate	DCPA	$CaHPO_4$	1.0
Octacalcium phosphate	OCP	$Ca_8(HPO_4)_2(PO_4)_4 \cdot 5H_2O$	1.33
α-Tricalcium phosphate	α-TCP	$Ca_3(PO_4)_2$	1.5
β-Tricalcium phosphate	β-TCP	$Ca_3(PO_4)_2$	1.5
Amorphous calcium phosphate	ACP	$Ca_x(PO_4)_y \cdot nH_2O$	1.2–2.2
Hydroxyapatite	HAp	$Ca_{10}(PO_4)_6(OH)_2$	1.67
Tetracalcium phosphate	TTCP	$Ca_4(PO_4)_2O$	2.0

As is well known, there are numerous kinds of enzymes in the body. Polymers that express their functions in response to enzymes in the body have been reported to date. In addition to polymers, certain ceramics have been known to react with enzymes. Hydroxyapatite (HAp) can be synthesized via artificial synthetic systems involving the reaction of calcium ions and phosphate ions, generated by hydrolyzation of phosphate esters, mediated by alkaline phosphatase (ALP) [4]. ALP mediates the decomposition reaction of phosphate esters to phosphoric acid and alcohol, and it is present in human serum. Therefore, salts of calcium ions and phosphate esters (SCPEs) are good candidates as novel bone substitutes that respond to ALP in vivo and form HAp.

On this basis, the transformation reaction of calcium methyl phosphate, ethyl phosphate, butyl phosphate, phenyl phosphate, and dodecyl phosphate, types of SCPEs, in simulated body fluid (SBF) modified with ALP was examined [5, 6]. Although the pH value of SBF was 7.4, which is outside of the optimal pH range for ALP, the obvious transformation from calcium methyl phosphate, ethyl phosphate, and phenyl phosphate to HAp with low crystallinity was observed. The morphological change of calcium phenyl phosphate following transformation is shown in Figure 2.1 [5]. The plate-shaped calcium phenyl phosphate changed to an aggregate of small HAp particles after incubation in SBF containing ALP. In contrast, the transformation reactions of calcium butyl phosphate and dodecyl phosphate did not obviously exhibit such a change due to their low solubility. In other words, the rate of the transformation reaction can be controlled by the solubility of the SCPEs. In addition, the solubility of SCPEs can be controlled through the design of the hydrocarbon group of phosphate esters.

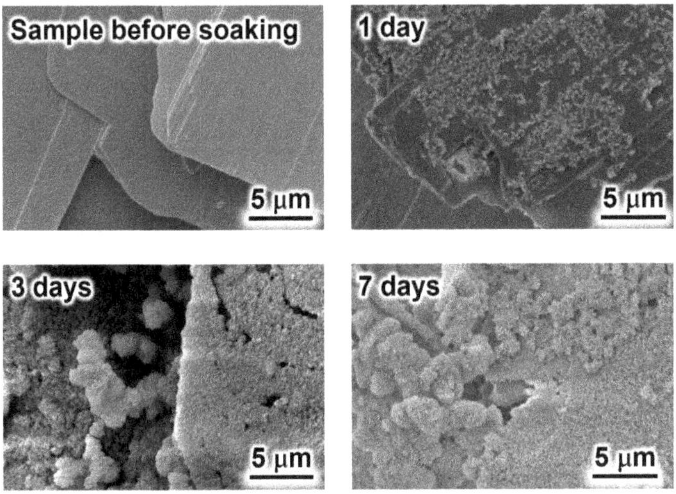

Figure 2.1 Scanning electron microscope images of calcium phenyl phosphate soaked in simulated body fluid containing alkaline phosphatase. Reprinted from reference [5] with permission.

In summary, it is becoming clear that SCPEs are credible candidates for bioresponsive ceramics that are likely to be absorbed by the action of ALP in vivo. For SCPEs that are intended to be gradually absorbed and replaced by bone tissue after implantation, the absorption and transformation rates of SCPEs into HAp after implantation in the body are most likely to be controllable. The concept of bioresponsive ceramics is undoubtedly one of the directions for future research into the development of ceramic biomaterials.

2.2.2 Antibacterial Materials

Fracture-related infection (FRI) is a devastating complication that can potentially lead to bone destruction and loss [7]. The incidence rate of FRI in complex open limb fractures is more than 15% [8]; thus, effective strategies are required to prevent FRI. The treatment for FRI is commonly performed by debridement, irrigation, dead space management using biomaterials such as scaffolds, and antibiotic administration. However, residual bacteria form biofilms that can resist antibiotics, owing to bacterial diversity and production of extracellular polymeric substances (EPS) on the scaffold and dead bone fragment (Figure 2.2 [9]); consequently, long-term hospitalization and antibiotic therapy are required, resulting in enormous treatment costs [8]. Antibacterial activity inhibits the initial stages of biofilm formation (i.e., bacterial adhesion and growth), and thereby may prevent biofilm formation. In other words, antibacterial materials are expected to be one of the effective strategies for preventing FRI and may achieve both bone regeneration and prevent biofilm formation simultaneously. In this section, we introduce the design of antibacterial scaffolds and surfaces based on biological responses, with the aim of both bone regeneration and infection prevention.

The composition of a scaffold governs both the osteogenic and antibacterial activities. For instance, carbonate apatite ($Ca_{10-a}(PO_4)_{6-b}(CO_3)_c$), which has a mineral composition similar to that of bone, exhibits compositional superiority in osteogenesis [10]; however, it does not show antibacterial activity. In contrast, silver (Ag) exhibits broad-spectrum antibacterial activity [11] against Gram-positive and -negative bacteria, including multi-drug resistant bacteria. However, it exhibits toxicity against cells and tissues in a concentration-dependent manner. Furthermore, the half-maximal inhibitory concentration (IC50) value of Ag ions against MC3T3-E1 cells was 2.77 μM [12], and thus low concentrations of Ag can impact osteogenesis. For these reasons, the composition of antibacterial scaffolds consisting of carbonate apatite and Ag must be optimized based on cell and tissue responses, in order to realize antibacterial and osteogenic activities without harmful effects on cells and tissues.

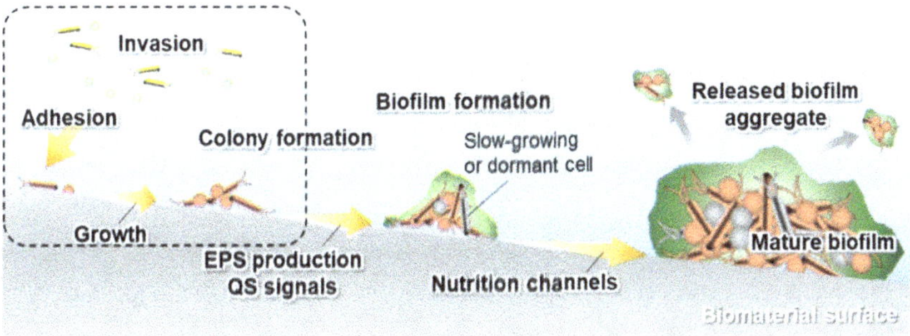

Figure 2.2 Schematic diagram of the biofilm formation process. The dashed area shows the initial stages of biofilm formation [9].

The no-observed-effect level (NOEL), which is the maximum level of a compound without any observed effect on biological and biochemical functions, is an important threshold for the composition of antibacterial scaffolds. To date, we have determined the NOEL of silver phosphate (Ag_3PO_4) in both in vitro and in vivo experiments using carbonate apatite scaffolds containing 0–6.8 wt.% Ag_3PO_4. The viability of *Staphylococcus epidermidis* and MC3T3-E1 cells decreased with increasing concentrations of Ag_3PO_4 in the carbonate apatite scaffolds. These results revealed that Ag_3PO_4 content of 0.1–0.3 wt.% was suitable to ensure antibacterial activity without cytotoxicity. Furthermore, Ag_3PO_4 content of 0.1–0.3 wt.% did not affect cellular adhesion, proliferation, ALP activity, calcification, and in vivo bone formation. However, an Ag_3PO_4 content of 0.3 wt.% caused an inflammatory reaction in the regenerated site (Figure 2.3 (C, F)), whereas a concentration of 0.1 wt.% did not (Figure 2.3 (B, E)).

In other words, the NOEL of Ag_3PO_4 was 0.1 wt.%, which was determined to be suitable for antibacterial scaffolds.

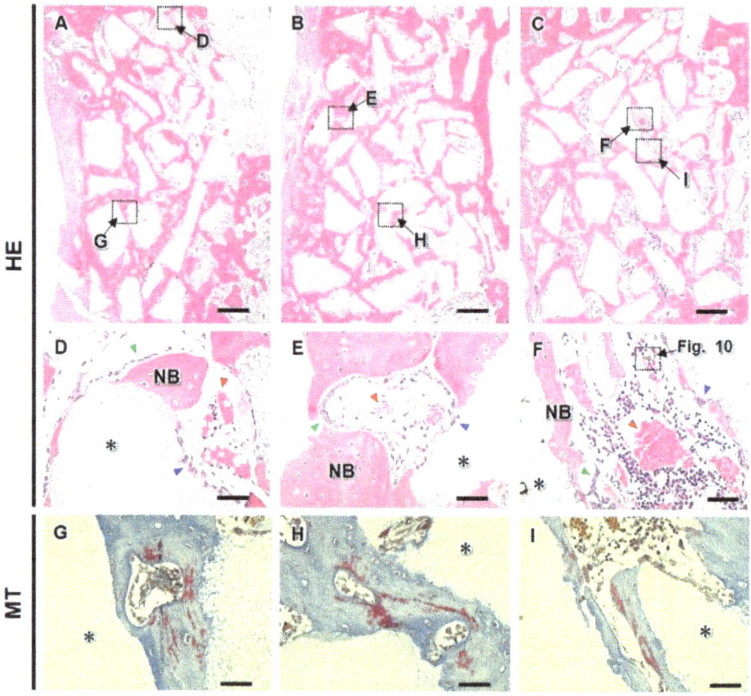

Figure 2.3 Hematoxylin-eosin-(A–F) and Masson's trichrome-stained (G–I) sections 4 weeks after implantation of carbonate apatite scaffolds containing 0 wt.% (A, D, G), 0.1 wt.% (B, E, H), and 0.3 wt.% (C, F, I); Ag_3PO_4 (D–I). Magnified views of the regions indicated by black squares in panels (A–C). "NB" and "*" in panels (D–I) indicate the newly formed bone and remaining materials, respectively. Scale bars in panels (A–C) and (D–I) represent 500 μm and 50 μm, respectively [15].

In addition to its composition, scaffold architecture is an important factor directly related to both bone regeneration and infection prevention. Honeycomb scaffolds have regularly aligned pores (so-called channels) that provide structural superiority in osteogenesis and angiogenesis [13]. Furthermore, this architecture allows the release of bacteria and necrotic bone through the scaffold channels, resulting in symptom improvement and bone formation [14]. Therefore, the honeycomb scaffold is an attractive architecture for achieving both bone regeneration and infection prevention. Based on its compositional and structural superiorities in bone regeneration and infection prevention, the surface of the carbonate apatite honeycomb scaffold was functionalized with Ag_3PO_4 at a concentration below its NOEL (0.1 wt.%) (Figure 2.4). The Ag_3PO_4-functionalized scaffold completely prevented bacterial infection in vivo in the presence of methicillin-resistant *Staphylococcus aureus*, formed new bone at 2 weeks after surgery, and was gradually replaced with new bone [14]. Hence, the use of optimal amounts of Ag in scaffolds can lead to simultaneous bone regeneration and infection prevention.

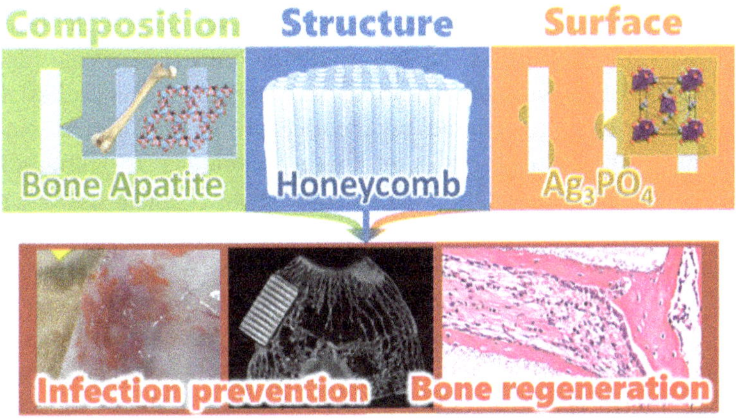

Figure 2.4 Schematic diagram of surface functionalization of carbonate apatite honeycomb scaffolds with Ag_3PO_4. Antibacterial honeycomb scaffolds achieved both bone regeneration and infection prevention [14].

In addition, copper (Cu) is another antibacterial element and is an essential trace element for humans. Furthermore, Cu ions upregulate bone-related genes, vascular endothelial growth factor, and hypoxia-inducible factor-1α [16, 17], resulting in the promotion of both osteogenesis and angiogenesis. Previously, we succeeded in the surface functionalization of carbonate apatite honeycomb scaffolds using Cu. Our results clearly demonstrated that an appropriate amount of Cu has beneficial roles in antibacterial activity, osteogenesis, and angiogenesis [18]. Thus, the design of antibacterial scaffolds based on cell and tissue responses can achieve both bone regeneration and infection prevention.

This concept is also applicable to titanium (Ti) surfaces and can prevent infectious diseases, such as peri-implantitis and prosthetic joint infection caused by biofilm formation, on medical devices made of Ti. Surface coating techniques have been used to control both the surface structure and composition of Ti surfaces, and they can be broadly divided into two groups: dry and wet processes. In general, dry processes, such as chemical vapor deposition, physical vapor deposition, and so on, mainly form dense ceramic layers with relatively high adhesive strength between the resulting layer and the substrate; however, these processes are limited by the target material, owing to high-temperature processing. The wet processes, such as chemical treatment, electrochemical treatment, and so on, mainly form porous ceramic layers at lower temperatures than the dry processes; however, the resulting layer shows lower adhesive strength than that formed by the dry processes. In this way, although the characteristics of these techniques are different, we introduce two coating techniques: alkaline heat treatment and micro-arc oxidation. Alkaline heat treatment, in which wet and dry processes are combined, forms a network-type porous oxide layer on Ti surfaces (Figure 2.5 (B)). Furthermore, micro-arc oxidation, an electrochemical surface treatment, forms a porous oxide layer consisting of electrolyte and substrate components (Figure 2.5 (C)). These surfaces show superior bioactivity to untreated Ti [19, 20]. Moreover, these coating techniques incorporate antibacterial elements such as Cu into the oxide layer. Previously, a Cu-doped porous oxide layer was formed on the Ti surface by alkaline-copper nitrate-heat treatment and exhibited antibacterial activity and bioactivity. Furthermore, the antibacterial activity of the resulting surface was enhanced by visible-light irradiation, owing to its photocatalytic activity [21]. In addition, antibacterial and pro-osteogenic activities without cytotoxicity were achieved on the Cu-incorporated porous oxide layer formed by micro-arc oxidation (MAO) [22, 23]. These coating techniques are attractive options for the design of antibacterial surfaces and are expected to prevent infection on Ti implants. Thus, antibacterial scaffolds and surfaces are effective strategies for preventing infection.

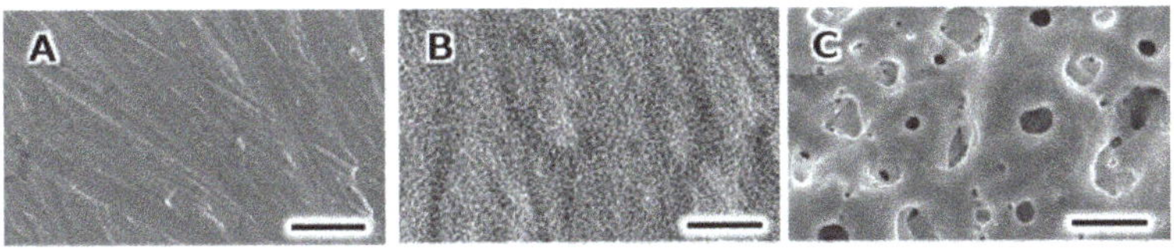

Figure 2.5 Scanning electron microscopy images of untreated Ti (A), alkaline-heat-treated Ti (B), and MAO-treated Ti (C). Scale bars represent 10 μm.

2.3 Ceramics for Cancer Therapy

As described in Section 2.1, radiotherapy is one of the cancer therapies that can be performed without surgical resection of the cancer. However, conventional radiotherapy is performed externally, and hence insufficient doses of radiation are often received by cancer, especially deep-seated cancer, and irradiation can also cause severe damage to healthy tissues. Stereotactic radiotherapy is a method of reducing radiation damage to normal tissues by delivering a narrowly focused low dose of radiation to the affected area from multiple directions. However, accurate irradiation is difficult when the location of the affected area fluctuates greatly with respiration. Further, because of the special nature of this treatment, there are currently only a limited number of facilities that provide the treatment in Japan. Radioactive ceramic microspheres that emit β rays can be used for intra-arterial radiotherapy for cancer, especially liver cancer (Figure 2.6).

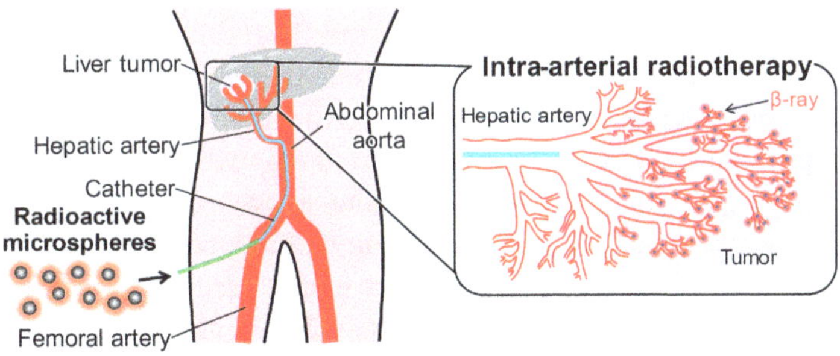

Figure 2.6 Schematic representation of intra-arterial radiotherapy using radioactive microspheres.

Cancerous tissues are heated more easily than normal tissues and cancer cells die at approximately 43 °C; a temperature that normal cells can tolerate. This is because blood vessels in normal tissues dilate when heated, increasing blood flow and allowing heat to escape, whereas blood vessels in cancerous tissues are thin and immature and cannot dilate to allow heat to escape when heated. Hyperthermia is a treatment method to kill cancer cells by heating the affected area. Magnetic materials can generate heat when exposed to an alternating current (AC) magnetic field. Therefore, when magnetic materials are loaded onto the cancer tissue and an AC magnetic field is applied, cancer cells can be heated and killed (magnetic hyperthermia). This section focuses on examples of ceramic microspheres for intra-arterial radiotherapy and ceramics for magnetic hyperthermia.

2.3.1 Ceramics for Radiotherapy

Since yttrium-89 (^{89}Y), holmium-165 (^{165}Ho), rhenium-185 (^{185}Re), and ^{187}Re can be β emitters (^{90}Y) and combined β-γ emitters (^{166}Ho, ^{186}Re, and ^{188}Re) by neutron bombardment, ceramic microspheres containing these elements have been developed for intra-arterial radiotherapy. Yttrium aluminosilicate (YAS) glass microspheres with 20–30 μm in size and composed of $17Y_2O_3{\cdot}19Al_2O_3{\cdot}64SiO_2$ (mol.%) (TheraSphere®) have been clinically used for intra-arterial radiotherapy for inoperable liver cancer [24, 25]. They are injected into the liver tumor by hepatic artery catheterization via the femoral artery. The controlled size of the microspheres enables embolization of the hepatic artery connected to the liver tumor. Since the radioactive isotope ^{90}Y is confined to the target organ by trapping it in chemically insoluble microspheres, it was necessary that the glass microspheres be highly durable as well as radioactive. Actually, glass microspheres with the above composition have shown excellent chemical durability. Radioactive ^{90}Y-loaded resin microspheres (SIR-spheres®) are also used in intra-arterial radiotherapy for inoperable liver cancer [26].

While both TheraSphere® and SIR-spheres® are revolutionary in that they enable intra-arterial radiotherapy using radioactive microspheres, the radiotherapeutic efficacy of the microspheres would be further improved by increasing the amount of yttrium in the microspheres. We found that pure yttrium oxide (Y_2O_3) microspheres 20–30 μm in size (Figure 2.7 (A)) with excellent chemical durability can be obtained by a high-frequency induction thermal plasma melting method, and administration of the radioactive Y_2O_3 microspheres could suppress tumor growth remarkably (Figure 2.7 (B)) [27]. It is expected that preclinical studies of Y_2O_3 microspheres will be initiated in the future.

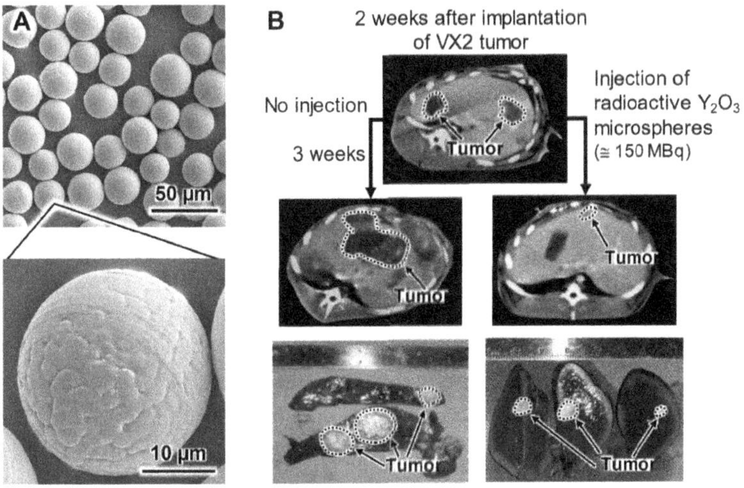

Figure 2.7 Scanning electron micrographs of Y_2O_3 microspheres (A), and representative CT and optical photographs of rabbit livers with and without infusion of radioactive Y_2O_3 microspheres (B). Modification of the figure from reference [27].

Since ^{166}Ho produced by neutron irradiation of ^{165}Ho emits not only β rays but also weak γ rays, the distribution of radioactive Ho-containing microspheres in the body can be visualized by single-photon radiation computed tomography (SPECT). Glass microspheres with a composition of $7Ho_2O_3{\cdot}52SiO_2{\cdot}21Al_2O_3{\cdot}20MgO$ (wt.%) [28] and ^{166}Ho-containing poly(lactic acid) (PLLA) microspheres have been developed to date. Clinical studies have been conducted on ^{166}Ho-containing PLLA microspheres [29]. Microspheres containing ^{186}Re and ^{188}Re, which emit β rays and weak γ rays, can be detected by SPECT, as for microspheres containing ^{166}Ho. Glass microspheres composed of metallic Re dispersed within a magnesium aluminoborate glass ($MgO-Al_2O_3-B_2O_3$) matrix have been proposed to date [30, 31]. These are produced by sintering ReO_2 powder and glass frit and then passing it through a propane/air flame. One advantage of the glass microspheres is that they can be activated for therapeutic action within 10 h by neutron bombardment, whereas several weeks are needed to activate YAS microspheres by neutron bombardment. Thus, they are considered a good candidate for in vivo radioembolization therapy because they are safe from the standpoint of radiation release in vivo, cost-effective in terms of neutron activation time, and can be directly imaged within the body [30].

2.3.2 Ceramics for Hyperthermia

Cancer cells generally perish at around 43 °C because of insufficient oxygen supply from blood vessels, whereas normal cells are not damaged at even higher temperatures. In addition, tumors are more easily heated than the surrounding normal tissues, since the blood vessels and nervous system of tumors are poorly developed. Therefore, hyperthermia is expected to be a very useful cancer treatment with a few side effects. Various techniques for heating tumors, such as treatments with hot water, infrared rays, ultrasound, and microwaves, have been investigated. However, deep-seated tumors cannot be heated effectively and locally using these techniques. Ferrimagnetic microspheres 20–30 μm in diameter are useful as thermoseeds to induce hyperthermia in deep-seated cancers. Following implantation using blood vessels, the spheres are entrapped in the capillary bed of tumors, similar to the radioactive microspheres described above, and the cancers can be heated locally by hysteresis loss when placed in an alternating magnetic field.

Iron oxide nanoparticles, such as magnetite (Fe_3O_4) and maghemite (γ-Fe_2O_3) nanoparticles, have been proposed as thermoseeds for magnetic hyperthermia [32]. Since the heat-generating ability of Fe_3O_4 nanoparticles depends largely on particle size as well as the AC magnetic field strength employed [33], fine-tuning the particle size of Fe_3O_4 nanoparticles is required to obtain high heat-generating ability [34]. Hyperthermia using Fe_3O_4 magnetic fluid [35, 36] has been developed and approved for the treatment of brain tumors in the EU since 2011, and pilot studies on patients with inter alia, pancreatic, prostate, breast, and esophageal cancers are being conducted.

Magnetic ceramic microspheres 20–30 μm in size may enable a new type of hyperthermia, intra-arterial hyperthermia. SiO_2 core-Fe_3O_4 shell microspheres (Figure 2.8) have been developed as thermoseeds for intra-arterial hyperthermia [27]. The next challenge is the further improvement of the heat-generating ability of these microspheres, by controlling the size of Fe_3O_4 and increasing the amount of Fe_3O_4 in the microspheres.

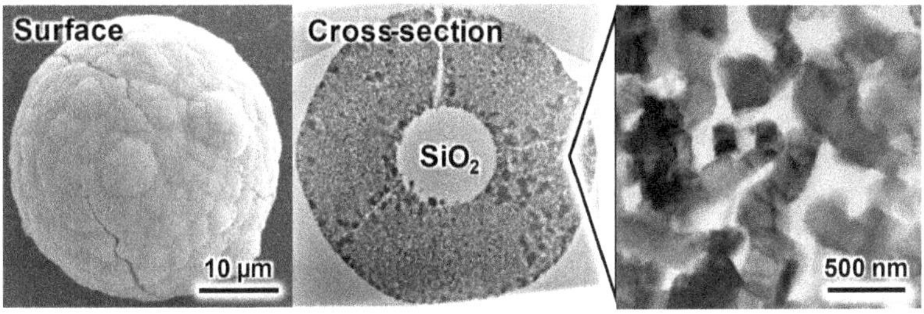

Figure 2.8 Scanning electron micrograph of a SiO_2 core-Fe_3O_4 shell microsphere and transmission electron micrographs of cross-sections of the microsphere. Modification of the figure from reference [27].

Besides Fe_3O_4 nanoparticles, iron nitride (Fe_xN_y) nanoparticles have recently been considered as next-generation thermoseeds because of their unique magnetic properties, such as high saturation magnetization and the potential to exhibit high heat generation capacity. $Fe_{16}N_2$ nanoparticles prepared by reduction and subsequent nitriding of Fe_3O_4 nanoparticles were estimated to show higher heat generation than Fe_3O_4 nanoparticles [37] and exhibited similar cytocompatibility as Fe_3O_4 nanoparticles [38]. These results indicate the high potential of Fe_xN_y as thermoseeds for more effective hyperthermia.

2.4 Summary

Ceramics have been developed mainly as bone substitutes, components of composites, and coating materials for metallic medical devices in biomedical fields. Additionally, as described in this chapter, some ceramics are useful for cancer therapy and have been developed as bioresponsive and antibacterial materials. It is expected that the excellent biofunctions of ceramics will continue to be exploited, and ceramic biomaterials will be developed for expanded medical applications in the future.

Acknowledgments

This work was partially supported by the JSPS KAKENHI grant numbers, JP21K18057, JP23H0464 and JP22H03949, and the Institute of Biomaterials and Bioengineering, Tokyo Medical and Dental University [Project "Design & Engineering by Joint Inverse Innovation for Materials Architecture"] of the Ministry of Education, Culture, Sports, Science, and Technology, Japan.

References

1. Hench, L. L., Splinter, R. J., Allen, W. C. and Greenlee, T. K. (1971) Bonding mechanisms at the interface of ceramic prosthetic materials, *J. Biomed. Mater. Res.*, **5**, pp. 117–141.
2. Hench, L. L. and Wilson, J. (1993) *An Introduction to Bioceramics*, World Scientific Publishing Co. Pte. Ltd., Singapore.
3. Dorozhkin, S. V. and Epple, M. (2000) Biological and medical significance of calcium phosphates, *Angew. Chem. Int. Ed.*, **41**, pp. 3130–3146.
4. Tanaka, H. and Ihata, D. (2010) Phase transformation of calcium phenyl phosphate in calcium hydroxyapatite using alkaline phosphatase at body temperature, *Mater. Res. Bull.*, **45**, pp. 103–108.
5. Yokoi, T., Ujiyama, T., Nakamura, J., Kawashita, M. and Ohtsuki, C. (2020) Behaviour of calcium phosphate ester salts in a simulated body fluid modified with alkaline phosphatase: a new concept of ceramic biomaterials, *Mater. Adv.*, **1**, pp. 3215–3220.
6. Yokoi, T., Mio, A., Nakamura, J., Sugawara-Narutaki, A., Kawashita, M. and Ohtsuki, C. (2022) Transformation behaviour of salts composed

of calcium ions and phosphate esters with different linear alkyl chain structures in a simulated body fluid modified with alkaline phosphatase, *Sci. Tech. Adv. Mater.*, **1**, pp. 341–351.

7. Metsemakers, W. J., Morgenstern, M., McNally, M. A., Moriarty, T. F., McFadyen, I., Scarborough, M., Athanasou, N. A., Ochsner, P. E., Kuehl, R., Raschke, M., Borens, O., Xie, Z., Velkes, S., Hungererm, S., Kates, L., Zalavras, C., Giannoudis, P. V., Richards, R. G. and Verhofstad, M. H. J. (2018) Fracture-related infection: a consensus on definition from an international expert group, *Injury*, **49**, pp. 505– 510.
8. Morgenstern, M., Kühl, R. Eckardt, H., Acklin, Y., Stanic, B., Garcia, M., Baumhoer, D. and Metsemakers, W. J. (2018) Diagnostic challenges and future perspectives in fracture-related infection, *Injury*, **49**, pp. S83–S90.
9. Shimabukuro, M. (2020) Antibacterial property and bio-compatibility of silver, copper, and zinc in titanium dioxide layers incorporated by one-step micro-arc oxidation: a review, *Antibiotics*, **9**, Article 716.
10. Hayashi, K., Kishida, R., Tsuchiya, A. and Ishikawa, K (2019) Honeycomb blocks composed of carbonate apatite, β-tricalcium phosphate, and hydroxyapatite for bone regeneration: effects of composition on biological responses, *Mater. Today Bio*, **4**, Article 100031.
11. Ruparelia, J. P., Chatterjee, A. K., Duttagupta, S. P. and Mukherji, S. (2008) Strain specificity in antimicrobial activity of silver and copper nanoparticles, *Acta Biomater.*, **4**, pp. 707–716.
12. Yamamoto, A., Honma, R. and Sumita, M. (1998) Cytotoxicity evaluation of 43 metal salts using murine fibroblasts and osteoblastic cells, *J. Biomed. Mater. Res.*, **39**, pp. 331–340.
13. Hayashi, K., Shimabukuro, M., Kishida, R., Tsuchiya, A. and Ishikawa, K. (2022) Structurally optimized honeycomb scaffolds with outstanding ability for vertical bone augmentation, *J. Adv. Res.*, https://doi.org/10.1016/j.jare.2021.12.010
14. Hayashi, K., Shimabukuro, M. and Ishikawa, K. (2022) Antibacterial honeycomb scaffolds for achieving infection prevention and bone regeneration, *ACS Appl. Mater. Interfaces*, **14**, pp. 3762–3772.
15. Shimabukuro, M., Hayashi, K., Kishida, R., Tsuchiya, A. and Ishikawa, K. (2022) No-observed-effect level of silver phosphate in carbonate apatite artificial bone on initial bone regeneration, *ACS Infect. Dis.*, **8**, pp. 159–169.

16. Dai, Q., Li, Q., Gao, H., Yao, L., Lin, Z., Li, Z., Zhu, S., Liu, C., Yang, Z., Wang, G., Chen, D. and Cao, X. (2021) 3D printing of Cu-doped bioactive glass composite scaffolds promotes bone regeneration through activating the HIF-1α and TNF-α pathway of hUVECs, *Biomater. Sci.*, **9**, pp. 5519–5532.
17. Ryan, E. J., Ryan, A. J., González-Vázquez, A., Philippart, A., Ciraldo, F. E., Hobbs, C., Nicolosi, C., Boccaccini, A. R., Kearney, C. J. and O'Brien, F. J. (2019) Collagen scaffolds functionalised with copper-eluting bioactive glass reduce infection and enhance osteogenesis and angiogenesis both in vitro and in vivo, *Biomaterials*, **197**, pp. 405–416.
18. Shimabukuro, M., Hayashi, K., Kishida, R., Tsuchiya, A. and Ishikawa, K. (2022) Surface functionalization with copper endows carbonate apatite honeycomb scaffold with antibacterial, proangiogenic, and pro-osteogenic activities, *Biomater. Adv.*, **135**, Article 212751.
19. Tsutsumi, Y., Niinomi, M., Nakai, M., Tsutsumi, H., Doi, H., Nomura, N. and Hanawa, T. (2012) Micro-arc oxidation treatment to improve the hard-tissue compatibility of Ti–29Nb–13Ta–4.6Zr alloy, *Appl. Surf. Sci.*, **262**, pp. 34–38.
20. Nishiguchi, S., Nakamura, T., Kobayashi, M., Kim, H. M., Miyaji, F. and Kokubo, T. (1999) The effect of heat treatment on bone-bonding ability of alkali-treated titanium, *Biomaterials*, **20**, pp. 491–500.
21. Suzuki, K., Yokoi, T., Iwatsu, M., Furuya, M., Yokota, K., Mokudai, T., Kanetaka, H. and Kawashita, M. (2021) Antibacterial properties of Cu-doped TiO_2 prepared by chemical and heat treatment of Ti metal, *J. Asian Ceram. Soc.*, **9**, pp. 1448–1456.
22. Shimabukuro, M., Tsutsumi, Y., Nozaki, K., Chen, P., Yamada, R., Ashida, M., Doi, H., Nagai, A. and Hanawa, T. (2020) Investigation of antibacterial effect of copper introduced titanium surface by electrochemical treatment against facultative anaerobic bacteria, *Dent. Mater. J.*, **39**, pp. 639–647.
23. Shimabukuro, M., Hiji, A., Manaka, T., Nozaki, K., Chen, P., Ashida, M., Tsutsumi, Y., Nagai, A. and Hanawa, T. (2020) Time-transient effects of silver and copper in the porous titanium dioxide layer on anti-bacterial properties, *J. Funct. Biomater.*, **11**, Article 44.
24. Ehrhardt, G. J. and Day, D. E. (1987) Therapeutic use of ^{90}Y micro-spheres, *Int. J. Rad. Appl. Instrum. B: Nucl. Med. Biol.*, **14**, pp. 233–242.
25. Salem, R., Lewandowski, R. J., Mulcahy, M. F., Riaz, A., Ryu, R. K., Ibrahim, S., Atassi, B., Baker, T., Gates, V., Miller, F. H., Sato, K. T., Wang,

E., Gupta, R., Benson, A. B., Newman, S. B., Omary, R., A., Abecassis, M. and Kulik, L. (2010) Radioembolization for hepatocellular carcinoma using yttrium-90 microspheres: a comprehensive report of long-term outcomes, *Gastroenterology*, **138**, pp. 52–64.

26. Kennedy, A., Cohn, M., Coldwell, D.M. Drooz, A., Ehrenwald, E., Kaiser, A., Nutting, C. W., Rose, S. C., Wang, E. A. and Savin, M. A. (2017) Updated survival outcomes and analysis of long-term survivors from the MORE study on safety and efficacy of radioembolization in patients with unresectable colorectal cancer liver metastases, *J. Gastrointest. Oncol.*, **8**, pp. 614–624.

27. Kawashita, M. (2018) Development and evaluation of the properties of functional ceramic microspheres for biomedical applications, *J. Ceram. Soc. Japan*, **126**, pp. 1–7.

28. Brown, R. F., Lindesmith, L. C. and Day, D. E. (1999) ^{166}Ho-containing glass for internal radiotherapy of tumors, *Int. J. Rad. Appl. Instrum. B: Nucl. Med. Biol.*, **18**, pp. 783–790.

29. Stella, M., Braat, A. J. A. T., van Rooij, R., de Jong, H. W. A. M. and Lam, M. G. E. H. (2022) Holmium-166 radioembolization: current status and future prospective, *Cardiovasc. Intervent. Radiol.* https://doi.org/10.1007/s00270-022-03187-y.

30. Conzone, S. D., Hafeli, U. O., Day, D. E. and Ehrhardt, G. J. (1999) Preparation and properties of radioactive rhenium glass microspheres intended for in vivo radioembolization therapy, *J. Biomed. Mater. Res.*, **42**, pp. 617–625.

31. Hafeli, U. O., Casillas, S., Dietz, D. W., Pauer, G. J., Rybicki, L. A., Conzone, S. D. and Day, D. E. (1999) Hepatic tumor radioembolization in a rat model using radioactive rhenium (^{186}Re/^{188}Re) glass microspheres, *Int. J. Radiat. Oncol. Biol. Phys.*, **44**, pp. 189–199.

32. Dadfar, S. M., Roemhild, K., Drude, N. I., von Stillfried, S., Knuchel, R., Kiessling, F. and Lammers, T. (2019) Iron oxide nanoparticles: diagnostic, therapeutic and theranostic applications, *Adv. Drug Deliv. Rev.*, 138, pp. 302–325.

33. Li, Z., Kawashita, M., Araki, N., Mitsumori, M., Hiraoka, M. and Doi, M. (2010) Magnetite nanoparticles with high heating efficiencies for application in the hyperthermia of cancer, *Mater. Sci. Eng. C*, **30**, pp. 990–996.

34. Jeyadevan, B. (2010) Present status and prospects of magnetite nanoparticles-based hyperthermia, *J. Ceram. Soc. Japan*, **118**, pp. 391–401.

35. Jordan, A., Wust, P., Fahling, H., John, W., Hinz, A. and Felix R. (1993) Inductive heating of ferrimagnetic particles and magnetic fluids: physical evaluation of their potential for hyperthermia. *Int. J. Hyperthermia*, **9**, pp. 51–68.

36. Thiesen, B. and Jordan, A. (2008) Clinical applications of magnetic nanoparticles for hyperthermia, *Int. J. Hyperthermia*, **24**, 467–474.

37. Shibata, M., Ogawa T. and Kawashita, M. (2019) Synthesis of iron nitride nanoparticles from magnetite nanoparticles of different sizes for application to magnetic hyperthermia, *Ceram. Int.*, **45**, pp. 23707–23714.

38. Shibata, M., Kanetaka, H., Furuya, M., Yokota, K., Ogawa, T. and Kawashita, M. (2021) Cytotoxicity evaluation of iron nitride nanoparticles for biomedical applications, *J. Biomed. Mater. Res.*, **109**, pp. 1784–1791.

Chapter 3

Hydrophilic Treatment Using Atmospheric Pressure Low-Temperature Plasma

Osawa Taiki, Liu Zhizhi, Fukuchi Kai, Yamauchi Motoaki, and Okino Akitoshi

FIRST, Tokyo Institute of Technology, Yokohama 226-8501, Japan

o-taiki@plasma.es.titech.ac.jp

3.1 Introduction

Currently, research on the development of treatment devices and artificial organs using biomaterials is being actively conducted in the medical field. The greatest advantage of biomaterials, such as silicone and some fluoropolymers, is that they do not cause rejection by the living body and can be used safely. However, they have the disadvantage of poor spreading of adhesives, due to their low hydrophilicity, making it difficult to bond with other materials. Therefore, it is generally necessary to perform pretreatment using primers or special solutions, but each material requires different solutions and pretreatment takes several tens of minutes to several hours.

Biomedical Engineering: Imaging Systems, Electric Devices, and Medical Materials
Edited by Akihiro Miyauchi and Hiroyuki Kagechika

ISBN 978-981-5129-16-8 (Hardcover), 978-1-003-46404-4 (eBook)
www.jennystanford.com

Recently, plasma treatment, which enables surface modification by generating various highly reactive chemical species, has been attracting attention. Atmospheric pressure plasma, which does not require vacuum equipment, is a low-cost and simple method. The author's group has developed several atmospheric pressure low-temperature plasma devices that can stably generate low-temperature plasma from room temperature to about 100 °C using various gases. This paper describes the results of plasma treatment of polyimide film, perfluoroalkoxy alkane (PFA) film, and silicon rubber sheet using the developed devices, and the evaluation of the hydrophilic effect.

3.2 Atmospheric Pressure Low-Temperature Plasma

Conventionally, low-pressure plasma has been used when plasma is used for the surface treatment or processing of materials. Low-pressure plasma is generated by applying a high voltage and a low pressure inside a container, like a fluorescent lamp. Since low-pressure plasma is generated in a vacuum chamber, plasma processing is possible in an environment with extremely low impurities. Therefore, low-pressure plasma has been used for the surface treatment of semiconductors. However, generating low-pressure plasma requires depressurization of the vessel, which requires a vacuum vessel and exhaust equipment, and the objects to be treated are limited to those that can be placed inside the vacuum vessel. In addition, if other processes are to be performed at atmospheric pressure, depressurization must be performed each time an object is loaded or unloaded into or out of the vacuum chamber, making it impossible to perform a series of operations efficiently.

In contrast, atmospheric pressure plasma does not require vacuum facilities because the inside of the vessel does not need to be depressurized as in the past, and plasma treatment of large objects, such as aircraft and biological tissue, which have been difficult to treat in low-pressure vessels, is now possible. In particular, atmospheric pressure low-temperature plasma can generate thermally non-equilibrium plasma in which plasma is repeatedly generated by short pulse discharges, which suppresses the slow temperature rise of the time constant and produces a large amount of reactive species such as radicals in spite of the low temperature. In other words, a field with high chemical activity can be formed even though the temperature is below about 100 °C. Therefore, applications such as surface treatment of heat-sensitive materials, irradiation of living organisms, sterilization, and virus inactivation are being investigated.

3.2.1 Direct and Remote Processing

Plasma processing methods can be broadly classified into two types: direct processing and remote processing. Direct processing is a method in which the object to be treated is directly treated in plasma, as shown in Figure 3.1. It is possible to treat thin objects uniformly, and the low temperature of the generated plasma makes it possible to irradiate even heat-sensitive materials. However, since plasma is generally generated in a strong electric field, this method generates electrical discharges on the treated object. Therefore, this method is not suitable for electronic devices that are vulnerable to electrical damage.

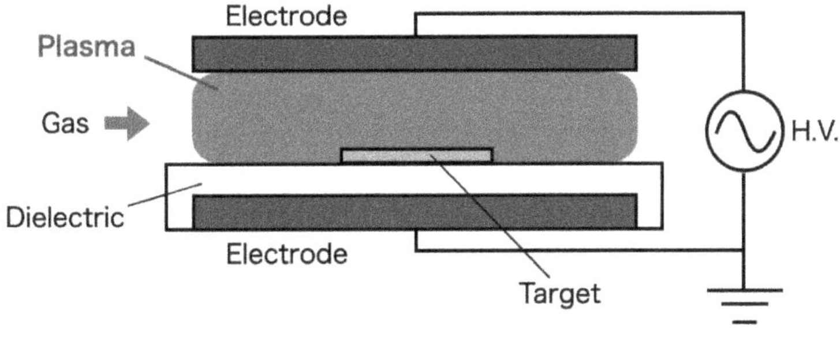

Figure 3.1 Direct processing method.

On the other hand, remote processing uses a gas stream to inject the generated plasma into the target object [1], as shown in Figure 3.2. In this method, the plasma generator and the target are separated from each other, so the target is not damaged by the discharge at all. In addition, the generated plasma reacts with the surrounding air to produce various reactive species, which can be expected to cause a variety of chemical reactions.

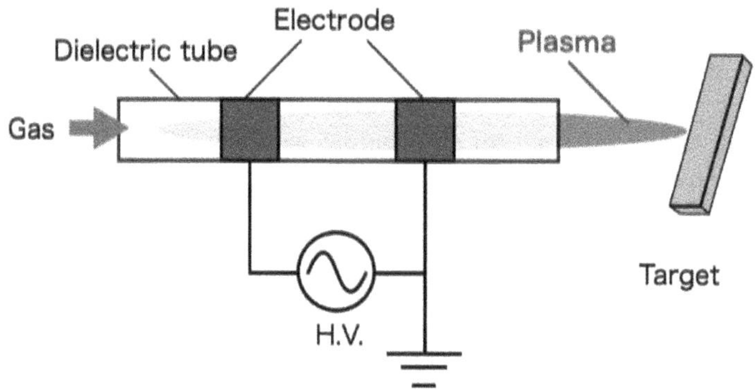

Figure 3.2 Remote processing method.

3.2.2 Dielectric Barrier Discharge

A typical plasma generation method for direct processing is dielectric barrier discharge (DBD). In DBD, a dielectric is placed on one or both surfaces of a pair of electrode plates, as shown in Figure 3.3, and a high AC voltage is applied between the electrode plates to generate plasma through discharge. When dielectrics are not placed on the surfaces of the electrode plates, a discharge is generated in a portion between the electrode plates, and a strong discharge is generated at that location thereafter. In contrast, when a dielectric is placed, even if a discharge is generated, an electric charge is accumulated on the surface of the dielectric and the discharge cannot be sustained at that location, so a discharge is generated at the next location. This is repeated at high speed to generate a uniform fine discharge between the electrode plates. Eventually, this charge accumulates over the entire surface of the dielectric, but by reversing the polarity of the voltage, a discharge in the opposite direction is generated. By repeating this process, plasma can be continuously maintained in the discharge space [2, 3]. Since the distance between the electrode plates is only a few millimeters, the thickness of the object to be treated is limited, but this discharge method is advantageous for the direct treatment of thin film-like materials.

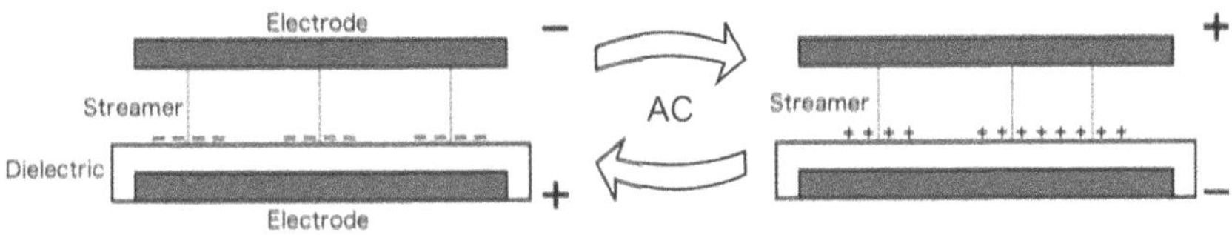

Figure 3.3 DBD method.

3.2.3 Multi-Gas Plasma Jet

A typical plasma generation method for remote processing is to inject the aforementioned DBD with a gas flow as shown in Figure 3.2. In this method, electrodes are placed outside a cylindrical dielectric, such as a glass tube, and a plasma generated by applying a high AC voltage to the electrodes while a certain flow rate of gas is flowing is injected. However, this method can only generate plasma with rare gases, such as argon and helium, which easily form plasma, limiting the fields of application.

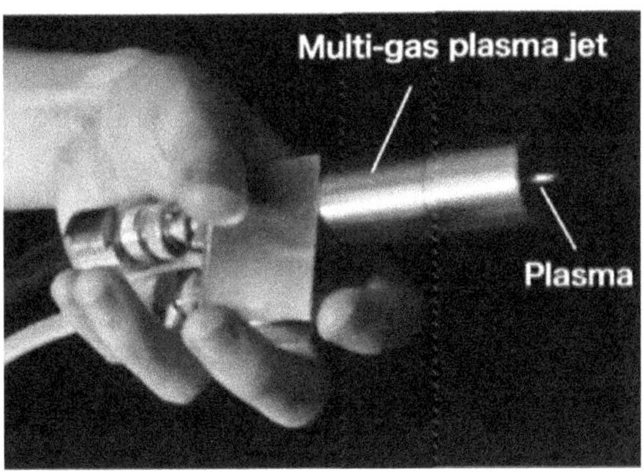

Figure 3.4 A multi-gas plasma jet device.

Therefore, the authors have developed a multi-gas plasma jet that can easily plasma not only rare gases such as argon and helium but also molecular gases such as nitrogen, oxygen, carbon dioxide, and mixed gases and air under atmospheric pressure (Figure 3.4). This plasma system is similar to the structure of the remote processing plasma described above, and stable atmospheric pressure low-temperature plasma can be generated by applying a high voltage of about 50 Hz to 40 MHz in the form of a sine wave or pulse between a pair of electrodes arranged in the plasma generator. Since a discharge occurs between the electrodes, high-density plasma can be generated.

3.3 Hydrophilic Treatment Using Atmospheric Pressure Low-Temperature Plasma

The hydrophilicity of a material surface is mainly determined by surface cleanliness, chemical properties, and surface roughness. In the hydrophilic treatment of polymeric compounds with plasma, the reactive species generated in the plasma are thought to contribute to the removal of surface deposits, or contaminants, and surface modification, or the addition of hydrophilic groups to the surface [4]. Substances adhering to the material surface are not chemically bonded to the surface but are weakly bound by intermolecular forces, so when the reactive species generated in the plasma strike the surface, the adhered substances are detached from the surface. This washes the adhered substances from the surface and improves the hydrophilicity. On the other hand, in surface modification, the reactive species generated in the plasma act on the surface of the material itself. In this case, the reactive species bind to the molecular chains of the polymeric material, forming carboxyl groups (–COOH), carbonyl groups (C=O), and hydroxy groups (–OH) on the surface. Since these functional groups have hydrophilic properties, the surface properties of the water-repellent material can be modified to be hydrophilic [5, 6].

Thus, the type and amount of reactive species generated in the plasma are thought to be involved in the hydrophilic treatment effect, and the treatment effect varies greatly depending on the type of gas used in the treatment and the plasma generation method [7]. As shown in Figure 3.5, various materials have been found to become hydrophilic when irradiated with plasma for 1 second using the developed multi-gas plasma jet. Since the plasma jet from the device is about room temperature, it is possible to irradiate heat-sensitive materials and living organisms.

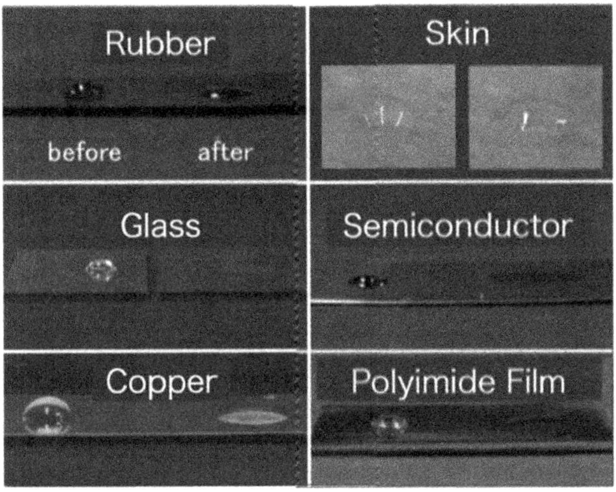

Figure 3.5 Plasma hydrophilic treatment for various materials.

3.3.1 Evaluation Method of Hydrophilicity

The contact angle of a drop of water on a horizontally placed specimen is often used to evaluate hydrophilicity. The higher the hydrophilicity of the material surface, the thinner the droplets spread and the smaller the contact angle of the droplets. The contact angle is measured to evaluate the hydrophilicity of the material surface, and the JIS (Japanese Industrial Standards) defines the contact angle measurement method in "JIS R 3257 Wettability Test Method for Glass Substrate Surfaces [8]. The principle is shown in Figure 3.6.

In the measurement of the contact angle, a stationary water droplet with a volume of 4 μL or less is considered to be part of a sphere. In this case, the following relationship holds between the contact angle θ, the height of the droplet h [mm], and the radius of the droplet r [mm].

$$\theta = 2\tan^{-1}(h/r) \tag{3.1}$$

Since the contact angle is difficult to measure visually, it is generally measured using a contact angle measuring device.

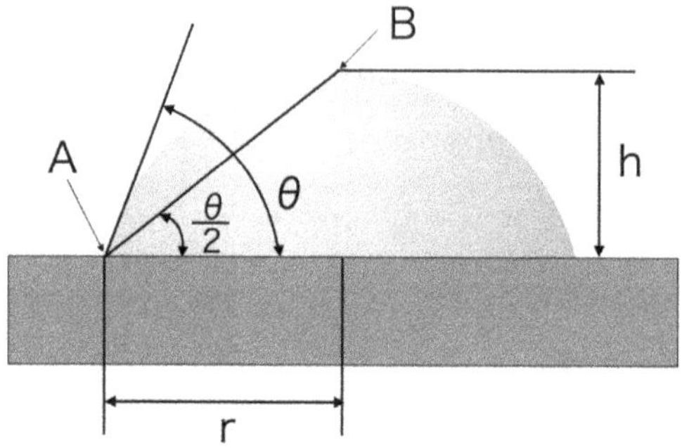

Figure 3.6 Contact angle measurement method.

3.3.2 Hydrophilization Effect on Polyimide Film

In this section, we describe the results of a comparison of direct and remote hydrophilization treatments of polyimide film, a thermally sensitive material, using various gas species. Kapton film (50 μm thick) from DuPont was used in the experiments.

In the experiment, a multi-gas plasma jet was used as shown in Figure 3.7 to irradiate the polyimide film at a distance of 5 mm from the plasma generator. In this process, the polyimide film is not damaged by heat or discharge because the plasma generator and the object to be treated are separated. However, since the plasma comes into contact with the surrounding atmosphere, it is affected by oxygen, nitrogen, carbon dioxide, and water vapor in the air. As mentioned above, the reactive species generated by the plasma remove surface deposits and modify the surface, resulting in a hydrophilic effect. By changing the gas used to generate the plasma, the type and concentration of the reactive species in the plasma can be greatly changed, resulting in different hydrophilic treatment effects.

Figure 3.8 shows the results of contact angle measurements of polyimide film irradiated with a plasma of each gas type (argon, helium, nitrogen, air, oxygen, and carbon dioxide) for 1 second [9]. The vertical axis shows the contact angle of a drop of 2 μL purified water. The contact angle before the treatment was 69.3°, but the contact angle decreased with plasma treatment of all gas types, indicating that the surface of the polyimide

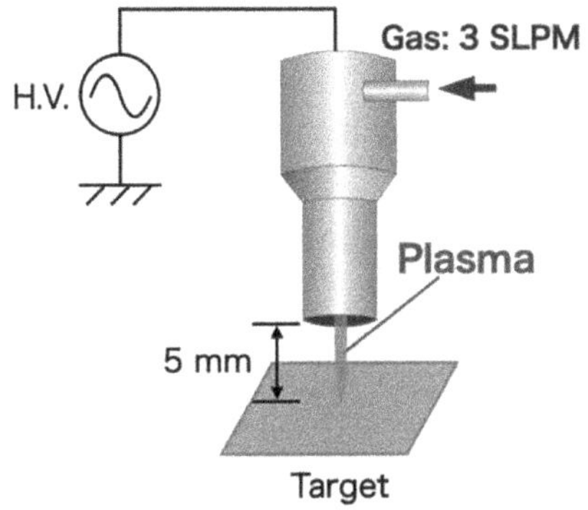

Figure 3.7 Remote processing using multi-gas plasma jet.

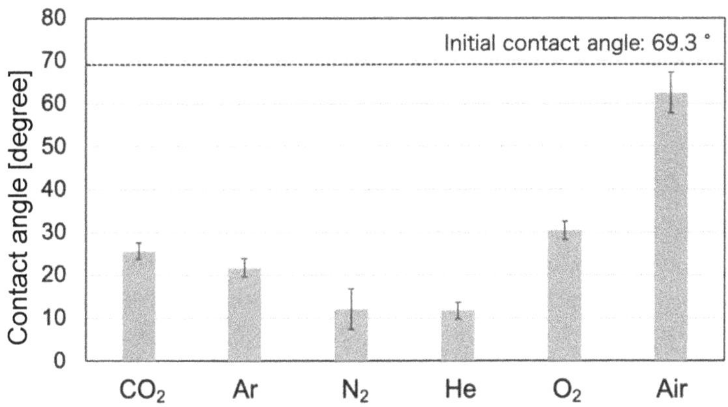

Figure 3.8 Hydrophilic effect of each gas plasma on polyimide film [8].

film became hydrophilic. In particular, the plasma treatment with helium and nitrogen showed a large hydrophilic effect. On the other hand, the air plasma did not cause much hydrophilic effect. In air plasma, N_xO_y is formed by the reaction of nitrogen and oxygen, whereas in nitrogen plasma, nitrogen radicals are formed. This suggests that nitrogen radicals contribute significantly to the hydrophilic treatment of polyimide film. Since helium and argon are rare gases, they cannot produce chemically reactive species by themselves, but they can be activated by collisions with nitrogen and oxygen in the air surrounding the plasma to produce reactive species. The ionization energy of helium is higher than that of argon, making it easier to activate molecules in the air. Therefore, the helium plasma is considered to have a large hydrophilic treatment effect. From the results shown in Figure 3.7, the selection of the gas types of the plasma is important to obtain a high hydrophilic effect.

3.3.3 Duration of Hydrophilic Effect by Nitrogen Plasma Treatment

The above results indicate that atmospheric pressure plasma treatment is a suitable technology for the hydrophilic treatment of polyimide film. However, the surface condition of polyimide changes over time, and the hydrophilic effect generally decreases. Therefore, we investigated the change in contact angle with time after plasma treatment. Nitrogen gas, which has a high hydrophilic effect, was used for plasma treatment, and treatment was performed for 1 second. The contact angles were then stored in air or purified water, and the contact angles were measured for each storage time. The results are shown in Figure 3.9. The contact angle increased rapidly with plasma treatment, and in the case of storage in air, the contact angle increased from 7° to 44° in 48 hours. On the other hand, when stored in purified water, the increase was limited to 29°. When stored in air, the increase in contact angle began to saturate after about 6 hours, while in purified water, the increase in contact angle began to saturate after about 1 hour. When polyimide film is placed in the air after plasma treatment, it is believed that the treatment effect is attenuated because the organic matter in the air adheres to the cleaned surface or segments containing hydrophilic groups imparted by the plasma invert and goes into the interior of the film. On the other hand, when the polyester was stored in purified water, there were few impurities in the water, and the binding of the hydrophilic groups to the water prevented the segments from burrowing into the interior, thus slowing down the decay rate of hydrophilicity.

In conclusion, the decay of the hydrophilic effect of plasma-treated polyimide film depends on the storage conditions, and storage in purified water is considered to be an effective method to prevent the decay of the hydrophilic treatment effect by plasma.

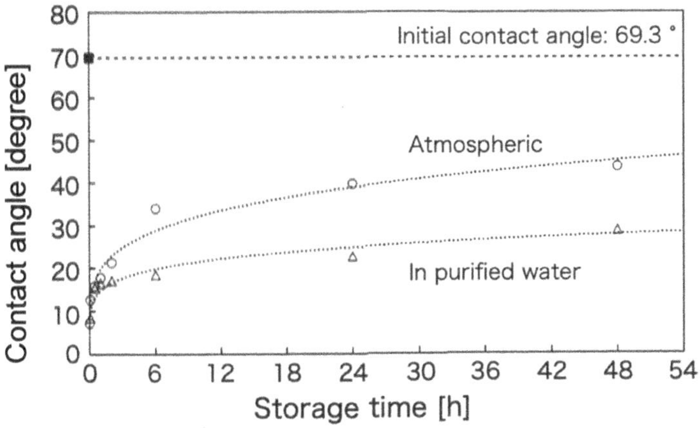

Figure 3.9 Change in contact angle with storage time [9].

3.4 Hydrophilization Effect on Biomaterials

Currently, silicone and fluorine-based resins, which are materials with high biocompatibility, are mainly used for artificial organs, artificial blood vessels, and dentures. These biomaterials are relatively soft and have high tensile strength, so they can be applied to any part of the body. However, they have very low hydrophilicity and are difficult to adhere to other materials. Fluorinated resins, in particular, cannot be easily surface modified because of the presence of fluorine on the surface of the material. Therefore, new treatment methods are required to improve the hydrophilicity and adhesion of biomaterials.

In this section, we present the results of our evaluation of the hydrophilic effect of atmospheric pressure low-temperature plasma irradiation on silicon, a biomaterial with very low hydrophilicity, and PFA, a fluorinated resin.

3.4.1 Hydrophilization Effect on PFA

For the hydrophilization experiment on PFA, plasma was generated in the same method as in Figure 3.7, and PFA was treated for 30 seconds. Then, 3 μL of purified water was dropped onto the PFA, and the contact angle was measured. Figure 3.10

shows the contact angle measurement results. The contact angle of PFA before plasma treatment was 85.7°. The contact angle remained almost unchanged even after treatment with argon and helium plasma, which are rare gases. Nitrogen plasma reduced the contact angle to about 60°, but it was equivalent to that of untreated polyimide film, so it could not be said that hydrophilic treatment was achieved. In contrast, carbon dioxide and oxygen plasma treatments showed a high hydrophilic effect, and especially oxygen plasma reduced the contact angle to about 10°.

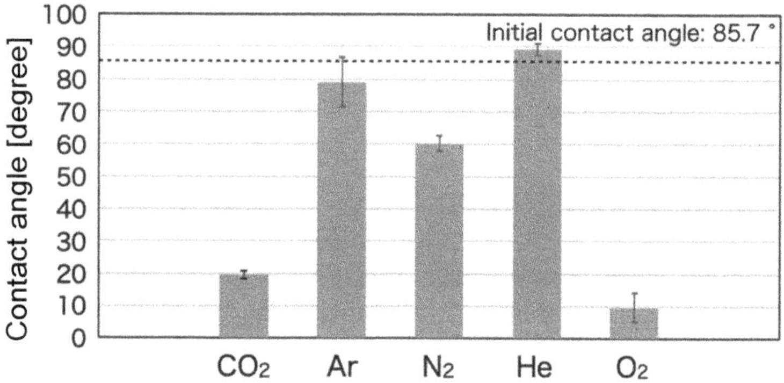

Figure 3.10 Hydrophilic effect of each gas plasma on PFA.

Figure 3.11 shows the change in the hydrophilic effect of PFA as a function of plasma irradiation time for each gas. The contact angle of helium plasma remained almost unchanged after 120 seconds of treatment. The contact angles of argon and nitrogen plasmas decreased to 63.3° and 40.5°, respectively, after 120 seconds of treatment. But the contact angles remained almost unchanged from those after 60 seconds of treatment, indicating that the hydrophilic effect tended to saturate. Carbon dioxide and oxygen plasmas were highly effective, and the contact angle decreased to less than 10° after 60 seconds of treatment with carbon dioxide plasma, and to less than 10° after 30 seconds of treatment with oxygen plasma. This suggests that fluorine atoms are attached to the surface of PFA and that the reactive species necessary for surface modification are generated in particularly large amounts by carbon dioxide and oxygen plasma. And that hydroxyl and carboxyl groups known as hydrophilic groups are attached instead of fluorine atoms. Hydroxyl and carboxyl groups, known as hydrophilic groups, are thought to be attached instead of fluorine atoms.

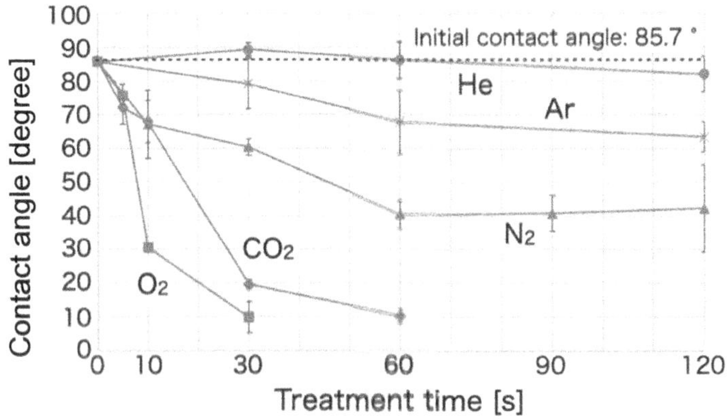

Figure 3.11 Hydrophilic effect of each gas plasma treatment time on PFA.

3.4.2 Hydrophilization Effect on Silicone Rubber Sheet

We conducted the same experiment as PFA on silicone rubber sheets, which are used as biomaterials in the same as PFA. The gases used were nitrogen, carbon dioxide, and oxygen, which have been shown to be highly effective in treating PFA. Figure 3.12 shows the change in hydrophilic effect with treatment time. All plasma treatments showed a high hydrophilic effect, especially nitrogen and carbon dioxide, which reduced the contact angle to less than 10° after 3 seconds of treatment. The contact angle of oxygen plasma was also reduced to 15.7° after 3 seconds of treatment, indicating that sufficient hydrophilic effect was obtained. Nitrogen, carbon dioxide, and oxygen plasma all showed high hydrophilic effects, suggesting that in addition to nitrogen radicals, hydrophilic groups such as carboxyl groups also contribute significantly to the hydrophilization of silicone rubber sheets. The fact that carbon dioxide plasma had a higher hydrophilic effect than oxygen plasma suggests that among the hydrophilic groups, carboxyl groups with carbon bonds contribute to the hydrophilicity of silicone rubber sheets.

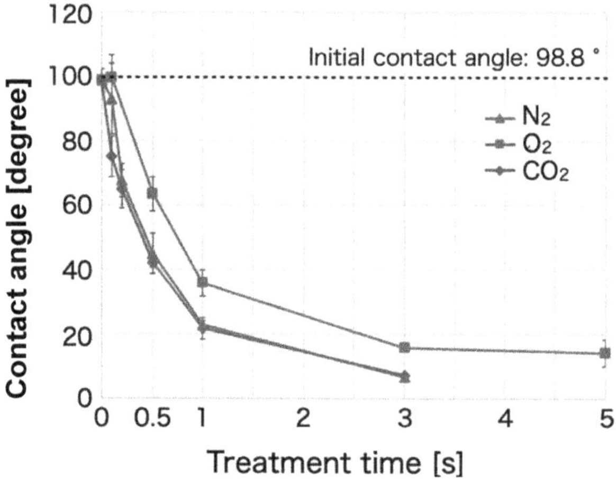

Figure 3.12 Hydrophilic effect of each gas plasma treatment time on silicone rubber sheets.

3.5 Summary

In this chapter, we introduce various methods of generating atmospheric pressure low-temperature plasma and describe the multi-gas plasma jet developed by our research group. The results of plasma hydrophilic treatment of various materials using the multi-gas plasma jet are presented. For polyimide film, irradiation with helium or nitrogen plasma for 1 second reduced the contact angle to about 12°, indicating a very high hydrophilic effect. This is thought to be due to the significant contribution of nitrogen radicals generated by nitrogen plasma and reactive species generated by the reaction between helium plasma and the surrounding air. On the other hand, carbon dioxide and oxygen plasma were particularly effective in treating PFA, a fluoropolymer. This can be attributed to the fact that fluorine atoms on the PFA surface were replaced by hydrophilic groups such as hydroxyl and carboxyl groups derived from oxygen. In addition, the hydrophilic effect of nitrogen and carbon dioxide plasma on silicone rubber sheets was very high, indicating that the surface of silicone rubber is relatively easy to hydrophilize.

It was also found that storage of polyimide film after plasma treatment in purified water was more effective to suppress the increase in contact angle than storage in air. The storage condition after treatment is also important to maintain the hydrophilic effect on the material surface.

In this study, plasma treatment was performed on a polyimide film, PFA, and silicon rubber sheet to evaluate the hydrophilic effect, and it was found that the gas type of plasma with high effect differed depending on the material. However, the mechanism of surface modification by plasma treatment has not yet been elucidated, and we intend to conduct surface analysis after plasma treatment to elucidate the mechanism.

References

1. Takamatsu, T., Hirai, H., Sasaki, R., Miyahara, H., Okino, A. (2013). Surface Hydrophilization of Polyimide Films Using Atmospheric Damage-Free Multigas Plasma Jet Source, *IEEE Transactions on Plasma Science*, **41**, 119.
2. Nozaki, T., Takagi, K., Namihira, T., Kitano, K., Kim, J., Nomura, S., Ichikawa, N., Tomita, H., Hayashi, N., Iwao, T. (2007). Let's Obtain an Atmospheric Pressure Plasma, *J. Plasma Fusion Res.*, **83**, 942 (in Japanese).
3. Ayan, H., Fridman, G., Gutsol, A. F., Vasilets, V. N., Fridman, A., Friedman, G. (2008). Nanosecond-Pulsed Uniform Dielectric-Barrier Discharge, *IEEE Transactions on Plasma Science*, **36**, 504.
4. Miyahara, H., Shibata, M., Oshita, T., Takamatsu, T., Okino, A. (2013). Hydrophilization of Polyimide Film using Damage-Free Multi-Gas Plasma Jet, *The Society of Chemical Engineers*, **39**, 372 (in Japanese).
5. Abdollah, S., Anton, Y. N., Nathalie, D. G., Rino, M., Christophe, L. (2011). Surface modification of polypropylene with an atmospheric pressure plasma jet sustained in argon and an argon/water vapor mixture, *Applied Surface Science*, **20**, 257, 8737.
6. Ono, S., Yamada, M. (2010). The Effect of Radicals on the Surface Treatment using Atmospheric Pressure Microwave Plasma, *IEEJ Trans FM*, **130**, 919 (in Japanese).
7. Suenaga, Y., Takamatsu, T., Iwai, T., Okino, A. (2020). Development and Application to Hydrophilization using Atmospheric Low Temperature Plasma, *Journal of the Institute of Electrostatics Japan*, **44**, 96 (in Japanese).

8. Japanese Standards Association (2007), JIS Handbook 33 Glass (in Japanese).
9. Liu, Z., Yamauchi, M., Taiki, O., Jo, M., Okino, A. (2022). High Performance Design and Application Technology of Polyimide, Technical Information Institute CO., LTD, pp. 354–366. (in Japanese).

Chapter 4

Microwave Imaging Algorithms for Breast Cancer Detection

Hang Song[a] and Takamaro Kikkawa[b]

[a]*Department of Transdisciplinary Science and Engineering, School of Environment and Society, Tokyo Institute of Technology, 2-12-1 Ookayama, Meguro-ku, Tokyo 152-8550 Japan*
[b]*Research Institute for Nanodevices, Hiroshima University, 1-4-2 Kagamiyama, Higashi-Hiroshima, Hiroshima 739-8527, Japan*

song.h.ac@m.titech.ac.jp

Microwave imaging has been studied for breast cancer detection as a non-invasive modality for the past decades. This technology is based on the fact that the dielectric properties of the tumor tissues are different from those of the normal tissues. Through years of effort, this technology has evolved from preliminary tests on phantoms to clinical trials. Several groups have developed the imaging system and applied it to clinical tests. Furthermore, encouraging results have also been obtained, which demonstrated the efficacy of this technology. It is promising that microwave breast imaging will be applied to practical usage and is expected to promote the frequent monitoring of breast health. In this

Biomedical Engineering: Imaging Systems, Electric Devices, and Medical Materials
Edited by Akihiro Miyauchi and Hiroyuki Kagechika

ISBN 978-981-5129-16-8 (Hardcover), 978-1-003-46404-4 (eBook)
www.jennystanford.com

chapter, the state-of-the-art of this technique is reviewed and the clinical results are presented.

4.1 Introduction

The widely used technology for breast health monitoring is X-ray mammography. However, this technology causes ionizing radiation and needs compression of the breast, which brings pain and harm to the women. Therefore, it cannot be utilized for frequent monitoring. Due to this issue, new methods are highly desired, which are non-invasive and easy to access for regular breast health monitoring. Through extensive measurements of the dielectric properties of the human breast tissues, it has been found that the dielectric properties of the tumor tissues are different from those of the normal tissues [1–3]. Based on this fact, microwave imaging has been studied for the purposes of breast cancer detection, breast health monitoring, breast tumor screening, and chemotherapy monitoring. There are generally two methodologies for breast imaging: the radar-based method and microwave tomography [4–12]. For the radar approach, the microwave pulse is emitted and the time-of-flight of the reflected wave is utilized to estimate the position of the tumor. On the other hand, microwave tomography aims at reconstructing the whole distribution of the dielectric property of the whole breast.

As state-of-the-art, both approaches have been applied to clinical trials. Among those, the radar-based approach is widely utilized for its computational simplicity and efficiency. There are also several systems, which have been applied to relatively large-scale clinical tests, and encouraging results have been obtained [9, 13–15]. In the following part, the radar-based approach will be concentrated. The fundamental principle of the radar-based approach and the algorithms utilized in recent progress are presented.

4.2 Fundamental Principle

In the electromagnetic theory, the behavior of the electromagnetic wave can be depicted by the Maxwell equations.

$$\nabla \cdot \boldsymbol{B} = 0$$

$$\nabla \times \boldsymbol{E} = -\frac{\partial \boldsymbol{B}}{\partial t}$$

$$\nabla \cdot \boldsymbol{D} = \rho$$

$$\nabla \times \boldsymbol{H} = \frac{\partial \boldsymbol{D}}{\partial t} + \boldsymbol{J} \tag{4.1}$$

where ***E***, ***H***, ***D***, and ***B*** are the electric field strength, magnetic field strength, electric displacement, and magnetic flux density, respectively. ρ and ***J*** are the electric charge density and electric current density. Additionally, there are two auxiliary constitutive equations to relate ***E*** and ***D***, ***H***, and ***B***. If the material is linear and isotropic, these relations are depicted as follows:

$$\boldsymbol{D} = \varepsilon \boldsymbol{E}$$

$$\boldsymbol{B} = \mu \boldsymbol{H} \tag{4.2}$$

where ε is the permittivity of the medium and μ is the permeability.

When the electromagnetic wave propagates on the same medium, the wave will be advancing without any hindrance. However, when the wave encounters the boundary between two different materials, there will be reflection and transmission occur. Figure 4.1 shows an image of the wave propagating at the boundary of two materials of medium 1 and medium 2. Here, the two media are assumed to have the permittivity and permeability of ε_1, μ_1 and ε_2, μ_2, respectively. At the boundary of the two media, the boundary conditions should be satisfied as follows:

$$\hat{n} \times (\boldsymbol{E}_2 - \boldsymbol{E}_1) = 0$$

$$\hat{n} \times (\boldsymbol{H}_2 - \boldsymbol{H}_1) = \boldsymbol{J}_s$$

$$\hat{n} \cdot (\boldsymbol{B}_2 - \boldsymbol{B}_1) = 0$$

$$\hat{n} \cdot (\boldsymbol{D}_2 - \boldsymbol{D}_1) = \rho_s \tag{4.3}$$

where $\boldsymbol{J}_s$ and ρ_s are the surface current density and surface charge density. $\boldsymbol{E}_2$, $\boldsymbol{H}_2$, $\boldsymbol{B}_2$, $\boldsymbol{D}_2$ and $\boldsymbol{E}_1$, $\boldsymbol{H}_1$, $\boldsymbol{B}_1$, $\boldsymbol{D}_1$ are the electric field, magnetic field, magnetic flux density, and electric displacement in medium 2 and medium 1 at the boundary. $\hat{n}$ is the surface normal pointing from medium 1 to medium 2. These equations imply that the tangential components of the electric field and the normal components of magnetic flux are continuous across the boundary. While the differential tangential component of the magnetic field is $\boldsymbol{J}_s$ and the differential normal component of electric displacement is ρ_s.

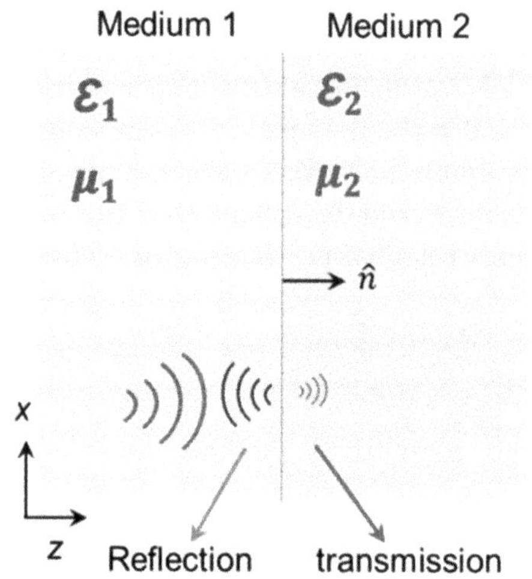

Figure 4.1 Schematic of the wave propagating from one medium to another.

Considering the planar wave case, which is normally incident, the components of electric and magnetic fields are all tangential to the boundary plane. Assume that the electric and magnetic fields are on the *x*- and *y*-axis and can be expressed as:

$$\boldsymbol{E}_i = \boldsymbol{x} \cdot E_i \cdot e^{i(k_1 z - \omega t)}$$

$$\boldsymbol{H}_i = \boldsymbol{y} \cdot H_i \cdot e^{i(k_1 z - \omega t)} \tag{4.4}$$

where $\boldsymbol{E}_i$ and $\boldsymbol{H}_i$ are the electric field and magnetic field of the incident wave. k represents the wave number in the medium. It can be related to the velocity v and angular frequency ω of the electromagnetic wave as $k = \omega/v$. Similarly, the reflected fields and the transmitted fields can be written as follows:

$$\boldsymbol{E}_r = \boldsymbol{x} \cdot E_r \cdot e^{i(-k_1 z - \omega t)}$$

$$\boldsymbol{H}_r = \boldsymbol{y} \cdot H_r \cdot e^{i(-k_1 z - \omega t)}$$

$$\boldsymbol{E}_t = \boldsymbol{x} \cdot E_t \cdot e^{i(k_2 z - \omega t)}$$

$$\boldsymbol{H}_t = \boldsymbol{y} \cdot H_t \cdot e^{i(k_2 z - \omega t)} \tag{4.5}$$

where $\boldsymbol{E_r}$, $\boldsymbol{E_t}$ and $\boldsymbol{H_r}$, $\boldsymbol{H_t}$ are the electric field and magnetic field of the reflected and transmitted waves, respectively. Here $-k$ means that the reflected wave propagates in the contrary direction of the incident wave. k_1 and k_2 are the wave numbers in the two media. Substitute the $\boldsymbol{E}$ and $\boldsymbol{B}$ in Eqs. (4.1) with (4.4), the relation between the amplitudes of incident electric and magnetic fields can be obtained as follows:

$$H_i = \frac{k_1}{\omega \mu_1} E_i \tag{4.6}$$

Similarly, the relationship between the reflected and transmitted fields can be expressed as:

$$H_r = -\frac{k_1}{\omega \mu_1} E_r$$

$$H_t = \frac{k_2}{\omega \mu_2} E_t \tag{4.7}$$

According to the boundary condition as given in Eq. (4.3), the tangential component of both the electric and magnetic fields are continuous at the interface between two non-conducting media with no free charges. Therefore, the relationship between the incident, reflected, and transmitted wave can be written as:

$$E_i + E_r = E_t$$

$$H_i + H_r = H_t \tag{4.8}$$

Substitute Eqs. (4.6) and (4.7) into Eq. (4.8), the following can be obtained:

$$\frac{k_1}{\omega\mu_1}E_i - \frac{k_1}{\omega\mu_1}E_r = \frac{k_2}{\omega\mu_2}E_t \tag{4.9}$$

Combining Eq. (4.8) and Eq. (4.9), the ratio between the incident and reflected, transmitted waves can be expressed as:

$$\frac{E_r}{E_i} = \left(\frac{\sqrt{\varepsilon_1} - \sqrt{\varepsilon_2}}{\sqrt{\varepsilon_1} + \sqrt{\varepsilon_2}}\right)$$

$$\frac{E_t}{E_i} = \left(\frac{2\sqrt{\varepsilon_1}}{\sqrt{\varepsilon_1} + \sqrt{\varepsilon_2}}\right) \tag{4.10}$$

Here, the two media are supposed to be non-magnetic. From Eq. (4.10), it can be known that when the dielectric property of the 2nd medium is large, there will be a large reflected wave from the interface. This gives an intuition of the basic principle of radar-based breast cancer detection. Since the breast tumor has larger dielectric properties compared to the normal tissue. When the electromagnetic wave propagates at the interface between the tumorous tissue and normal tissues, there will be reflected waves. By collecting the reflected waves, the position of the tumor tissues can be estimated.

Figure 4.2 shows the concept of radar-based confocal imaging for breast cancer detection. The basic principle of this method is as follows. The input pulse is emitted by the emitter antenna (Tx) and will be reflected by the target. Then the reflection will be received by the detector (Rx). From the delay time of the target reflection, the length of the propagation path can be calculated. Since the position of the emitter and detector is known, the possible target position can be drawn as an ellipse. By summing the ellipse from different channels, the target position is added coherently and can be estimated.

In the implementation of the confocal imaging algorithm, the procedure is as follows. As shown in Figure 4.3, the area that will be reconstructed is selected and this area will be divided into many cells. Here, we call it pixels. Then a certain pixel $\boldsymbol{P}$ is selected and the distance between the center of the pixel and a certain antenna pair (e.g., Ant1–Ant2) is calculated. The distance is denoted as L. Next, the delay time for this point is calculated as $\Delta t = L/v$.

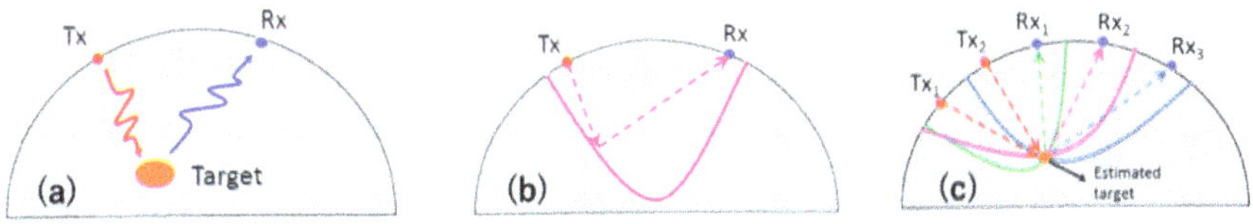

Figure 4.2 The principle of confocal imaging. (a) Wave propagation. (b) Possible position by one channel. (c) Target position estimation by numerous channels [16].

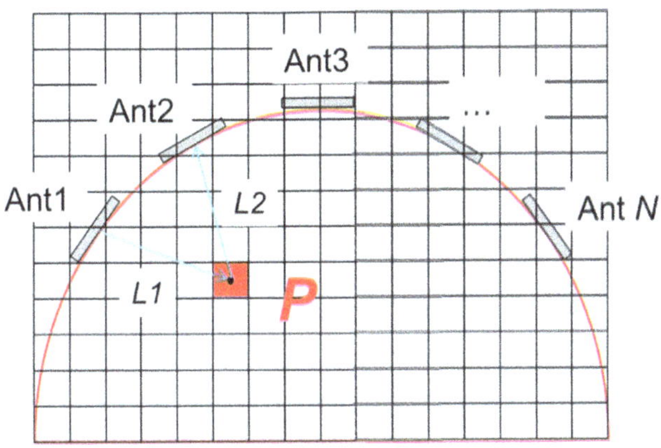

Figure. 4.3 The calculated imaging area and the pixels.

Suppose the signal emitted from Ant1 and received by Ant2 is $S_{12}(t)$. Then, the energy from $S_{12}(t)$ for this pixel P is assigned as $I_{12}(P) = S_{12}(\Delta t)$. Next, move the pixel and use the same procedure as depicted above, the time-domain signal amplitude is mapped to the space as the ellipsoidal orbit as shown in Figure 4.4.

By mapping all the signals to space and add together, an energy distribution can be obtained. The maximum point is regarded as the target estimated position.

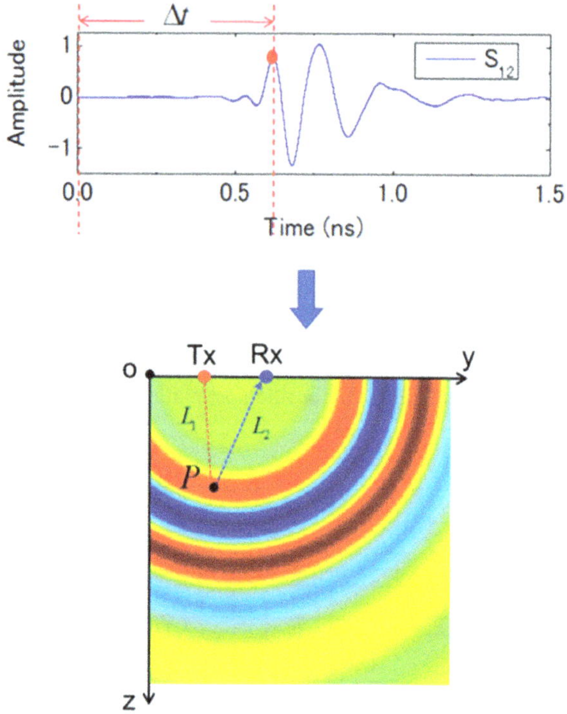

Figure 4.4 Mapping the time-domain signal into the spatial domain.

4.3 Imaging Algorithm for Breast Cancer Detection

In the hand-held microwave imaging device, complementary metal oxide semiconductor (CMOS) circuits were designed and utilized to generate and receive the pulse signals. Generally, the functional modules that compose the main part of the detector are the Gaussian monocycle pulse (GMP) generator, the switching matrix, and the sampling circuits [17–20]. As shown in Figure 4.5, from the signal generator module, the GMP is generated as the pulse train with a repetition rate of 100 MHz. The pulse width is around 160 ns.

When the pulse signals encounter an area, which has large dielectric properties such as tumor tissues, there will be reflections from the area. The sampling circuit can capture and digitize the analog signals into digital form and save the data into the computer for post-processing. Figure 4.6 shows an example of the received signals from a certain antenna pair measured at different positions. It can be observed that although the shape of the signals is similar, they have offsets along the time axis at different positions. This is caused by the system jitter and this offset should be compensated. The compensation for the phase shift is conducted in the following procedure. First, the baseline signal is chosen, which is the one measurement at the initial position. Then, the other signals are adjusted in time to let them align with the baseline signal. The alignment procedure is basically to find the best time shift factor, which can minimize the difference between the compensated signal and the baseline signal. As shown in Figure 4.7, the range for determining the time shift factor is defined as the t_s and t_e. This range is chosen as three times the interval between the t_{min} and t_{max}, which are the maximum peak and minimum peak of the received signal.

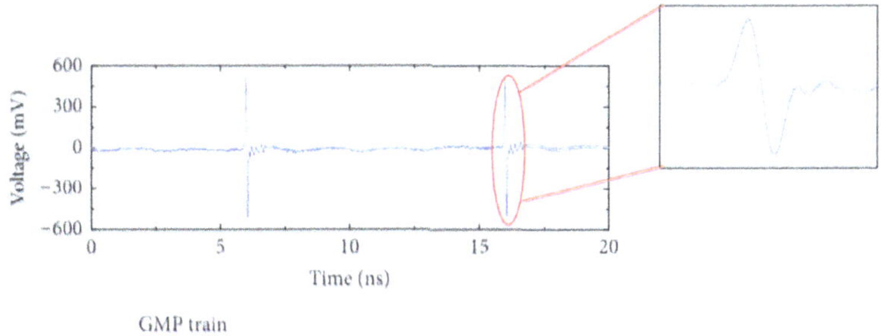

Figure 4.5 The Gaussian monocycle pulse train with a pulse width of 160 ps and a repetition period of 10 ns [19].

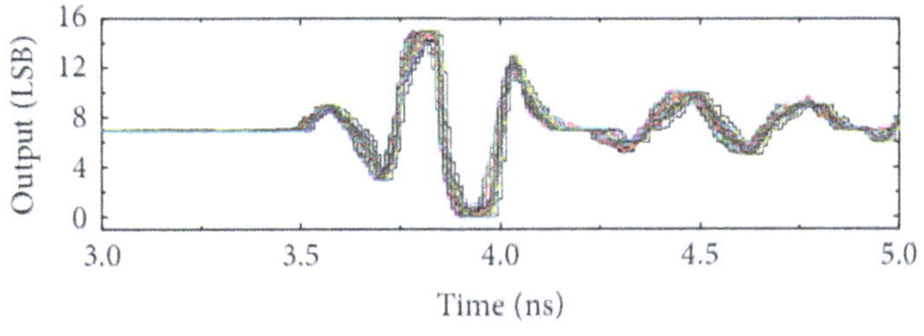

Figure 4.6 The received signals at different positions from the same antenna pair [19].

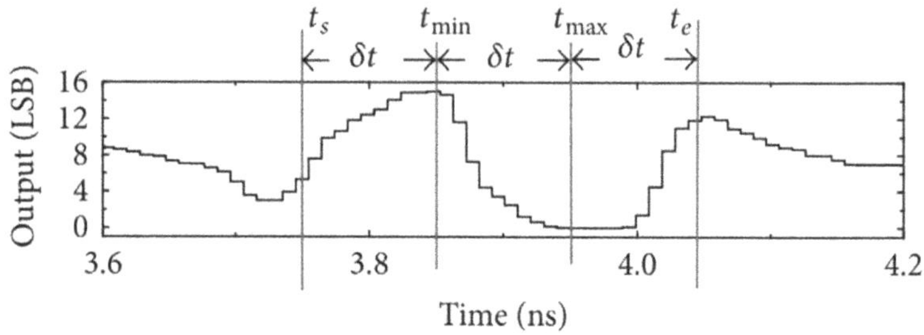

Figure 4.7 The time range for signal phase shift compensation [19].

The processing is depicted as equations in the following. Define all the received signals from the measurement as:

$$\boldsymbol{S} = \{\boldsymbol{S}_1, \ldots, \boldsymbol{S}_1, \ldots, \boldsymbol{S}_N\} \tag{4.11}$$

where N indicates the total antenna pairs and $\boldsymbol{S}_i$ means the signals measured at all positions from the ith antenna pair. Here, the antenna pair is also named a channel. Then, the $\boldsymbol{S}_i$ can be further depicted as:

$$\boldsymbol{S}_i = \{\boldsymbol{S}_{i1}[n], \ldots, \boldsymbol{S}_{ij}[n], \ldots, \boldsymbol{S}_{iM}[n]\} \tag{4.12}$$

where M indicates the total positions during the measurement. Here n is utilized to represent the discrete time because the signals are digitized. After receiving the signals, the phase shift is compensated first. The compensation factor Δn_{ij} to each signal is determined by the following optimization problem:

$$\min_{\Delta n_{ij}} \sum_{n=t_s}^{t_e} \left| S_{i1}[n] - S_{ij}[n + \Delta n_{ij}] \right|^2 \tag{4.13}$$

The signals after the compensation are shown in Figure 4.8. Compared with those in Figure 4.6, it can be observed that the offset between signals is reduced significantly.

After the compensation, the extraction of the target signals is carried out. As a basic method, the averaging method is utilized to get a reference signal by averaging all the received signals from the same channel. Since during the measurement, the relative positions of the antennas are not changed, the shape of the direct wave is similar to each other. On the other hand, the relative position of the antenna to the target is changed. Therefore, by averaging the direct waveform part will almost remain and the signals from the target will be suppressed. The reference signals can be obtained as:

$$S_{i,\text{ave}} = (S_{i1}[n] + \cdots + S_{iM}\,[n + \Delta n_{iM}])/M \tag{4.14}$$

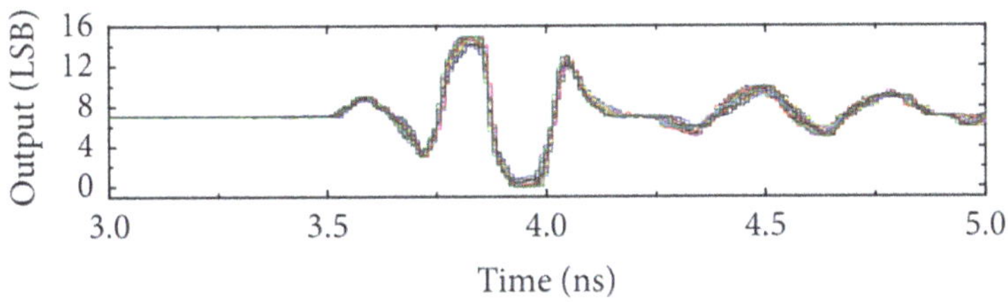

Figure 4.8 The signals after phase shift compensation [19].

Then, by subtracting the reference signals from the original received ones, the target signal can be extracted. Figure 4.9 shows an example of the target signal extraction by using the averaging method. The part marked by the red rectangle is the reflection from the target.

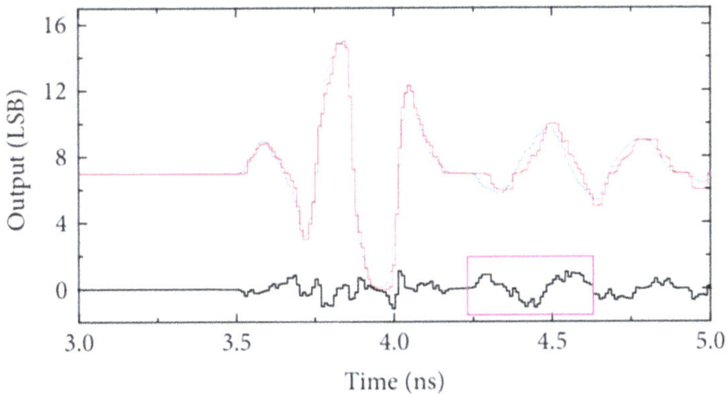

Figure 4.9 Extraction of the target signal by the averaging method [19].

After the extraction of the target signals from the received signal, it can be observed that there is some high-frequency noise in the target signal. This is caused by the imperfect subtraction between the reference signal and the original signals. In order to suppress the noise, the bandpass filter is applied as follows:

$$y_{ij}[n] = \sum_{k=0}^{l} h[k] \cdot D_{ij}[n-k] \tag{4.15}$$

where h is the filter coefficients and l is the filter order. Figure 4.10 shows the results after the bandpass filtering of the extracted target signal. It can be observed that the filtered signal is much smoother than the original one.

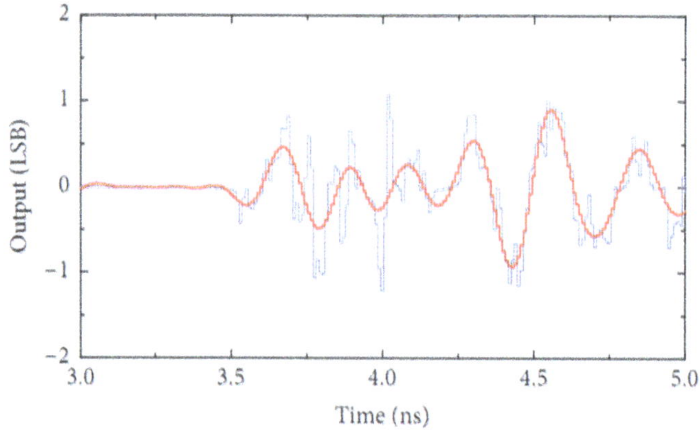

Figure 4.10 Extraction of the target signal by the averaging method [19].

Except for the averaging method, there is also an advanced algorithm to process the data when the measurement condition is more irregular. The averaging method is based on the assumption that the direct waves from different positions are the same. However, in the real case, this assumption cannot hold because the surface condition is quite different at different positions. Therefore, the averaging method cannot remove the direct signals effectively. The two-stage rotational (TSR) method was proposed to deal with this problem [21]. This method consists of two parts: the signal selection part and the adaptive filtering part. In the first part, the signals, which have large similarities, are grouped and then the adaptive filtering is carried out within the group to remove the direct waveform and extract the target signal. During the adaptive filtering, the TSR introduces a prior constraint to facilitate the filtering process as follows:

$$\min_{w}\left[\left\|b_{k,i}-Hw\right\|^{2}+\lambda\left\|w-\bar{w}\right\|^{2}\right] \tag{4.16}$$

where the $\bar{w}$ is the average weight. With this prior constraint, the target signals can be subtracted and the direct wave can also be suppressed. The detail of the TSR method is given in reference [21].

4.4 Review of Recent Progress

As the state-of-the-art of microwave breast imaging technology, recent progresses show encouraging results for practical usage. This section reviews these progresses and the algorithms utilized in that system.

Fear et al. developed a mono-static radar-based system, where the single Vivaldi antenna with a director is utilized [22, 23]. With the antenna, there is also a laser equipped and attached to a movable arm. By moving the antennas and laser, the signals from different positions can be obtained and the shape of the breast can also be depicted [24]. This system has been applied to several patients and the results show that the tumorous tissue area can be identified [6]. In this system, the delay-and-sum (DAS) method is utilized [4], which is depicted as:

$$I(\boldsymbol{x})=\left[\sum_{n=1}^{N}s_{n}(\tau_{n}(\boldsymbol{x}))\right]^{2} \tag{4.17}$$

where $I(\boldsymbol{x})$ is the energy at the point $\boldsymbol{x}$ · $\tau_n(\boldsymbol{x})$ is the estimated delay time from the antenna to the focal point $\boldsymbol{x}$ · s_n is the received signal and N is the total antenna position number. The reflections from the skin surface are removed by a neighborhood-based algorithm [25]. In this algorithm, to remove the reflection from a certain position, the signals from at least nine neighborhood positions are chosen. The skin reflection removed signal is expressed as:

$$\vec{r}_{\tau}[n]=\vec{s}_{\tau}[n]-\vec{q}^{T}\vec{b}_{patch,\tau}[n] \tag{4.18}$$

where $\vec{q}^{T}$ is the weight of the filter. This weight is calculated by:

$$\vec{q}^{T} = (\boldsymbol{R}_{GCV})^{-1}\vec{p} \tag{4.19}$$

where $(\boldsymbol{R}_{GCV})^{-1}$ is the inverse of the low-rank estimation of $\boldsymbol{R}$, which is the autocorrelation matrix of the input vector $\vec{b}_{patch,\tau}[n]$ · $\vec{p}$ is the cross-correlation vector between the target signal and the $\vec{b}_{patch,\tau}[n]$. The rank of R is estimated by the generalized cross-validation (GCV) method, which can be expressed as the minimization of the following function:

$$g(k) = \frac{\|\boldsymbol{I} - \boldsymbol{R}\boldsymbol{R}^{-1}(k)\vec{p}\|^{2}}{|trace(\boldsymbol{I} - \boldsymbol{R}\boldsymbol{R}^{-1})|} \tag{4.20}$$

where $\boldsymbol{I}$ is the identity matrix.

Craddock et al. developed a multi-static radar-based imaging system [9]. In this system, the antennas are fixed as the hemispherical dome. During the detection, the vector network analyzer is utilized to generate the signal and synthesize it as a short pulse. In order to remove reflection from the skin, the differential method is utilized, which rotates the antenna array at a certain angle [26]. This method assumes that the distance between the antenna and skin, skin properties, and normal tissue properties are consistent at the two angles. Therefore, the direct waves are the same. By taking the differential of these two datasets, the tumor signal is expected to be extracted. Then, an improved delay-and-sum imaging algorithm is utilized to reconstruct the breast interior image [8]. In this algorithm, in addition to the original DAS method, a quality factor (QF) is added as follows:

$$F_{e}(x,y,z) = QF(x,y,z)\int_{0}^{\tau}\Big(\sum_{i=1}^{M} w_{i}(x,y,z)\cdot y_{i}(t - T_{i}(x,y,z))\Big)^{2} dt \tag{4.21}$$

where $M = N(N-1)/2$ in which N is the number of the antenna array. w_i is the weight. y_i is the radar signal and the T_i is the delay time. The QF factor is calculated with the following procedures. First, an energy curve is plotted with the coherent signal summation. Then, the energy curve is rescaled to the standard energy deviation. Finally, the energy curve is fitted by a second-order polynomial $y = ax^2+bx+c$. Then, the a is assumed to be the QF. This method gives greater weight to those signals that more closely resemble the desired case of equal energy.

The MARIA system was developed which is toward the clinical trials [9]. It has been applied to 86 patients and the total sensitivity is large than 74%. Also, the cases for pre/peri-menopausal and post-menopausal are analyzed separately. While no significant difference is observed between these two kinds. These results show that radar-based microwave imaging is promising for future clinical examination.

MammoWave is a system that is composed of two antennas and the VNA [13]. This system operates in the frequency range of 1–9 GHz. During the measurement, the S21 is recorded and the antennas are moved around the breast. In this system, the imaging method based on Huygens Principle (HP) is utilized [27–29]. The HP method is described as follows. Consider an object in the free space. When it is illuminated by the transmitter antenna (Tx) at the frequency of f, the received signal measured along the surface of the object at the points $rx_{np} \equiv (a0, \varnothing_{np}) \equiv \vec{\rho}_{np}$ can be expressed as:

$$E_{tx_m}^{known}\big|_{rx_{np}} = E_{np,\,tx_m}^{known} \tag{4.22}$$

Based on the Huygens Principle, if the $E_{np,\,tx_m}^{known}$ is applied as a locus of a wave, the field inside the object can be calculated as the superposition of the fields radiated by the observation points on the surface as:

$$E_{HP,2D}^{rcstr}(\rho,\varphi;tx_m;f) = \Delta_s \sum_{np=1}^{N_{PT}} E_{np,tx_m}^{known} G(k_1 \,|\, \vec{\rho}_{np} - \vec{\rho}\,|) \tag{4.23}$$

where $(\rho,\ \varphi)$, Δ_s, and k_1 are the observation point, spatial sampling, and wave number of the internal media, respectively. Then the inside field calculated is utilized to generate an image to represent the map of the dielectric property. Assume that there are frequencies f_l in the measurement band, then the intensity of the reconstructed image can be calculated as follows:

$$I_{2D}(\rho,\varphi) = \frac{1}{B}\sum_{m=1}^{M}\sum_{l=1}^{F}\Delta_f \,|\, E_{HP,2D}^{rcstr}(\rho,\varphi;tx_m;f_l)\,|^2 \tag{4.24}$$

The MammoWave system has been applied to 58 patients with 103 breasts. Also, the distinction between benign and malignant lesions is investigated. Within the 103 breasts, 52 are considered to be benign and 51 are malignant through the radiologist study review. The total sensitivity is 74% and the value increases to 82% if the rule of thumb is used [13].

The Wavelia system is a low-power microwave imaging device [14]. The Wavelia system consists of 18 wideband Vivaldi-type probes forming a circle in the horizontal plane. The coupling fluid is utilized in this system. The probes will emit signals in turn and the other probes are utilized to receive the signal at different angles. This system is a multi-static radar-based type. In the Wavelia system, the data pre-processing is conducted to remove the strong coupling between antennas. Also, the processing is carried out to obtain the target echoes from the breast interior. The imaging algorithm utilized is the time-reversal multiple signal classification (TR-MUSIC) [30, 31].

Since the existence of the breast will influence the coupling condition between probes, the calibration is conducted to correct the drift as follows:

$$\mathrm{Dat}_{CAL,Txi/Rxj,Hn}(f) = (\mathrm{Dat}_{Driftcorr,Txi/Rxj,Hn}(f) - \mathrm{DCal}_{CAL,Txi/Rxj,Hn}(f)) \cdot \mathrm{PhCen}_{corr,Txi/Rxj}(f, e_{r,trans}(f)) \tag{4.25}$$

where $\mathrm{DCal}_{CAL,Txi/Rxj,Hn}(f)$ and $\mathrm{Dat}_{Driftcorr,Txi/Rxj,Hn}(f)$ are the estimated coupling signal and the drift-corrected raw data, respectively. $\mathrm{PhCen}_{corr,Txi/Rxj}(f,\ e_{r,trans}(f))$ is the multiplicative compensation factor. The principal component analysis (PCA) is utilized to extract the target signal based on the assumption that the antennas are identical. The TR-MUSIC is originally utilized for the detection of the radar target in heavily cluttered environments. The implementation of the TR-MUSIC into Wavelia is detailed in reference [30].

The Wavelia system has been applied to 24 patients [14]. The results that the system can successfully localize the benign breast lesion with a rate of 12/13. Meanwhile, the detectability of malignant breast cancer is 9/11. These results also show the promise of microwave imaging for breast tumor detection.

The above-mentioned systems are radar-based ones. SAFE is developed as a microwave tomography system [15]. In SAFE, there are 36 antennas, and one of them is utilized to illuminate the breast in turn. The remaining antennas are used for received signals. The operation frequency band is chosen between 1.4 GHz and 8 GHz with the step of 200 MHz to obtain the data. The measurement time for one patient is about 20 minutes and the image processing time is about 5 seconds. The inverse scattering algorithm is utilized to reconstruct the breast interior and the detail of the algorithm is depicted in reference [32]. SAFE has been applied to 115 patients and a sensitivity of 63% is obtained. It is also found that the breast size influences the results. The larger breast has higher sensitivity than the smaller one.

In this section, the recent progress of microwave breast cancer detection is reviewed mainly focusing on the system, which has been applied to a relatively large number of patients. From the results, it can be observed that the sensitivity is good and this technology is promising to be applied to clinical usage.

4.5 Conclusion

In this chapter, the microwave breast imaging algorithms were reviewed from the fundamental principles toward the state-of-the-art of clinical applications. Both radar-based systems and tomography systems have been developed through clinical trials that were carried out. From the recent progress, several groups have reported encouraging results, which demonstrate sensitivities in the range of 60–80%. These results show that microwave breast imaging is promising for clinical usage.

References

1. M. Lazebnik, D. Popovic, L. McCartney, C. Watkins, M. Lindstrom, J. Harter, S. Sewall, T. Ogilvie, A. Magliocco, T. Breslin, W. Temple, D. Mew, J. Booske, M. Okoniewski, and S. Hagness, "A large-scale study of the ultrawideband microwave dielectric properties of normal, benign and malignant breast tissues obtained from cancer surgeries," *Phys. Med. Biol.*, vol. 52, pp. 6093–6115, 2007.

2. M. Lazebnik, L. McCartney, D. Popovic, C. B. Watkins, M. J. Lindstrom, J. Harter, S. Sewall, A. Magliocco, J. H. Booske, M. Okoniewski, and S. C. Hagness, "A large-scale study of the ultrawideband microwave dielectric properties of normal breast tissue obtained from reduction surgeries," *Phys. Med. Biol.*, vol. 52, pp. 2637–2656, 2007.

3. T. Sugitani, S. Kubota, S. Kuroki, K. Sogo, K. Arihiro, M. Okada, T. Kadoya, M. Hide, M. Oda, and T. Kikkawa, "Complex permittivities of breast tumor tissues obtained from cancer surgeries," *Applied Physics Letters*, vol. 104, no. 25, pp. 253702, 2014.

4. E. C. Fear, X. Li, S. C. Hagness, and M. Stuchly, "Confocal microwave imaging for breast cancer detection: Localization of tumors in three dimensions," *IEEE Trans. Biomed. Eng.*, vol. 49, no. 8, pp. 812–822, 2002.

5. X. Li, E. J. Bond, B. D. Van Veen, and S. C. Hagness, "An overview of ultrawideband microwave imaging via space-time beamforming for early-stage breast cancer detection," *IEEE Antennas Propag. Mag.*, vol. 47, no. 1, pp. 19–34, Feb. 2005.

6. E. C. Fear, J. Bourqui, C. Curtis, D. Mew, B. Docktor, and C. Romano, "Microwave breast imaging with a monostatic radar-based system: A study of application to patients," *IEEE Trans. Microw. Theory Tech.*, vol. 61, no. 5, pp. 2119–2128, 2013.

7. J. M. Sill and E. C. Fear, "Tissue sensing adaptive radar for breast cancer detection-experimental investigation of simple tumor models," *IEEE Trans. Microw. Theory Tech.*, vol. 53, no. 11, pp. 3312–3319, 2005.

8. M. Klemm, I. J. Craddock, J. A. Leendertz, A. Preece, and R. Benjamin, "Improved delay-and-sum beamforming algorithm for breast cancer detection," *Int. J. Antennas Propag.*, vol. 2008, 2008.

9. A. W. Preece, I. Craddock, M. Shere, L. Jones, and H. L. Wintond, "MARIA M4: Clinical evaluation of a prototype ultrawideband radar scanner for breast cancer detection," *J. Med. Imaging*, vol. 3, no. 3, 2016, pp. 033502-1–7.

10. P. M. Meaney, M. W. Fanning, D. Li, S. P. Poplack, and K. D. Paulsen., "A clinical prototype for active microwave imaging of the breast," *IEEE Trans. Microw. Theory Tech.* 48, pp. 1841–1853, 2000.

11. P. M. Meaney, P. A. Kaufman, L. S. Muffly, M. Click, S. P. Poplack, W. A. Wells, G. N. Schwartz, R. M. di Florio-Alexander, T. D. Tosteson, Z. Li, S. D. Geimer, M. W. Fanning, T. Zhou, N. R. Epstein, and K. D. Paulsen, "Microwave imaging for neoadjuvant chemotherapy

monitoring: Initial clinical experience," *Breast Cancer Res.*, vol. 15, no. 2, pp. R35, 2013.

12. P. Meaney, A. Hartov, S. Bulumulla, T. Raynolds, C. Davis, F. Schoenberger, S. Richter, and K. Paulsen, "A 4-channel, vector network analyzer microwave imaging prototype based on software defined radio technology," *Rev. Sci. Instrum.*, vol. 90, pp. 044708-1–044708-14, 2019.
13. L. Sani, A. Vispa, R. Loretoni, M. Duranti, N. Ghavami, D. Alvarez, Sánchez-Bayuela, S. Caschera, M. Paoli, A. Bigotti, M. Badia, and M. Scorsipa, "Breast lesion detection through MammoWave device: Empirical detection capability assessment of microwave images' parameters," *Plos one*, 16(4), e0250005, 2021.
14. B. M. Moloney, P. F. McAnena, S. M. A. Elwahab, A. Fasoula, L. Duchesne, J. D. Gil Cano, C. Glynn, A. O'Connell, R. Ennis, A. J. Lowery, and M. J. Kerin, "Microwave imaging in breast cancer: Results from the first-in-human clinical investigation of the Wavelia system," *Acad. Radiol.*, 2021.
15. A. Janjic, M. Cayoren, I. Akduman, T. Yilmaz, E. Onemli, O. Bugdayci, and M. E. Aribal, "SAFE: A novel microwave imaging system design for breast cancer screening and early detection—clinical evaluation," *Diagnostics*, vol. 11, no. 3, pp. 1–10, 2021.
16. H. Song, "Time-domain impulse radar imaging for breast cancer detection using CMOS integrated circuits", Doctoral thesis of Electrical and Electronic Engineering, Graduate School of Advanced Sciences of Matter, Hiroshima University, Higashi-Hiroshima, Japan, 2018.
17. H. Song, H. Kono, Y. Seo, A. Azhari, J. Somei, E. Suematsu, Y. Watarai, T. Ota, H. Watanabe, Y. Hiramatsu, A. Toya, X. Xiao, and T. Kikkawa, "A radar-based breast cancer detection system using CMOS integrated circuits," *IEEE Access*, vol. 3, pp. 2111–2121, 2015.
18. H. Song, S. Sasada, T. Kadoya, M. Okada, K. Arihiro, X. Xiao, and T. Kikkawa, "Detectability of breast tumor by a hand-held impulse-radar detector: Performance evaluation and pilot clinical study," *Scientific Reports*, vol. 7, pp. 16353, 2017.
19. H. Song, A. Azhari, X. Xiao, E. Suematsu, H. Watanabe, and T. Kikkawa, "Microwave imaging using CMOS integrated circuits with rotating 4 × 4 antenna array on a breast phantom," *Int. J. Antennas Propag.*, vol. 2017, article no. 6757048, 2017.
20. T. Kikkawa, Y. Masui, A. Toya, H. Ito, T. Hirano, T. Maeda, M. Ono, Y. Murasaka, T. Imamura, T. Matsumaru, M. Yamaguchi, M. Sugawara,

A. Azhari, H. Song, S. Sasada, and A. Iwata, "CMOS Gaussian monocycle pulse transceiver for radar-based microwave imaging," *IEEE Transactions on Biomedical Circuits and Systems*, vol. 14, no. 6, pp. 1333–1345, Dec. 2020.

21. H. Song, S. Sasada, N. Masumoto, T. Kadoya, M. Okada, K. Arihiro, X. Xiao, T. Kikkawa, "A two-stage rotational surface clutter suppression method for microwave breast imaging with multistatic impulse-radar detector," *IEEE Transactions on Instrumentation and Measurement*, vol. 69, no. 12, pp. 9586–9598, 2020.
22. J. Bourqui, M. Sill, and E. C. Fear, "A prototype system for measuring microwave frequency reflections from the breast," *International Journal of Biomedical Imaging*, vol. 2012, Article ID 851234, 2012.
23. J. Bourqui, M. Okoniewski, and E. C. Fear, "Balanced antipodal Vivaldi antenna with dielectric director for near-field microwave imaging," *IEEE Transactions on Antennas and Propagation*, vol. 58, no. 7, pp. 2318–2326, 2010.
24. T. C. Williams, J. Bourqui, T. R. Cameron, M. Okoniewski, and E. C. Fear, "Laser surface estimation for microwave breast imaging systems," *IEEE Transactions on Biomedical Engineering*, vol. 58, no. 5, pp. 1193–1199, May 2011.
25. B. Maklad, C. Curtis, E. C. Fear, and G. G. Messier, "Neighborhood-based algorithm to facilitate the reduction of skin reflections in radar-based microwave imaging," *PIER B*, vol. 39, pp. 115–139, 2012.
26. M. Klemm, I. J. Craddock, J. A. Leendertz, A. Preece, and R. Benjamin, "Radar-based breast cancer detection using a hemispherical antenna array—Experimental results," *IEEE Transactions on Antennas and Propagation*, vol. 57, no. 6, pp. 1692–1704, June 2009.
27. A. Vispa, L. Sani, M. Paoli, A. Bigotti, G. Raspa, N. Ghavami, S. Caschera, M. Ghavami, M. Duranti, and G. Tiberi, "UWB device for breast microwave imaging: Phantom and clinical validations," *Measurement*, vol. 146, pp. 582–589, 2019.
28. N. Ghavami, G. Tiberi, D. J. Edwards, and A. Monorchio, "UWB microwave imaging of objects with canonical shape," *IEEE Transactions on Antennas and Propagation*, vol. 60, no. 1, pp. 231–239, Jan. 2012.
29. L. Sani, N. Ghavami, A. Vispa, M. Paoli, G. Raspa, M. Ghavami, F. Sacchetti, E. Vannini, S. Ercolani, A. Saracini, M. Duranti, and G. Tiberi, "Novel microwave apparatus for breast lesions detection: Preliminary clinical results," *Biomed. Signal Process. Control*, vol. 52, pp. 257–263, Jul. 2019.

30. A. Fasoula, L. Duchesne, J. Gil Cano, P. Lawrence, G. Robin, and J.-G. Bernard, "On-site validation of a microwave breast imaging system, before first patient study," *Diagnostics*, vol. 8, no. 3, p. 53, Aug. 2018.
31. A. Fasoula, B.M. Moloney, L. Duchesne, J.D.G. Cano, B.L. Oliveira, J. Bernard, and M.J. Kerin, "Super-resolution radar imaging for breast cancer detection with microwaves: The integrated information selection criteria," *Conf. Proc. IEEE Eng. Med. Biol. Soc.*, 2019, pp. 1868–1874.
32. M. N. Akıncı, T. Çağlayan, S. Özgür, U. Alkaşı, H. Ahmadzay, M. Abbak, M. Çayören, and İ. Akduman, "Qualitative microwave imaging with scattering parameters measurements," *IEEE Transactions on Microwave Theory and Techniques*, vol. 63, no. 9, pp. 2730–2740, Sept. 2015.

Chapter 5

Synergy of Data Glove-Based Motion Tracking and Functional Electrical Stimulation for Rehabilitation and Assisted Learning

Hidenori Mimura, Soichi Takigawa, Kamen Kanev, and Katsunori Suzuki

Research Institute of Electronics, Shizuoka University, 3-5-1 Johoku, Naka-ku, Hamamatsu 432-8011, Japan

mimura.hidenori@shizuoka.ac.jp

This chapter introduces some advanced methods and technologies for tracking fine hand and finger motions and postures employing data gloves (DG), coupled with specialized functional electrical stimulation (FES) equipment for computer-assisted training and stimulation of the upper limb motor functions. The core of the chapter covers the design and development of specialized hardware and assistive applications for post-stroke rehabilitation with the accelerated recovery of the affected hand and finger motor functions. The chapter concludes with a discussion of a specialized system for communication support of users with sight and hearing

Biomedical Engineering: Imaging Systems, Electric Devices, and Medical Materials
Edited by Akihiro Miyauchi and Hiroyuki Kagechika

ISBN 978-981-5129-16-8 (Hardcover), 978-1-003-46404-4 (eBook)
www.jennystanford.com

impairments, hosting FES-based enhancements to facilitate the employment of the mobile Malossi alphabet.

5.1 Introduction

Tracking of hand and arm motions and postures in research, education, and training environments is common and their adoption in various practical application areas continues to expand [1, 2]. The early wired glove designs [3] employed embedded optical sensors constructed from a light emitter and a photocell connected by a flexible rubber tube that bends following the motions of the human fingers [4]. In such sensors, the light reaching the photocell decreases proportionally to the tube bend, which controls the output voltage of the photocell. In a similar manner, more performant and easy-to-handle sensors have been constructed from optical fiber with an intentionally damaged surface that attenuates the light propagation proportionally to the bend [5]. More advanced fiber-optic sensors based on double-cladding fiber have also been reported [6]. Such sensors tend to be employed in high-end wired gloves, (e.g., the virtual programming languages (VPL) DataGlove [7]), while lower-cost capacitive [8], and resistive bend sensors are commonly used in consumer-grade products (e.g., the Nintendo Power Glove [9]). Bendable resistive sensors for wired gloves can also be produced by applying conductive inks to a flexible substrate [10]. With respect to high-fidelity finger motion tracking and the detection of subtle finger movements, optimal results are obtained with stretchable sensors. Currently, stretchable sensors are built employing either capacitive [11–13], or resistive [14–16] technologies. In the work discussed in this chapter, advanced, rapid-response, widely stretchable carbon nanotube (CNT)-based sensors, specialized for human motion tracking, have been used [17–19].

The focus of this chapter is on exploring different possibilities for the integration of hand and finger motion tracking with techniques for stimulation and controlled movement of the human limbs. With respect to this, we consider the FES method, which is often used to help restore the motor functions of patients, paralyzed as a result of a stroke or spinal injury [20]. This method activates the nerve tissue connected to the muscle groups thus contracting the muscles and inducing movement of the hands or feet [21]. The FES method is susceptible to different specializations, for example, the contralaterally controlled functional electrical stimulation (CCFES) method regulates the opening and closing of a paralyzed hand following the movements of the contralateral hand [22]. Such bilateral work in patients with chronic motor disorders after stroke allows the interhemispheric facilitation of a limb [23]. The symmetrical movement has been found to further reduce upper limb disability in some stroke patients [24–26] and is deemed more advantageous than the cyclic electrical stimulation for motor function recovery [27, 28]. Other FES specializations integrate myoelectric sensing of the movements of the non-paralyzed hand [29, 30] with mirror therapy [31]. Such specializations employ the detected movements of the reference hand as triggers for the applied electrical stimulation.

In all FES-related methods, the construction and the placement of the electrodes are of utmost importance for the proper delivery of the stimulation signals. Modern signal delivery methods rely on multi-pad electrodes organized in easy-to-attach arrays of individually controllable non-invasive electrodes capable of selectively producing muscle contraction in a paralyzed hand [32]. The search for the optimal stimulation points is performed by detecting the kinetic response provoked by the electrical stimulation and comparing it with predefined movements [33, 34]. In the work discussed in this chapter, a direct kinetic response detection method employing high-fidelity data gloves for reliable tracking of the fine hand and finger motions is employed [35, 36]. A different approach to detect electrophysiological responses caused by electrical stimulation uses surface electromyography (sEMG) of the forearm [37, 38]. While this method can detect responses to low levels of stimulation, it requires more precise positioning of the individual electrodes that are usually carried out by trained professionals.

Data glove-based motion tracking coupled with FES can be also integrated into an assistive system to facilitate the communication of users with sight and hearing impairments using the Malossi alphabet [39, 40]. It is estimated that approximately 1.5 million people globally are completely deafblind, compared to 150 million people with different levels of blindness associated with deafness [41]. Given the importance placed on vision and hearing in our daily activities, including communication [42], accessing information, and mobility, those with deafblindness face many complex challenges that may hinder their functioning and participation in daily events and activities and require a variety of assistive, educational, and therapeutic services [43]. Communication based on the sense of touch (i.e., tactile-based) is a fundamental aspect of social life for deafblind people who heavily rely on this, given their inability to communicate using audio and visual cues [44]. Advancements in communication and haptic technologies create opportunities for innovative assistive solutions for the deafblind. Such technology-assisted interactions could provide the deafblind community with a functional communication base in the absence of a caretaker and/or in social distancing or isolation situations as imposed by the COVID-19 pandemic [45]. In the work discussed in this chapter, an extended version of the traditional Malossi alphabet, tailored for single-hand signing in mobile setouts is employed [39].

5.2 Components, Devices, and Equipment

With respect to motion and posture tracking, this section covers the construction of the highly-stretchable CNT sensors (5.2.1), and their employment in the design of the specialized data gloves for high-fidelity hand and finger motion tracking (5.2.2). With respect to FES, it covers the construction of arrays of belt-shaped multi-pad electrodes (5.2.3), and their employment in the specialized multichannel FES equipment for interactive muscle stimulation (5.2.4).

5.2.1 Rapid Response Widely Stretchable CNT-Based Strain Sensors

The widely stretchable CNT sensors [17–19] are indispensable components of the work discussed in this book chapter. The CNT sensor structure is illustrated in Figure 5.1. In the stretchable sensor, millimeter-long multi-walled carbon nanotubes (MWCNTs) are aligned in the direction of the strain axis and sandwiched between elastomer layers.

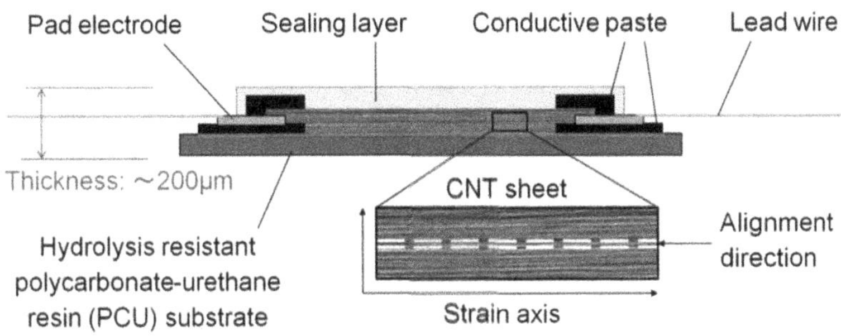

Figure 5.1 The CNT sensor structure.

A urethane resin with special properties is synthesized to make an elastomer exhibiting low elasticity and good affinity to the human skin. The aligned CNT layer is formed by stacking CNT webs drawn from a spinnable CNT forest. The electrical resistance of the sensor increases with strain and returns back to its initial value when the strain is removed. The sensor can be stretched up to 200%, it operates at frequencies up to 30 Hz, and its gauge factor exceeds 10, which makes it a perfect fit for human motion tracking. The final product is thin and soft as human skin, employing highly flexible material ideally suited for wearable sensors, including textile-based wearables, often used in real-time human body motion-sensing applications.

5.2.2 High-Fidelity Data Gloves with Embedded CNT Strain Sensors

High-fidelity motion tracking data gloves with embedded widely stretchable CNT strain sensors [35, 36] have been employed in the work discussed in this chapter to track the motions and detect the postures of the user's hands. The top and the bottom views of the data glove are shown in Figure 5.2(a) while the internal layout of the embedded CNT strain sensors is depicted in Figure 5.2(b).

The data glove incorporates 11 CNT strain sensors, positioned over the carpometacarpal (CMC), the metacarpophalangeal (MP), and the interphalangeal (IP) joints of the thumb and over the MP and the proximal interphalangeal (PIP) joints of the remaining four fingers. The resistance of the CNT strain sensor changes proportionally to the amount of stretching. As a finger joint bends, the CNT strain sensor stretches and the resistance increases. In contrast, when the finger joint stretches, the sensor shrinks and the resistance decreases. Based on this, the degree of the bending of each joint is individually measured. This process inflicts minimal strain on the fingers as the stretchable CNT sensors are highly flexible. In addition, the data glove is made of breathable fabric, so it can be worn comfortably for long periods of time.

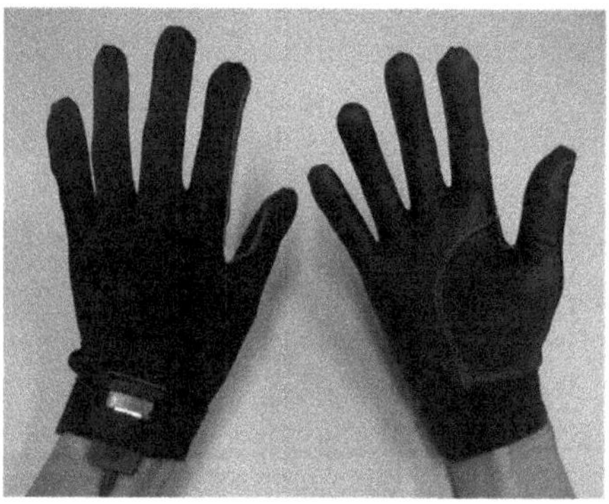

(a)

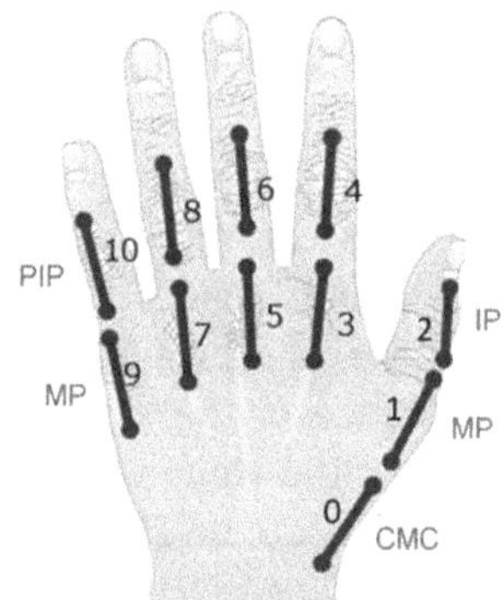

(b)

Figure 5.2 Top and bottom views of the data glove (a) and the layout of the embedded CNT strain sensors (b).

While both a wired [35] and a wireless [46] version of the data glove are available, only the wired version was employed in the discussed work. The data glove was connected to a PC through a USB interface for serial communication. Sensor resistance measurements were recorded at 100 ms intervals with 12-bit resolution. The resistance R_j of each sensor was calibrated using the resistance $R_{j_{closed}}$ of the fully closed hand posture and the resistance $R_{j_{open}}$ of the relaxed, open posture to define the rate of flexion P_j for each of the finger joints as follows:

$$P_j = \frac{R_j - R_{j_{open}}}{R_{j_{closed}} - R_{j_{open}}} \tag{5.1}$$

In this work, the sensor placed over the CMC of the thumb was not used, so the values of j were from 1 to 10, as shown in Figure 5.2(b).

5.2.3 Belt-Shaped Multi-Pad Electrodes

The multi-pad electrodes for muscle stimulations are constructed from wet gel electrodes (Omron Corporation, HV-LLPAD) aligned in a row. As shown in Figure 5.3(a), the individual electrodes are 20 mm wide and 30 mm long and are equally spaced with a pitch of 24 mm.

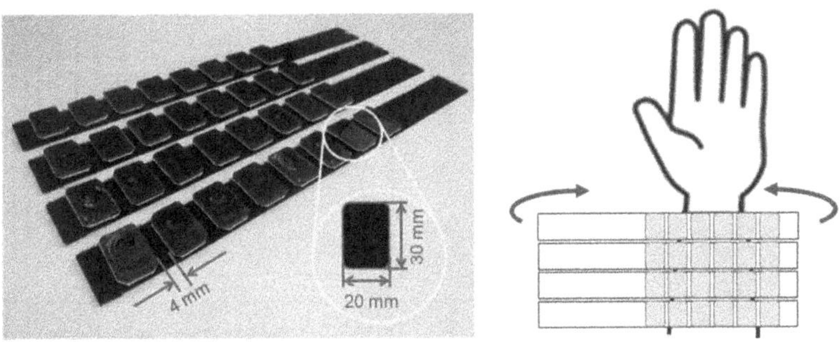

(a) (b)

Figure 5.3 The belt-shaped multi-pad electrodes (a) and their placement on the target arm (b).

While up to eight gel electrodes could be mounted on a single hook-and-loop fastener belt, in this experiment, belts with six electrodes were used. The placement of the four belts with a total of 24 electrodes on the forearm as employed in the experiments is illustrated in Figure 5.3(b).

5.2.4 Multichannel FES Equipment

A simplified block diagram of the multichannel FES system [47] employed in this work is shown in Figure 5.4. A dedicated host PC is used for controlling the FES equipment through specialized application software developed in Microsoft Visual C#. The system incorporates a USB connection unit, a microcontroller unit (MCU), a constant current circuit, and an electrode switching circuit with connectors to the multi-pad electrodes. Electric isolation is ensured by employing a local power supply with eight nickel metal hydride (Ni-MH) batteries (1.2 V, 2400 mAh). The battery output is transformed to 50V by a DC–DC converter and passed through a constant current unit (0–50 mA, controllable in 1 mA increments) that feeds the drive electrode switching circuit.

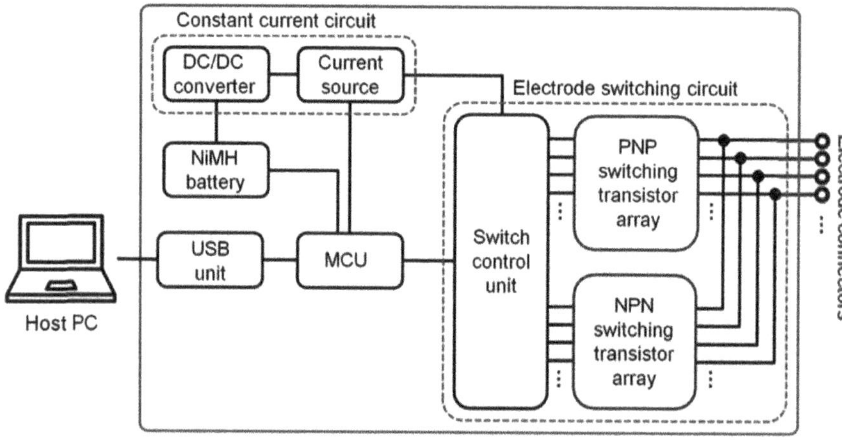

Figure 5.4 A simplified block diagram of the multichannel FES equipment.

Based on the USB control input from the host PC, each of the 24 pads is dynamically configured either as an active or as a return electrode, and currents are applied as prescribed.

5.3 Data Processing Framework

The developed data processing framework employs two data gloves – one for the reference hand and another one for the target hand. The tracking data obtained from the data glove on the reference hand is analyzed and converted to hand postures that are mirrored to map the target hand. The data glove on the target hand is then used to track and detect the postures of the target hand resulting from the applied FES.

In the experiment, the reference hand was the right hand of the subject, so it presented the required motions and finger bending postures used as targets. During the experiments, subjects sat in a chair with their elbow bent and forearms placed on a desk with palms facing up. The subjects wore the two data gloves on their hands and the 24 gel electrodes placed on four belts were attached to the inside of the left forearm for the electrical stimulation. In addition, a camera was used for video recording of the hand motions and postures during the experiment for further analysis. The subjects were specifically instructed not to resist the motions of the target hand evoked by the electrical stimulation.

5.3.1 Registering the Set of Target Finger Bending Postures Provided by the Reference Hand (Step 1)

In this step, multiple-finger bending postures were recorded by the PC employing the data glove worn on the reference (right) hand of the subject. Six different postures were employed - the relaxed open hand posture (i = 0), and the five finger bending postures (i = 1,...,5) as shown in Figure 5.5.

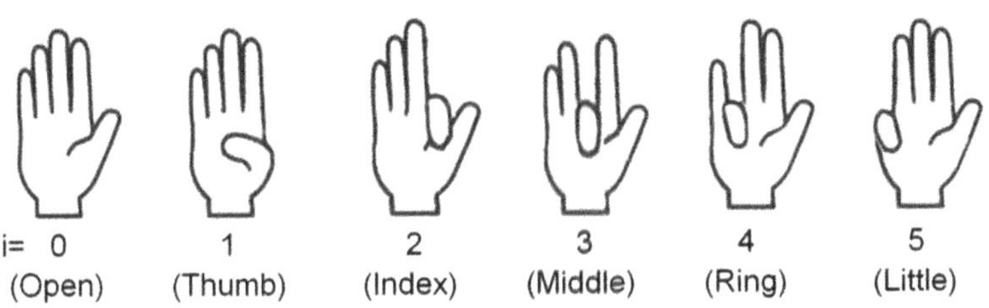

Figure 5.5 The relaxed open hand posture (i = 0), and the five single-finger bending hand postures (i = 1,...,5) were employed as targets.

The recorded data was organized in a two-dimensional posture reference array for subsequent hand posture identification in real-time. This array is essential for the proper evaluation of the hand postures during the search through the electrode pairs stimulating the target hand and for the identification of the hand postures of both the reference and the target hands.

5.3.2 Identifying the Optimal Stimulation Electrode Combinations by Pairing and Scanning (Step 2)

In this step, the stimulation electrodes attached to the target hand of the subject were activated in pairs, in order to identify the best possible combinations of active and return electrodes based on the feedback obtained through the data glove. More specifically, the objective was to identify the electrical stimulation patterns applied to the target hand, which produced mirror-symmetric finger bending postures as close as possible to those registered with the reference hand in advance. For this, an exhaustive sequence of electrode pairs was generated by the controlling PC. In each of those pairs, one electrode served as an active electrode while the other electrode was connected as a return electrode. For each pair, biphasic pulses with a period of 30 ms and a pulse width of 200 μs were applied for 1 sec with the current level adjusted as needed to minimize the user discomfort. Immediately after the stimulation, the finger posture data of the target hand was retrieved by the data glove and stored as a resulting pattern vector.

The obtained resulting pattern vectors $\overrightarrow{P_{Tn}}$ and the reference patterns vectors $\overrightarrow{P_{Oi}}$ of the respective six previously recorded target hand postures are evaluated using the normalized Euclidean distance $d_{NE}\left(\overrightarrow{P_{Oi}},\overrightarrow{P_{Tn}}\right)$ [48] as follows:

$$R_{in} = 1 - d_{NE}\left(\overrightarrow{P_{Oi}},\overrightarrow{P_{Tn}}\right) = 1 - \frac{1}{10}\sqrt{\sum_{j=1}^{10}\left(P_{Oi,j} - P_{Tn,j}\right)^2} \tag{5.2}$$

As a result, the optimal electrode combination for producing the finger bending posture pattern i is determined as the one with the largest R_{in} value.

5.3.3 Applying Electrical Stimulation Patterns to the Target Hand to Match Finger Bending Postures of the Reference Hand (Step 3)

The objective of this step is to induce postures of the target hand that are mirror-symmetric to the postures exposed by the reference hand. The process begins with presenting one of the six postures shown in Figure 5.5 by the reference hand. The reference pattern vector $\overrightarrow{P_O}$ obtained from the data glove is then compared to the six posture pattern vectors $\overrightarrow{P_{Oi}}$ and the similarity distance R_i is calculated as follows:

$$R_i = 1 - d_{NE}\left(\overrightarrow{P_{Oi}}, \overrightarrow{P_O}\right) = 1 - \frac{1}{10}\sqrt{\sum_{j=1}^{10}\left(P_{Oi,j} - P_{Oj}\right)^2} \tag{5.3}$$

Based on this, the posture i with the largest R_i value is selected and used as a target finger bending posture. The optimal electrode combination corresponding to the selected target posture as identified in Step 2 is then employed for stimulating the target hand. Finally, the posture of the target hand resulting from the applied stimulation is tracked by the data glove and analyzed for mirror-symmetric similarity to the target posture.

5.3.4 Possible Optimizations of the Electrode Selection Process

The exhaustive search described in the previous subsections is time-consuming and tiresome for users so possible optimizations reducing the number of explored electrode combinations should be considered. Indeed, if the search is confined to sufficiently small subsets of electrodes, it can be conducted on-the-fly and thus the search time can be greatly reduced. To achieve this, surface electromyography (sEMG) techniques [37, 38] can be applied to the reference hand to identify the neural activity areas associated with the specific finger motions and postures detected by the data glove. Such areas can be identified on-the-fly with the minimal computational effort since the finger motions and postures are tracked by the data glove and do not have to be inferred from the collected sEMG data. The electrode search process on the target hand could then be optimized by imposing area limitations based on an appropriate mirror-symmetric pairing with the reference hand.

5.4 Application Examples

This section describes two applications of the generic FES-based approach and the related components, devices, and equipment discussed so far. The first application targets the FES-assisted rehabilitation of the hand and finger motor functions affected by a stroke or injury. The second application explores possibilities for assisted learning and FES-enhanced practice of the mobile Malossi alphabet for users with sight and hearing difficulties.

The outline of the employed integrated system is shown in Figure 5.6. The controlling PC employs two USB connections – one to track the finger motions of the reference and the target hands, and another one to send the target stimulation signals to the FES system. More specifically, the data glove input obtained from the reference hand is used as a search pattern for identifying the most similar posture within a set of predefined target postures. A prerecorded electrical stimulation pattern, corresponding to the selected target posture is then extracted and sent to the FES system for activating the electrodes attached to the target hand. The finger movements of the target hand resulting from the stimulation are finally tracked by the second data glove and used for analyzing the stimulation responses.

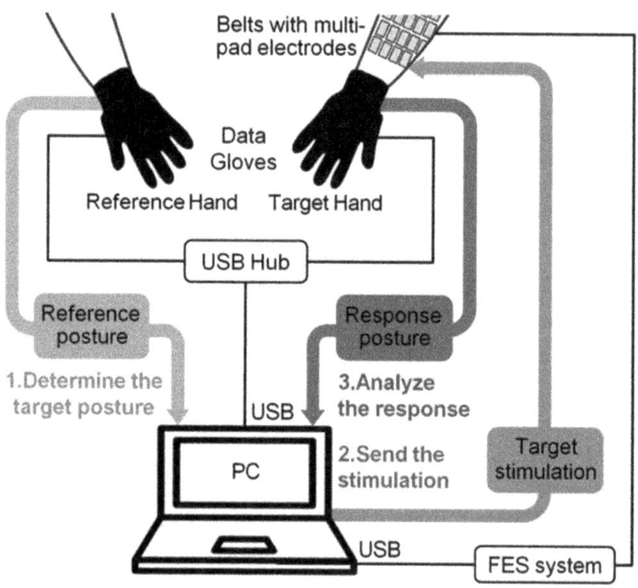

Figure 5.6 The integrated system, based on the equipment and the methods presented in Sections 5.2 and 5.3 and employed in the application experiments.

5.4.1 Employing FES for Restoring the Hand and Finger Motor Functions

The equipment and the methods presented in Sections 5.2 and 5.3 have been used in the construction of an experimental environment for facilitating the exercising and rehabilitation of the hand and finger motor functions. Four healthy right-handed male subjects in their 30–50's were admitted to the experiments. This study was performed in accordance with the declaration of Helsinki and was approved by the Research Ethics Committee of Shizuoka University in compliance with the Regulations on Research Involving Human Subjects at Shizuoka University. During the initialization phase, subjects were asked to exercise in a sequence the relaxed open posture followed by the five-target finger bending postures with their reference hand, as shown in Figure 5.5. Simultaneous real-time recording of the corresponding hand and finger motions was carried out through the data glove worn on the reference hand, and searches in the posture reference array were made. More specifically, each of the 24 electrodes was designated as an active electrode and paired with the remaining 23 return electrodes producing 552 different stimulation patterns altogether that were scanned in about 20 min. The optimal electrode combinations that produced the closest approximations to the target finger bending postures were identified by the employed search algorithm and look-up arrays were created for each subject.

To illustrate the above-described process, we refer to Figure 5.7 where the tracking of the finger bending motions and the respective hand posture evaluation functions are shown. The blue curves in Figure 5.7(a) correspond to the measured bending rates of the MP and PIP joints of the index finger. Note the good synchronization of the registered changes in the MP (top graph) and the PIP (bottom graph) values that indicate a natural finger bending motion. The changes in the evaluation function values for all six hand postures (i = 0,...,5) during the index finger bending motion are shown in Figure 5.7(b). The function producing the highest value at a given time point is used to determine the current hand posture. The recording begins with an open hand posture confirmed by the highest recorded values registered for $i0$. The index finger bending motion takes place in the time interval t = (2, 3) where the recorded $i0$ values decrease while the $i2$ values increase. The reverse effect is observed in the interval t = (9, 10) when the index finger is stretched back. The current hand pose can, therefore, be tracked by determining the evaluation function that currently produces the highest value.

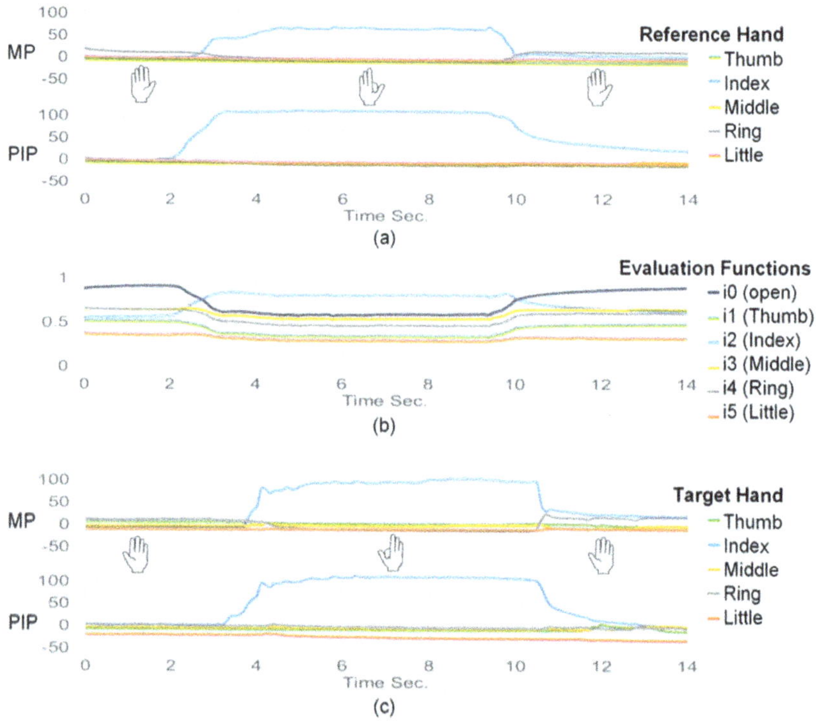

Figure 5.7 MP and PIP finger bending rates on the reference hand (a), the respective posture evaluation function values (b), and the resulting finger bending rates on the target hand (c).

Given the above, the function values in Figure 5.7(b) allow us to detect an open hand posture $i0$ in the time interval t = (0, 3), an index finger bent posture $i2$ in the time interval t = (3, 10), and again an open hand posture $i0$ in the time interval t = (10, 14). Once the transition from $i0$ to $i2$ is detected at t = 3, the prerecorded optimal stimulation electrode combination for hand posture $i2$ is retrieved from the corresponding look-up array and electrical stimulation is applied to the target hand accordingly. The finger motions of the target hand resulting from the applied stimulation as tracked by the data glove are shown in Figure 5.7(c). Note the gradual increase of the recoded MP and PIP flexion rates within the interval t = (3, 4), right after the electrical stimulation was applied. The stimulation was discontinued at t = 10 when the transition back to an open hand posture of the reference hand was detected. Following a small delay, the target hand also returned to an open hand posture at t = 11.

Figure 5.8 shows the postures presented by the reference hand, and the resulting postures of the target hand induced by the electrical stimulation selected in response to the posture of the reference hand. Note the close approximation demonstrated by the obtained postures of the target hand when compared to the postures of the reference hand with a mirror-symmetry applied.

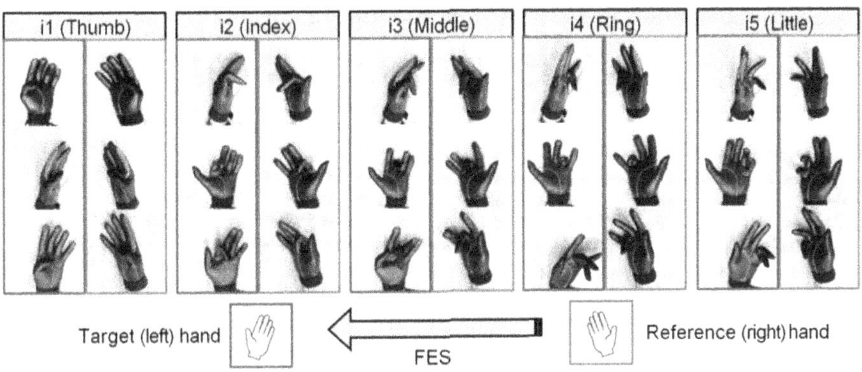

Figure 5.8 Postures of the reference hand and the corresponding postures of the target hand induced by the applied electrical stimulation.

5.4.2 Employing FES for Facilitating the Mobile Malossi Alphabet Learning

The integrated system shown in Figure 5.6 offers generic functionality that is not confined to the exercising and rehabilitation discussed in Section 5.4.1. In this section, we will discuss the applicability of the system in FES-assisted learning setouts.

The advanced CNT-based stretchable sensors embedded in the data glove ensure highly reliable tracking of the subtle motions of the user's fingers. This allows for precise pose estimation and recognition of the Malossi alphabet signs at high speed thus providing a solid base for novel data glove-based applications in the digital world. Based on this, different communications scenarios could be envisaged where the parties are not in direct physical contact to accommodate, for example, social distancing and remote and mobile communications. In the traditional Malossi alphabet, signing messages are received by sensing the touches on the recipient's hand. Supportive devices can, therefore, employ embedded pressure sensors to identify the touches and convert them to digital signals. However, the high-fidelity finger motion tracking of the data glove allows for identifying such touches without additional pressure sensors. In this scenario, the touches are derived from the tracked finger motions and postures.

This approach can be extended to accommodate single-hand signing in mobile setouts by minimal adjustments of the traditional Malossi alphabet as shown in Figure 5.9. The specific changes [39] are enlisted below:

- Pressed letters A–O, excluding A, F, and K are signed by touching the designated spots with the tip of the thumb of the same hand (letters L, M, N, and O that require touches on the palm could be signed by touching the proximal phalange of the corresponding finger if easier to reach).
- Pressed letters F and K are signed by touching the designated spots with the tip of the index finger.
- Pinched letters Q, R, S, T, V, X, Y, and Z are signed by touching next to the designated spots on the side of the corresponding finger phalanges using the index finger.
- The remaining letters A, P, U, and W are signed by touching with the thumb the side of the middle phalange of the index, middle, ring, and small fingers, respectively.

The extension attempts to preserve the touch sensations associated with the traditional Malossi alphabet letters as much as possible. Indeed, almost all pressed letters retain their original sensations since the pressure is exercised on the original Malossi spots as shown in Figure 5.9(a). This also applies to most of the pinched letters since they are signed by pressing the side of the finger phalanges where the original Malossi pinching takes place as shown in Figure 5.9(b). Finally, the remaining four letters, shown in red in Figure 5.9(b), are reallocated to the unused spots on the middle phalanges in a consistent and easy-to-remember way.

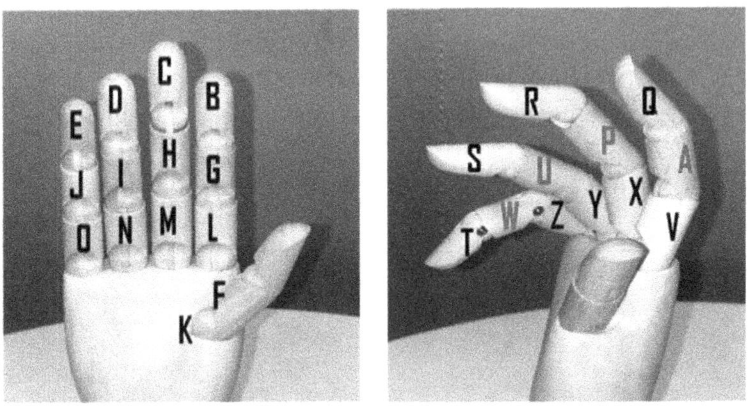

(a) (b)

Figure 5.9 The mobile Malossi alphabet with the adjusted letter positions shown in red.

While the transition from the traditional Malossi alphabet to its mobile version is fairly straightforward, the differences in the letter signing still have to be properly taught to the learners. For mastering the mobile version of the alphabet, some practice exercises and supervised training will certainly be instrumental, so the integrated system depicted in Figure 5.6 can be used in the process.

The sample application discussed in Section 5.4.1 focused on hand and finger exercises for rehabilitation purposes where the motor functions of the individual fingers were addressed separately. In the mobile Malossi alphabet, however, hand postures involving more than one finger are used for signing the different letters. As shown in Figure 5.10(a), for example, the signing of the letter I involves both the thumb and the ring fingers. Therefore, a more complex search, for identifying larger sets of active and return electrodes for simultaneous stimulation is required. However, given the closeness of the hand postures for signing letters such as I (Figure 5.10(a)) and U (Figure 5.10(b)), the reproducibility and the reliable discrimination of the FES-induced letter signing might suffer. While the implementation of a fully automated system overcoming such issues will require further experimental work and possible functional enhancements, the outlined approach could still be used in semi-automated mode when a caretaker is engaged in the process. In such situations, the caretaker can act as an instructor wearing a data glove on their reference hand and demonstrating with it the hand postures corresponding to the mobile Mallosi letters taught.

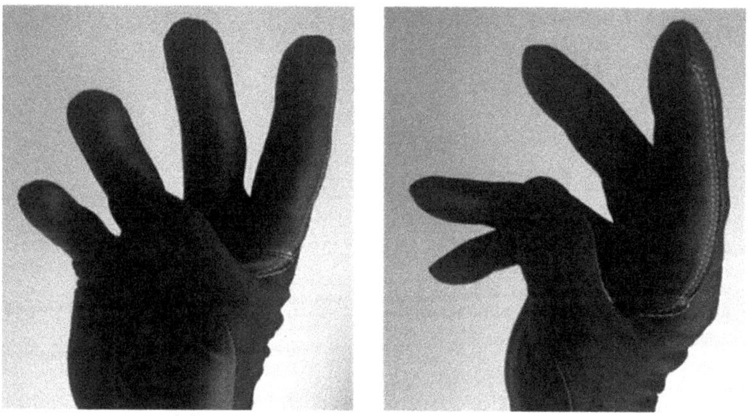

(a) (b)

Figure 5.10 Single-hand signing of the letters I (a) and U (b).

5.5 Conclusion and Further Developments

In this chapter, we have presented some methods and technologies for data glove-based finger motion tracking and hand posture recognition integrated into an FES system for computer-assisted stimulation and exercising of the upper limb motor functions both for rehabilitation and assisted learning.

While it has been reported that the optimal stimulation positions for different subjects are reproducible [32], the reliable recording of the electrode placement positions and the subsequent reinstallation are quite challenging. In the conducted experiments, complications arose from the use of the one-dimensional electrode arrays organized as individual belts that were positioned and fastened one by one. This incurred fluctuations in the relative positioning of the electrodes on the different belts impeded the reproducibility of the electrode reattachment. To address this problem, we are planning rearrangements of the one-dimensional electrode arrays into two-dimensional structures that will minimize the electrode reattachment discrepancies.

It was also observed that some stimulation patterns incurred unintended wrist motions that interfered with the FES-assisted motor function exercising. While such patterns were manually removed from the look-up arrays, the pattern identification could be automated through the gyro and the accelerometer functionality of the data glove. The physical gyro and accelerometer are embedded in the communication box positioned at the wrist (refer to the top view of the data glove in Figure 5.2(a)). While absolute wrist tracking is not possible, large wrist motions are successfully detected based on the accelerometer and the gyro readings.

References

1. D. J. Sturman, D. Zeltzer, A survey of glove-based input, *IEEE Computer Graphics and Applications*, Vol. 14, no. 1, Jan. 1994, pp. 30–39.
2. L. Dipietro, A. M. Sabatini, P. Dario, A survey of glove-based systems and their applications, *IEEE Transactions on Systems, Man, and Cybernetics, Part C: Applications and Reviews*, 2008, pp. 461–482.
3. T. DeFanti, D. J. Sandin, Sayre glove final project report, *US NEA R60-34-163 Final Project Report*, Nov. 10, 1977.
4. T. G. Zimmerman, Optical flex sensor, *US Patent 4 542 291*, Sept. 17, 1985.
5. Y. L. Harvill, T. G. Zimmerman, J. G. Grimaud, Motion sensor which produces an asymmetrical signal in response to symmetrical movement, *US Patent 5 097 252*, Mar. 17, 1992.
6. O. Ivanov, A. Chertoriyskiy, Fiber-optic bend sensor based on double cladding fiber, *Journal of Sensors*, 2015, pp. 1–6.

7. T. Zimmerman, J. Lanier, C. Blanchard, S. Bryson, Y. Harvill, A hand gesture interface device, *ACM Sigchi Bulletin*, Vol. 17, 1986, pp. 189–192.
8. J. S. Neely, P. J. Restle, Capacitive bend sensor, *US Patent 5 610 528*, Mar. 11, 1977.
9. D. L. Gardner, Inside story on: The power glove (Cover), *Design News*, Vol. 45, No. 23:63, Dec. 4, 1989.
10. G. B. Langford, Flexible potentiometer, *US Patent 5 583 476*, Dec. 10, 1996.
11. I. Hirata, H. Nakamoto, H. Ootaka, M. Tada, The flexible interface using a stretch sensor, *Procedia Manufacturing*, Vol. 3, 2015, pp. 845–849.
12. A. Tairych, I. Anderson, Capacitive stretch sensing for robotic skins, *Soft Robotics*, Vol. 6, 2019.
13. O. Glauser, D. Panozzo, O. Hilliges, O. Sorkine-Hornung, Deformation capture via soft and stretchable sensor arrays, *ACM Transactions on Graphics*, Vol. 38, 2019, pp. 1–16.
14. A. Firouzeh, J. Paik, The design and modeling of a novel resistive stretch sensor with tunable sensitivity, *IEEE Sensors Journal*, Vol. 15, 2015, pp. 6390–6398.
15. L. Sbernini, A. Pallotti, G. Saggio, Evaluation of a stretch sensor for its inedited application in tracking hand finger movements, *Proceedings of the IEEE International Symposium on Medical Measurements and Applications* (MeMeA), Benevento, 2016, pp. 1–6.
16. H. Lee, H. Cho, S. Kim, Y. Kim, J. Kim, Dispenser printing of piezo-resistive nanocomposite on woven elastic fabric and hysteresis compensation for skin-mountable stretch sensing, *Smart Materials and Structures*, Vol. 27, 2018.
17. Y. Inoue, K. Kakihata, Y. Hirono, T. Horie, A. Ishida, H. Mimura, "One-step grown aligned bulk carbon nanotubes by chloride mediated chemical vapor deposition, *Applied Physics Letters*, Vol. 92, 2008.
18. Y. Inoue, Y. Suzuki, Y. Minami, J. Muramatsu, Y. Shimamura, K. Suzuki, A. Ghemes, M. Okada, S. Sakakibara, H. Mimura, K. Naito, Anisotropic carbon nanotube papers fabricated from multiwalled carbon nanotube webs, *Carbon*, Vol. 49, 2011.
19. K. Suzuki, K. Yataka, Y. Okumiya, S. Sakakibara, K. Sako, H. Mimura, Y. Inoue, Rapid-response, widely stretchable sensor of aligned MWCNT/elastomer composites for human motion detection, *ACS Sensors*, 2016.

20. P. H. Peckham, J. S Knutson, Functional electrical stimulation for neuromuscular applications, *Annual Review of Biomedical Engineering*, Vol. 7, 2005, pp. 327–360.

21. S. Micera, T. Keller, M. Lawrence, M. Morari, D. B. Popovic, Wearable neural prostheses, *IEEE Engineering in Medicine and Biology Magazine*, vol. 29, No. 3, May–June 2010, pp. 64–69.

22. J. S. Knutson, M. Y. Harley, T. Z. Hisel, J. Chae, Improving hand function in stroke survivors: A pilot study of contralaterally controlled functional electric stimulation in chronic hemiplegia, *Archives of Physical Medicine and Rehabilitation*, Vol. 88, No. 4, pp. 513–520, 2007.

23. A. R. Luft, S. McCombe-Waller, J. Whitall, L. W. Forrester, R. Macko, J. D. Sorkin, J. B. Schulz, A. P.Goldberg, D. F. Hanley, Repetitive bilateral arm training and motor cortex activation in chronic stroke: A randomized controlled trial, *Journal of the American Medical Association*, Vol. 292, No. 15, 2004, pp. 1853–1861.

24. K. Lin, Y. Chen, C. Chen, C. Wu, Y. Chang, The effects of bilateral arm training on motor control and functional performance in chronic stroke: A randomized controlled study, *Neurorehabilitation and Neural Repair*, Vol. 24, No. 1, 2010.

25. R. Sleimen-Malkoun, J. J. Temprado, L. Thefenne, E. Berton, Bimanual training in stroke: How do coupling and symmetry-breaking matter?, *BMC Neurology*, Vol. 11, January 2011.

26. J. Metrot, D. Mottet, I. Hauret, L. van Dokkum, H.-Y. Bonnin-Koang, K. Torre, I. Laffont, Changes in bimanual coordination during the first 6 weeks after moderate hemiparetic stroke, *Neurorehabilitation and Neural Repair*, Vol. 27, No. 3, 2013.

27. J. S. Knutson, M. Y. Harley, T. Z. Hisel, S.D. Hogan, M. M. Maloney, J. Chae, Contralaterally controlled functional electrical stimulation for upper extremity hemiplegia: An early-phase randomized clinical trial in subacute stroke patients, *Neurorehabilitation and Neural Repair*, Vol. 26, No. 3, 2012.

28. J. S. Knutson, D. D. Gunzler, R. D. Wilson, J. Chae, Contralaterally controlled functional electrical stimulation improves hand dexterity in chronic hemiparesis: A randomized trial, *Stroke*, Vol. 47, No. 10, October 2016, pp. 2596–2602.

29. J. H. Kim, B. H. Lee, Mirror therapy combined with biofeedback functional electrical stimulation for motor recovery of upper extremities after stroke: A pilot randomized controlled trial,

Occupational Therapy International, Vol. 22, No. 2, June 2015, pp. 51–60.

30. G. J. Yun, M. H. Chun, J. Y. Park, B. R. Kim, The synergic effects of mirror therapy and neuromuscular electrical stimulation for hand function in stroke patients, *Annals of Rehabilitation Medicine*, Vol. 35, No. 3, 2011, pp. 316–321.
31. G. Yavuzer, R. Selles, N. Sezer, S. Sutbeyaz, J. B. Bussmann, F. Koseoglu, M. B. Atay, H. J. Stam, Mirror therapy improves hand function in subacute stroke: A randomized controlled trial, *Archives of Physical Medicine and Rehabilitation*, Vol. 89, No. 3, 2008, pp. 393–398.
32. A. D. Koutsou, J. C. Moreno, A. J. del Ama, E. Rocon, J. L. Pons, Advances in selective activation of muscles for non-invasive motor neuroprostheses, *Journal of NeuroEngineering and Rehabilitation*, Vol. 13, 56, 2016.
33. D. B. Popovic, M. B. Popovic, Automatic determination of the optimal shape of a surface electrode: Selective stimulation, *Journal of Neuroscience Methods*, Vol. 178, No. 1, 2009, pp. 174–181.
34. S. B. O'Dwyer, D. T. O'Keeffe, S. Coote, G. M. Lyons, An electrode configuration technique using an electrode matrix arrangement for FES-based upper arm rehabilitation systems, *Medical Engineering & Physics*, Vol. 28, No. 2, 2006, pp. 166–176.
35. F. Gelsomini, P. C. K. Hung, B. Kapralos, A. Uribe-Quevedo, M. Jenkin, A. Tokuhiro, K. Kanev, M. Hosoda, H. Mimura, Specialized CNT-based sensor framework for advanced motion tracking, *The 54th Hawaii International Conference on System Sciences (HICSS-54), Symposium: Computing in Companion Robots and Smart Toys*, Grand Wailea, Maui, Hawaii, January 7–10, 2021, pp. 1898–1905.
36. K. Wilcocks, A. Perivolaris, B. Kapralos, A. Quevedo, M. Jenkin, K. Kanev, H. Mimura, M. Hosoda, F. Alam, A. Doubrowski, Work-in-progress: A novel data glove for psychomotor-based virtual medical training, *2021 IEEE Global Engineering Education Conference (EDUCON)*, Vienna, Austria, April 21–23, 2021, pp. 1318–1321.
37. C. De Marchis, T. S. Monteiro, C. Simon-Martinez, S. Conforto, A. Gharabaghi, Multi-contact functional electrical stimulation for hand opening: Electrophysiologically driven identification of the optimal stimulation site, *Journal of NeuroEngineering and Rehabilitation*, Vol. 13, No. 22, 2016.
38. H. Shin, Y. Zheng, X. Hu, Variation of finger activation patterns post-stroke through non-invasive nerve stimulation, *Frontiers in Neurology*, No. 9, 2018.

39. F. Gelsomini, E. Tomasuolo, M. Roccaforte, P. Hung, B. Kapralos, A. Doubrowski, A. Quevedo, K. Kanev, H. Makoto, H. Mimura, Communicating with humans and robots: A motion tracking data glove for enhanced support of deafblind, *The 55th Hawaii International Conference on System Sciences (HICSS-55)*, Grand Wailea, Maui, Hawaii, Jan. 4–7, 2022, pp. 2056–2064.

40. R. Raavi, K. Kanev, P. C. K. Hung, Integration of optical and data gloves input for improved sign language analysis and interpretation through machine learning, *The 8th International Symposium toward the Future of Advanced Research in Shizuoka University (ISFAR-SU2022)*, Shizuoka, Japan, March 1, 2022, pp. 52.

41. N. Caporusso, L. Biasi, G. Cinquepalmi, G. F. Trotta, A. Brunetti, V. A. Bevilacqua, Wearable device supporting multiple touch- and gesture-based languages for the deaf-blind, *Advances in Human Factors in Wearable Technologies and Game Design*, pp. 32–41, 2018.

42. N. Olson, J. Urbanski, N. Krister Persson, J. Starosta-Sztuczka, M. Fuentes, Sensor technology, gamification, haptic interfaces in an assistive wearable, *Journal on Technology and Persons with Disabilities*, pp. 80–87, 2019.

43. A. Jaiswal, H. M. Aldersey, W. Wittich, M. Mirza, Finlayson, M., Participation experiences of people with deafblindness or dual sensory loss: A scoping review of global deafblind literature. *PLOS ONE*, Vol. 13, No. 9, Article e0203772, 2018.

44. F. Sorgini, R. Calio, M. C. Carrozza, C. M. Oddo, Haptic-assistive technologies for audition and vision sensory disabilities, *Disab. Rehabil., Assistive Technol.*, vol. 13, no. 4, pp. 394–421, 2018.

45. G. Goggin, K. Ellis, Disability, communication, and life itself in the COVID-19 pandemic: Health sociology review, *The Journal of the Health Section of the Australian Sociological Association*, Vol. 29, No. 2, pp. 168–176, 2020.

46. K. Kanev, H. Mimura, P. C. K. Hung, Data gloves for hand and finger motion interactions. *Encyclopedia of Computer Graphics and Games*, SpringerLink, Cham, Switzerland, 2022.

47. S. Takigawa, H. Mimura, Development of contralaterally controlled functional electrical stimulation to realize multiple finger bending postures with data glove, *Sensor and Materials*, Vol. 33, pp. 3645–3656, 2021.

48. M. M. Deza, E. Deza, *Encyclopedia of Distances*, Springer Berlin, Heidelberg, pp. 590, 2009.

Chapter 6

Motion Estimation from Surface EMG Signals Using Multi-Array Electrodes

Yasuharu Koike

Institute of Innovative Research, Tokyo Institute of Technology, 4259-J3-11, Nagatsuta, Midori-ku, Yokohama 226-8503, Japan

koike@pi.titech.ac.jp

6.1 Introduction

When we want to manipulate a multi-degree-of-freedom robot as we wish, it is difficult to perform sufficient manipulation with the current human interface. Although it may be possible to operate the robot by measuring body movements with motion capture, the motion part must be within the camera's field of view. However, when grasping an object, for example, problems occur such as the fingers being occluded by the grasped object.

One of the most positively moving parts of the body is the finger. It can grasp objects, write letters, and perform a variety of other movements. The muscles that generate this movement are the muscles that move the fingers. Most of the muscles that move

Biomedical Engineering: Imaging Systems, Electric Devices, and Medical Materials
Edited by Akihiro Miyauchi and Hiroyuki Kagechika

ISBN 978-981-5129-16-8 (Hardcover), 978-1-003-46404-4 (eBook)
www.jennystanford.com

the fingers are located in the forearm. However, because the forearm contains muscles associated with wrist movements as well as finger movements, it is difficult to separate the activity of the muscles associated with wrist and finger movements from the surface sensor signals.

This chapter outlines a device for estimating wrist and finger motion simultaneously with good accuracy and an algorithm for motion estimation.

6.2 Human Interface

Consider the control of a robot with five fingers. Assuming that each finger has three joints, a total of 15 joint angles must be controlled simultaneously.

- Control the gripping and opening by pressing the button. The way to move the fingers should be programmed in advance.
- Continuously control the opening angle by using a 1-DOF joystick or other means. One command moves all fingers in the same way.
- Continuously control the joint angles of all fingers. For all finger joints to move independently, 15 devices are controlled continuously and simultaneously.

As described above, there are several possible control methods, and the devices and input methods to be used for each control are determined accordingly.

The human interface is described in Figure 6.1. A human interface is something that sits between humans and machines and has a certain function. In response to the input given by a person, it realizes that function and controls a machine such as a robot. In the case of a computer mouse, the input is hand movements, and the left/right and front/back movements are detected by sensors to move the cursor on the computer screen left/right and up/down. In this case, the left and right hands' movements are reflected on the screen as they are, but the back-and-forth movements become up-and-down movements on the screen, which means that a coordinate transformation of about 90 degrees is applied. The function of the human interface is to convert the hand movement so that the cursor movement at the screen size is as intended by the operator by magnifying or reducing the hand movement.

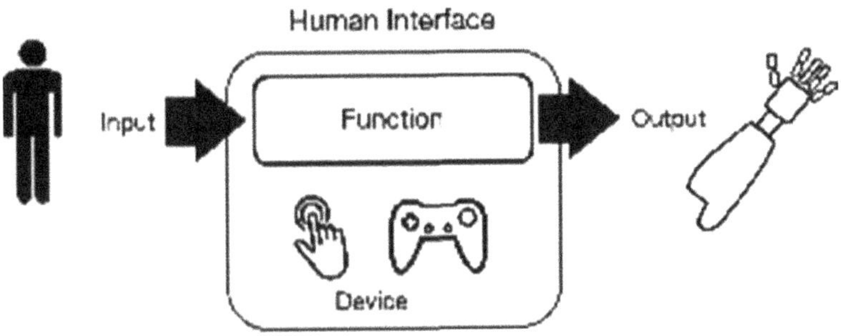

Figure 6.1 Human Interface.

At this point, if you hold the mouse rotated 90 degrees and manipulate the cursor, it becomes difficult to move it as you wish. However, as for the output, it is already rotated 90 degrees around the horizontal axis, but it does not feel so difficult. And even if it is further rotated 90 degrees around the vertical axis, the operation will not be so difficult. Thus, the usability differs greatly between the case where a transformation is applied to the input and the case where a transformation is applied to the output of the function as shown in Figure 6.1. The reason for this may be that the input-output relationship (internal model) learned during the use of the human interface is broken, making it difficult to predict the output when a transformation is applied to the input.

When considering the control of a prosthetic hand, a person has already acquired an internal model that uses his or her muscles to move the fingers. They can move their fingers as they wish without being aware of which muscles to move when moving them. If the same functionality can be extracted from this model, it will be possible to implement it in a human interface and move the prosthetic hand in the same way as one's hand has moved in the past. The input to the human interface is the activity of the muscles involved in the hand movement.

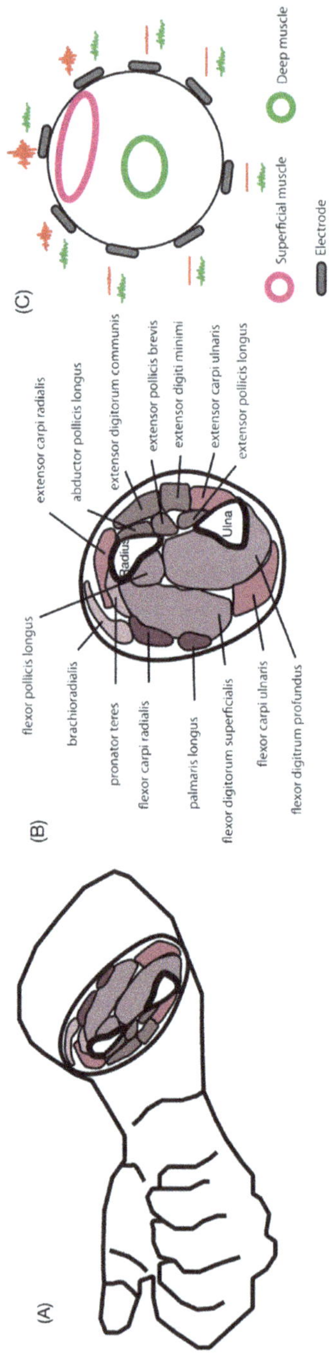

Figure 6.2 Muscle location in the forearm.

Many of the associated muscles are located on the forearm, as shown in Figure 6.2 (A, B). Muscles associated with wrist movements, such as the flexor/extensor carpi radialis and flexor/extensor carpi ulnaris, are located on the surface, while the flexor pollicis longus, the thumb flexor, is located inside the forearm. As shown in Figure 6.2 (C), when the activity of these muscles is measured with electrodes on the skin surface, superficial muscle activity is measured as a large amplitude signal at electrodes close to the muscle location, while deep muscle activity is measured as a small amplitude signal at many electrodes.

If the interface is to estimate wrist movement only, it is thought that the desired muscle activity can be obtained by attaching electrodes directly above the surface muscles, but in reality, deep muscle activity is mixed in as cross-talk. For this reason, muscle activity is often measured by opening and closing the fingers without moving the wrist, and the wrist is perceived as having moved. To avoid this, where should the sensor be attached?

Even if electrodes are attached directly above the muscles based on anatomical knowledge, unwanted muscle activity is also measured due to crosstalk, as mentioned earlier. In addition, if we try to measure not only wrist activity but also finger activity, the number of related muscles will increase and the time required to attach the electrodes will also increase. Considering the general human interface, such preparation time should be as short as possible. Furthermore, it needs to be accessible to anyone without requiring anatomical knowledge, etc.

A typical electric-powered prosthetic hand measures about two channels of muscle activity to achieve finger opening and closing. One reason why few prosthetic hands are capable of motorized movement of both the wrist and fingers is that the additional degrees of freedom make the prosthetic hand heavier, but another reason is that it is necessary to measure a large number of muscle activities to control them independently [1].

To solve these problems, we developed a multi-array electrode.

6.3 Multi-Array Measurement System

6.3.1 Multi-Array Electrode System

In order to find the innervation points to estimate muscle fiber conduction velocity, linear array electrodes have been developed. High-density sEMG electrodes, two-dimensional grid electrodes, are also developed for finding the localization and size estimation of motor units (MUs) [2, 3]. The size of an array electrode fits for one muscle because the purpose of this electrode is to detect the characteristics of each muscle.

We are developing a multi-channel multi-array electrode that can be used as a human interface to install a large number of electrodes in a short time without requiring anatomical knowledge. Figure 6.3 shows the current multi-array electrodes, which have eight electrodes in the circumferential direction and five electrodes in the longitudinal direction of the forearm, for a total of 40 electrodes made of cloth sewn on, and can measure EMG of eight channels in the circumferential direction and four channels in the longitudinal direction of the forearm for a total of 32 channels by differential amplification. Signals are transmitted wirelessly via Bluetooth, with a sampling frequency of up to 500 Hz.

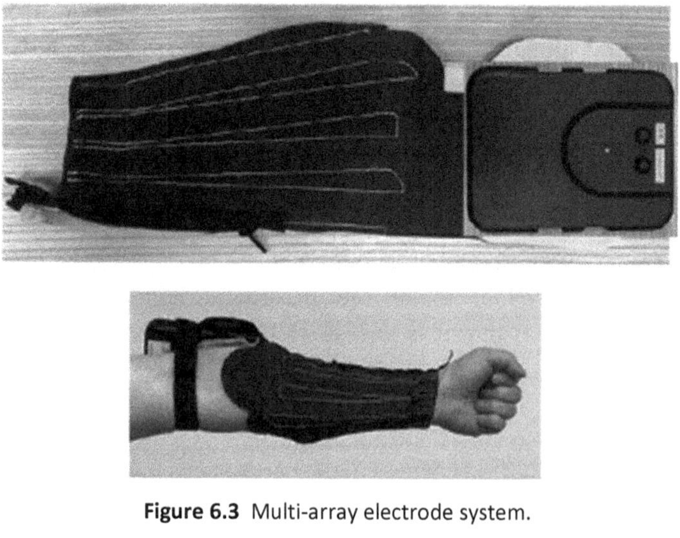

Figure 6.3 Multi-array electrode system.

6.3.2 Independent Component Analysis

Figure 6.2 (C) shows the relationship between EMG and array electrodes. Superficial muscle is easy to measure from surface electrodes, but deep muscle is hard. The adjacent electrode measures the EMG signal from the same superficial muscle (red signals), but several electrodes receive signals from deep muscle (green signals). Independent component analysis (ICA) is a signal processing method to separate independent signals, which are linearly mixed in multiple sensors. The problem of blind signal separation is solved by the ICA technique in various research fields, such as speech recognition, data communication, and sensor signal processing.

$$x(t) = As(t)$$

$$Y(t) = Wx(t) \tag{6.1}$$

where A, $s(t)$, and $x(t)$ is an unknown mixing matrix, source signal, and observation, respectively.

It is hard to recover the original signals $s(t)$, but matrix W tries to recover the original signals to minimize the error between $s(t)$ and $y(t)$. Figure 6.4 shows an example of independent components (ICs), indicated by the weight value of matrix W [4].

The number of independent components is equal to that of the input, as shown in Eq. (6.1). Since some of these components are noise components, the number of components actually related to muscle activity is less than the number of inputs. The independent components include muscle activities as well as various noise components. Currently, the muscle activation components are manually selected.

6.3.3 Non-Negative Matrix Factorization

The number of ICs as same as the number of electrodes are computed. Some of the ICs are noise components, such as power supply. The rest components are mainly related to muscle activities.

Mathematically, muscle synergy is obtained by Non-negative matrix factorization (NMF) (Figure 6.5).

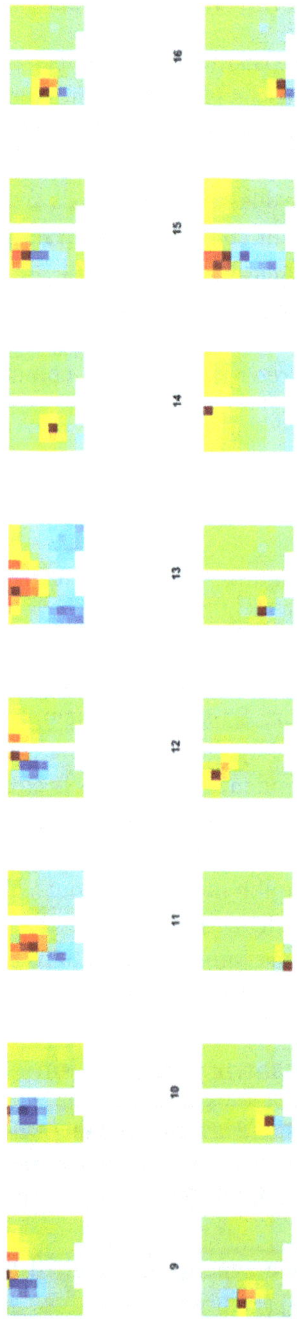

Figure 6.4 Independent components.

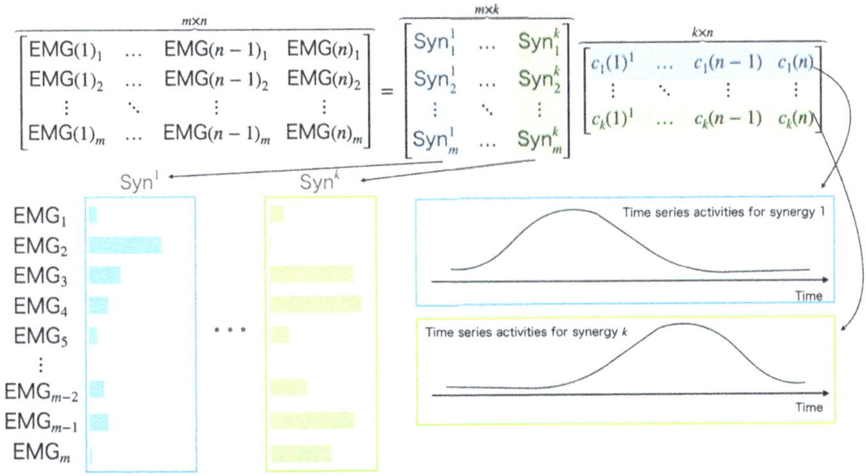

Figure 6.5 Muscle synergy.

$$\mathrm{EMG}(t) = \mathrm{Syn}c(t) \tag{6.2}$$

Suppose there are m muscle time patterns (EMG (t)) and sampled at n points in the time direction; by decomposing this $m \times n$ matrix into $m \times k$ spatial patterns of muscle activity (Syn) and $k \times n$ temporal patterns ($c(t)$), we can represent muscle activity patterns with k ($< m$) synergies, which are less than the number of muscles. This means that k ($< m$) synergies can be used to represent muscle activity patterns. This matrix decomposition is possible because muscle activity patterns can be represented by non-negative values.

6.4 Motion Control

6.4.1 Motor Control Issue

Consider reaching for a cup in front of you and lifting it. The position of the handle of the cup is recognized visually, and the brain sends appropriate motor commands to the muscles of the upper limbs to move the hand to that position. At this time, it is necessary to control not only the position of the hand but also the direction of the hand appropriately according to the direction of the handle. Even now, it is still not fully understood how the brain actually gives commands to the muscles, even in actions that we normally perform without thinking. A contributing factor to the difficulty is redundancy. The shoulder, elbow, and wrist can be thought of as having 3-DOF, 1-DOF, and 3-DOF joints, respectively. A DOF is an axis of a joint, and a ball joint, such as the shoulder joint, has three DOFs because the angles can be defined by the three axes x, y, and z. The elbow has one degree of freedom because it has only one joint that can be bent and extended. The wrist has 1 DOF of twisting the radius and ulna, and the rest are 2 DOFs of wrist bending, flexion, and ulnar flexion, making a total of 3 DOFs. The position of the hand can be defined in the Cartesian coordinate system by six variables: x, y, and z, the three-dimensional position, and R_x, R_y, R_z, the rotation angle of each axis. Since these six variables are represented by joints with seven degrees of freedom, the position of the elbow can be freely changed even if the position and orientation of the hand are determined, which means that the number of joints is redundant. This causes the problem that even if the position and orientation of the hand are determined, the posture of the entire arm is not uniquely determined. This is what is known as the faulty configuration problem, and it is a problem that must be solved even when the action is as simple as lifting a cup in front of one's eyes.

Furthermore, when lifting the cup, if the contents of the cup are heavier than expected, the same posture must be lifted with a great deal of force. Even if the same posture is used immediately before lifting, different forces will be generated depending on the weight of the cup's contents. Even if the posture is determined, there are multiple possible motor commands to the muscles to maintain that posture, so redundancy exists here as well.

Thus, by controlling position and force simultaneously, it is possible to control a robot that is used in a real environment, such as a prosthetic hand. We will also explain how the robot is controlled below from the information obtained by the muscle activity measurement device and signal processing described so far.

6.4.2 Posture Control

When considering the trajectory of the current hand position and velocity to the endpoint position, it is necessary to consider dynamics, including the weight of the arm. On the other hand, when controlling posture at the starting point and end point, it is necessary to consider statics as the balance between the main muscles and antagonist muscles at each joint.

Each joint involves multiple primary and antagonist muscles, and each muscle activity can be controlled independently. For example, considering the upper extremity motion of the shoulder and elbow, more than 20 muscles are used to control three degrees of freedom of the shoulder and one degree of freedom of the elbow. There are monoarticular muscles related only to the shoulder and bi-articular muscles related to the shoulder and elbow, and they can remain in the same posture even if they apply different amounts of force. How, then, do we determine the activity of these muscles?

The forward statistics model can be represented by the following using the musculoskeletal model. Figure 6.6 shows the schematic picture to estimate hand force from EMG signals. Muscle force is estimated from the musculoskeletal system and joint torque can be calculated from muscle force and moment arm. We have been developing the musculoskeletal model and joint torques were estimated from only EMG activities,

$$
\begin{aligned}
& f_{muscle_j}(\theta, u_j) = (k_0 + k_1 u_j)\left(l_o + l_1 u_j - \sum_i a_{ij}\theta_i\right) \\
& \tau_i = \sum_j a_{ij} \times f_{muscle_j} \\
& R_{ij} = -\frac{\partial \tau_i}{\partial \theta_j} = a_{ij}^2(k_0 + k_1 u_j) \\
& \theta_{eq} = \left.\frac{\sum_j a_{ij}(k_0 + k_1 u_j)(l_o + l_1 u_j)}{\sum_j a_{ij}^2(k_0 + k_1 u_j)}\right|_{\tau_i(u,\theta)=0},
\end{aligned}
\tag{6.3}
$$

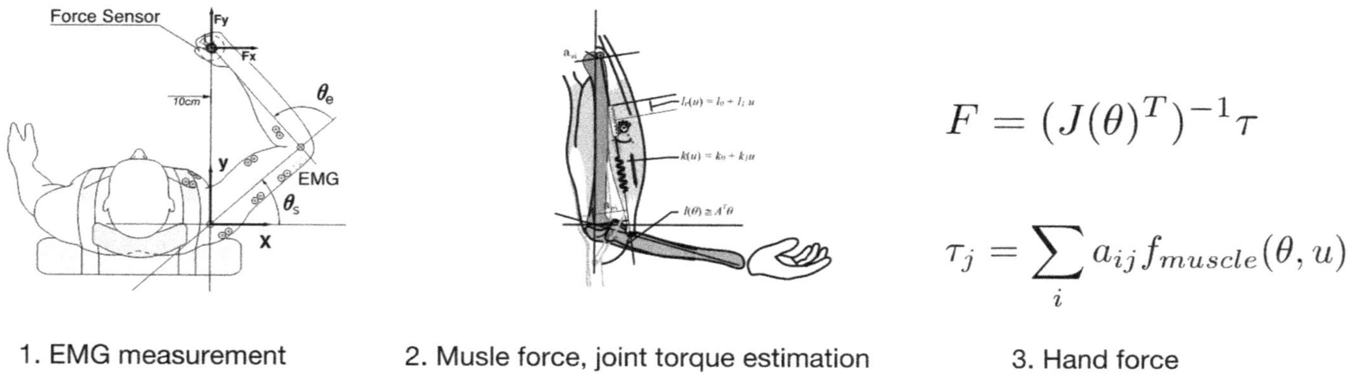

Figure 6.6 Hand force estimation by musculoskeletal model.

where $f_{musclej}$, $k_0 + k_1 u_j$, and $l_0 + l_1 u_j$ are muscle force, muscle stiffness, and changes in the natural length of the muscle, respectively. a_{ij} is the moment arm, which is the length from the line of muscle to the joint center and θ_j is the joint angle [8]. Joint torques are calculated from muscle force and moment arm as shown in Figure 6.6.

Thus, the tension generated by the muscle is defined by the stiffness and elongation from the natural length of the muscle as in the case of a spring. Muscles are actuators whose stiffness and elongation from their natural length vary with the motion command u from the brain, and joint torque is calculated as the combined force of several antagonistic muscle tensions. The equilibrium position is where the net torque of the joint is 0, taking into account gravity and forces from the outside world. In addition, when the joint is θ, a force to return to the original position is generated, and this ratio is the stiffness. The joint stiffness is defined by $\partial\tau/\partial\theta$, the equilibrium angle is calculated using Eq. (6.3).

Both motion and force control can be performed by controlling the robot with a force proportional to the magnitude of the stiffness toward the angle calculated as the equilibrium position.

6.4.3 Muscle Synergy

The idea of control by reducing the degrees of freedom in this way is called synergy, which was proposed by Bernstein. As mentioned earlier, reducing the degrees of freedom of a joint does not reduce the degrees of freedom of muscle activity. This is because there are an infinite number of combinations of muscle activities in which the difference between the active and antagonist muscles is equal, even in a posture with the same joint angle. To reduce the degree of freedom of muscle activity, it is necessary to combine muscle groups that are active at the same time into one. Giszter et al. found that when the frog's spinal cord is stimulated, the legs converge to different equilibrium positions depending on the location of stimulation. In this experiment, they also measured muscle activity at the same time and showed that changing the posture of the foot in response to constant stimulation produced specific patterns of muscle activity for each posture. Tresch et al. also found that different muscle synergy patterns are generated depending on the location of the skin of the frog's foot, and they claim that these muscle synergy patterns can generate many different movement patterns. In fact, d'Avella et al. have shown that there are different muscle synergy patterns for each motor pattern, such as frog jumping and walking. Furthermore, Overduin et al. successfully induced muscle synergies in gripping different objects by stimulating the primary motor cortex in monkeys [7]. This series of studies by Bizzi's group suggests that there is neural activity related to muscle synergy in the spinal cord and primary motor cortex.

However, it is not known whether these muscle activities are innate or acquired by learning. Since complex finger postures such as grasping a cup, like upper limb movements, require appropriate adjustments according to the weight of the object being held, it seems more appropriate to assume that they were acquired by learning rather than being innate. While we do not know where and how this is learned, differences at the level of muscle activity are evident through experimentation.

Depending on the task, muscle synergies are often required [9]. For example, if the wrist is moved up and down or left and right, muscle synergies are calculated according to the orientation (Figure 6.7).

In this experiment, electromyograms were measured from seven muscles involved in the wrist movement, when the wrist was moved up and down and left and right. The muscle synergies (S1–S4) obtained by NMF are those shown in the figure and are related to the direction of the wrist. If one calculates which synergies are manifested during the movement and to what extent, the movement can be calculated as the combined force of the synergies. This method does not require the creation of a sequential model and allows for simple control. Furthermore, by using muscle synergies, even if noise is introduced into each muscle, synergy is identified at the synergy level, and the movement itself is generated with high accuracy.

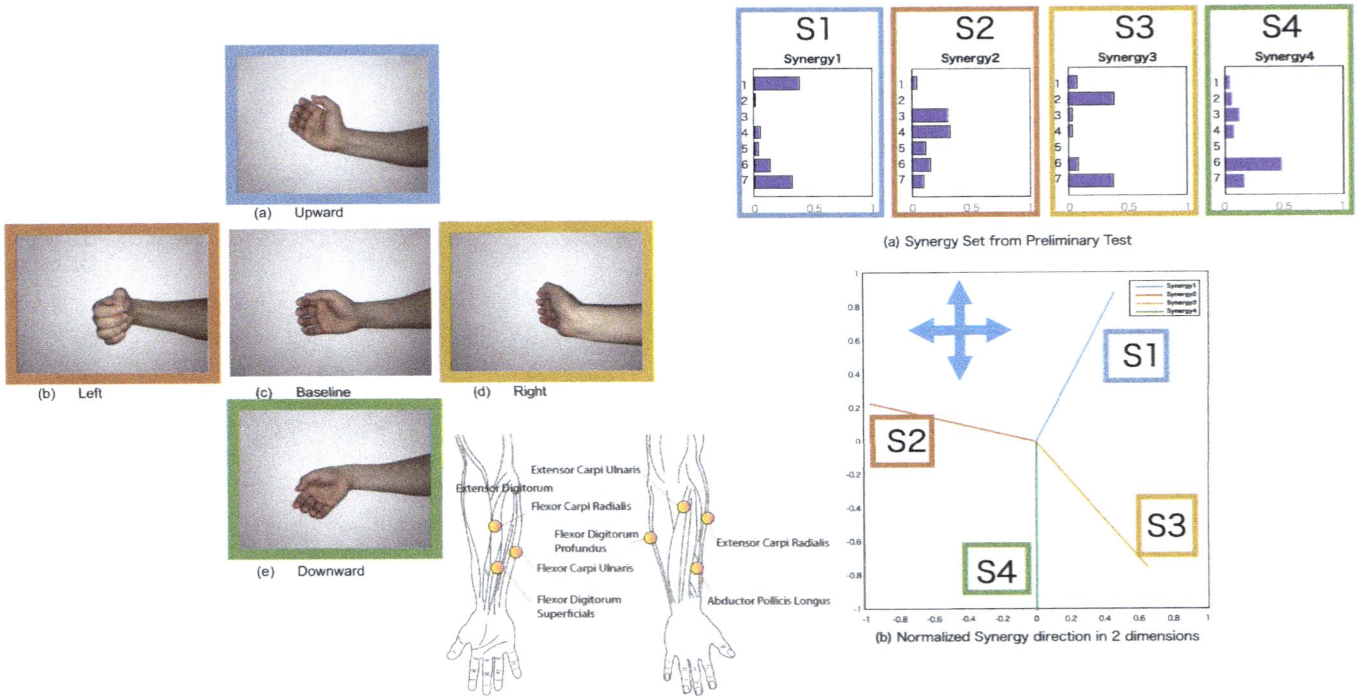

Figure 6.7 Muscle synergy for wrist motion.

6.5 Applications

6.5.1 Prosthetic Hand

In commercial multi-DOF prosthetic hands, finger opening/closing, and wrist rotation are mainly controlled by 2-channel EMG. The 2-channel EMG has difficulty controlling these two DOFs simultaneously, so the user switches between modes of finger opening/closing and wrist rotation and performs one of the two movements in each mode. This is a good method for stable control using multi-degree of freedom, but it requires learning to operate the prosthetic hand because it cannot control multiple degrees of freedom at the same time.

By using multi-array electrodes to measure muscle activity in the deep as well as the superficial layers of many muscles, and by reducing the degrees of freedom while maintaining the information of the human interface input through muscle synergy, it is possible to control the movement of each joint at the same time [4, 10, 11].

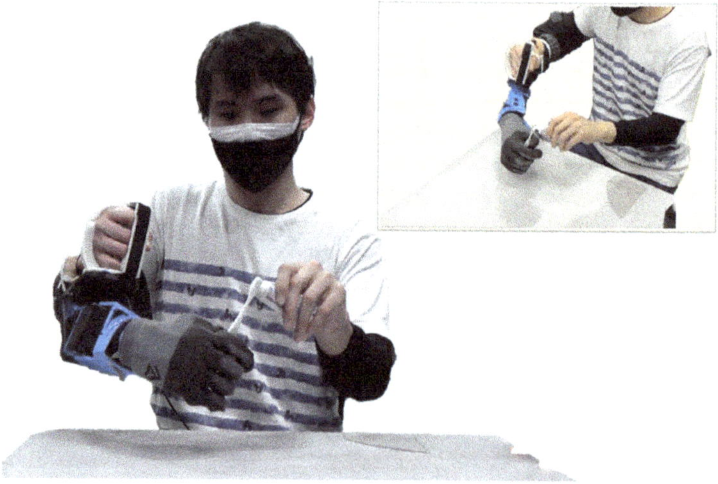

Figure 6.8 3 DOF myoelectric control.

In Figure 6.8, the multi-degree-of-freedom prosthetic hand is being used in everyday activities, with no training required. The able-bodied person fixates the hand as if gripping a stick and controls the prosthetic hand in a state of isometric contraction. The prosthetic hand is capable of controlling three degrees of freedom: opening and closing of the fingers, wrist extension and flexion, and internal and external rotation.

6.5.2 Rehabilitation

In areas such as rehabilitation, consider comparing the muscle activity of a patient with that of a healthy person. It is often observed that the patient's exercise time is longer and the muscle activity is more active than that of a healthy person, even if the same exercise is attempted. However, when muscle synergies are calculated, the patterns of muscle synergies show some similarity. Rather than examining how much each muscle activity differs, it is possible to extract more functional differences by comparing differences in the synergy patterns of how the muscle activities fit together.

In addition, by examining the muscle activity patterns of skilled persons in skill training, it becomes easier to quantitatively evaluate what muscle activity patterns express the elements of the skill and how many there are, as well as to understand the differences more clearly by visualizing a large number of muscle activities with a small number of synergies. The visualization of a large number of muscle activities with a small number of synergies makes it possible to understand the differences more clearly.

6.6 Summary

This chapter outlines the human interface that can be used to control prosthetic hands and other devices, including multi-channel multi-array electrodes and signal processing using them.

For a good human interface, it is important that the user can move the device as intended. Furthermore, it is not a good interface if it takes time to learn to use. Our bodies can be moved as we wish. We also outlined an algorithm that uses this body to move the control target as if it were our own body. By separating superficial and deep muscle activity from the signals of the multichannel multi-array electrodes currently under development, and using muscle synergy, which summarizes groups of similarly active muscles from numerous muscle activities, control can be achieved with fewer degrees of freedom depending on the task. Since adding conversions to the input signals of the human interface makes control difficult, the degree of freedom for control could be reduced by using muscle synergy, while still having the same degree of freedom for muscles as the body. In addition, it is said that each individual muscle activity contains noise according to the magnitude of the muscle activity, but by using muscle synergy, we were able to reduce this variability and thus control can be said to be stable.

In addition, in order to perform effective exercise within a limited time, such as in rehabilitation, the equipment must be easy and quick to put on and take off. For this reason, he also demonstrated the need for a device that can measure a large number of electromyograms just by putting it on.

In the future, it is necessary to continue the development of the device so that it can be applied not only to hands but also to arms, legs, and other sports.

References

1. Dario Farina, Ning Jiang, Hubertus Rehbaum, Ales Holobar, Bernhard Graimann, Hans Dietl, and Oskar C Aszmann. The extraction of neural information from the surface EMG for the control of upper-limb prostheses: Emerging avenues and challenges. *IEEE Transactions on Neural Systems and Rehabilitation Engineering*, 22(4):797– 809, 2014.
2. Tadashi Masuda, Hisao Miyano, and Tsugutake Sadoyama. A surface electrode array for detecting action potential trains of single motor units. *Elec- troencephalography and Clinical Neurophysiology*, 1985. doi: 10.1016/0013- 4694(85)91018-1.
3. Tadashi Masuda and Carlo J. De Luca. Recruitment threshold and muscle fiber conduction velocity of single motor units. *Journal of Electromyography and Kinesiology*, 1991. doi: 10.1016/1050-6411(91)90005-P.
4. Sorawit Stapornchaisit, Yeongdae Kim, Atsushi Takagi, Natsue Yoshimura, and Yasuharu Koike. Finger angle estimation from array EMG system using linear regression model with independent

component analysis. *Frontiers in Neurorobotics*, 2019. doi: 10.3389/fnbot.2019.00075.

5. Matthew C. Tresch, Philippe Saltiel, and Emilio Bizzi. The construction of movement by the spinal cord. *Nature Neuroscience*, 1999. ISSN 10976256. doi: 10.1038/5721.
6. Andrea d'Avella and Emilio Bizzi. Shared and specific muscle synergies in natural motor behaviors. *Proceedings of the National Academy of Sciences*, 2005. ISSN 0027-8424. doi: 10.1073/pnas.0500199102.
7. Simon A. Overduin, Andrea d'Avella, Jose M. Carmena, and Emilio Bizzi. Muscle synergies evoked by microstimulation are preferentially encoded during behavior. *Frontiers in Computational Neuroscience*, 8(March):1–10, 2014. ISSN 1662-5188. doi: 10.3389/fncom.2014.00020.
8. D Shin, J Kim, and Y Koike. A myokinetic arm model for estimating joint torque and stiffness from EMG signals during maintained posture. *J Neurophysiol*, 101(1):387–401, 2009. doi: 00584.2007 [pii] 10.1152/jn.00584.2007.
9. Yeongdae Kim, Sorawit Stapornchaisit, Hiroyuki Kambara, Natsue Yoshimura, and Yasuharu Koike. Muscle synergy and musculoskeletal model-based continuous multi-dimensional estimation of wrist and hand motions. *Journal of Healthcare Engineering*, 2020.
10. Yeongdae Kim, Sorawit Stapornchaisit, Makoto Miyakoshi, Natsue Yoshimura, and Yasuharu Koike. The effect of ICA and non-negative matrix factorization analysis for EMG signals recorded from multi-channel EMG sensors. *Frontiers in Neuroscience*, 14(December):1–10, 2020.
11. Zixuan Qin, Sorawit Stapornchaisit, Zixun He, Natsue Yoshimura, and Ya- suharu Koike. Multi-joint angles estimation of forearm motion using a regression model. *Frontiers in Neurorobotics*, 15(August): 1–18, 2021.

Chapter 7

Low-Power Wireless Transmitter with Quadrature Backscattering Technique

Hiroyuki Ito

Nano Sensing Unit, Tokyo Institute of Technology,
4259-J2-31 Nagatsuta-cho, Midori-ku, Yokohama, Kanagawa 226-8503, Japan

ito@pi.titech.ac.jp

This chapter introduces quadrature backscattering as a wireless communication technology that can achieve both low power consumption and Mbps-class data rates required for some biomedical applications. After introducing the principle of backscatter technology, the principle of the proposed technology and its implementation in integrated circuits are explained. Finally, measurements of the prototype show that the proposed technology is realized in principle.

7.1 Introduction

In biomedical applications such as brain-machine computing, there is a strong demand for wireless power supply and high-speed wireless data transmission to eliminate cables connecting

Biomedical Engineering: Imaging Systems, Electric Devices, and Medical Materials
Edited by Akihiro Miyauchi and Hiroyuki Kagechika

ISBN 978-981-5129-16-8 (Hardcover), 978-1-003-46404-4 (eBook)
www.jennystanford.com

inside and outside the body. Wireless communication circuits are required to operate at ultra-low power consumption of less than 100 μW and data rates of Mbps or higher. Recent trends in wireless integrated circuits show that impulse-radio ultra-wideband (IR-UWB) [1] and backscattering methods [2] have been the mainstream. Especially, the backscattering technology, which can eliminate the use of RF active circuits and can consist of low-frequency active circuits and RF passive circuits, has the possibility to provide lower power consumption because RF active circuits operating at high frequencies consume more power as a general matter. The backscattering technology has originally been used in radio frequency identification (RFID) [3], which does not require large amounts of data transmission. In this chapter, after explaining the principle of backscattering, an idea of increasing the data rate by enabling quadrature amplitude modulation in backscattering is presented. Then, implementation in integrated circuits is explained, and measurement results are shown.

7.2 Basics of Backscattering

First, let us understand the principle with a simple example of backscattering. The wireless system consists of a reader that outputs a high-frequency signal (usually a sine wave) and receives and demodulates the signal sent by the tag, and a tag or edge that uses the signal sent by the reader to generate power and sends ID and sensor data by backscattering.

Consider the case where a wireless signal is supplied from the reader terminal and received by the antenna in the tag as shown in Figure 7.1. Furthermore, suppose that the nature of the signal as a wave is not negligible. In other words, the reflection of the wave occurs at the impedance mismatch. Let ν_{m} be the voltage of the input wave, ν_{out} be the voltage reflected by the load, and Γ be the reflection coefficient, then the following relationship obtains.

$$\nu_{\mathrm{out}} = \Gamma \nu_{\mathrm{in}} \tag{7.1}$$

Suppose the output impedance of the source is Z_S and the impedance of the load is Z_L, the reflection coefficient is

$$\Gamma = \frac{Z_L - Z_S}{Z_L + Z_S}. \tag{7.2}$$

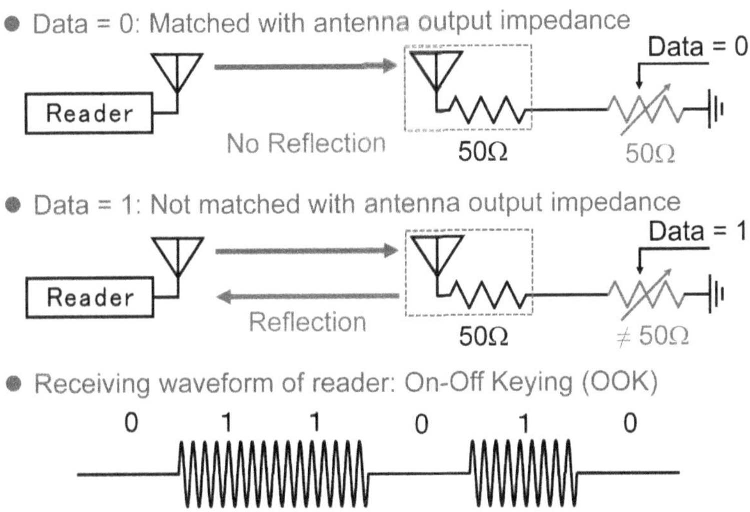

Figure 7.1 Example of amplitude modulation by backscattering.

As shown in Figure 7.1, when a load impedance Z_L = 50 Ω is matched to the output impedance of an antenna Z_S = 50 Ω, no reflection occurs because all the power of the signal coming in from the antenna is consumed by the load, and the reflection coefficient is zero. On the other hand, when the load impedance $Z_L \neq 50$ Ω is not matched to the antenna output impedance Z_S = 50 Ω, the signal from the antenna is reflected by the load and radiated from the antenna again. Thus, if the load impedance is matched when the tag device wants to send signal "0" of binary and not matched when it wants to send signal "1" of binary, e.g., set to a very high impedance, a type of amplitude shift keying (ASK) called on-off keying (OOK) can be achieved, in which reflection signals exist only for signal "1", as shown in Figure 7.1.

As another example, if a binary signal is sent with the load open, i.e., very high impedance, and short, i.e., 0 Ω, binary phase shift keying (BPSK) can be realized because the open and short loads produce full reflection signal with phase 0 degrees ($\Gamma = 1$) and with phase 180 degrees rotation ($\Gamma = -1$), respectively.

The above examples are the cases where there is no imaginary part in the load impedance, but if inductors and capacitors are combined appropriately, arbitrary phase rotation can be achieved for the reflected signal, enabling quadrature phase shift keying (QPSK) [4]. However, inductors are large area-consuming devices in integrated circuits, so they should be used as little as possible. Our motivation is to achieve multi-level modulation such as quadrature amplitude modulation (QAM), which can give a higher data rate, using only MOS transistors and resistors with relatively small areas in silicon CMOS integrated circuit technology.

7.3 Quadrature Backscattering

The following is an explanation of the concept of how QAM is achieved with backscattering. The top of Figure 7.2 shows a block diagram of a superheterodyne transmitter, which is the general transmitter architecture. The baseband signals I and Q are upconverted with local signals $\cos\omega_{\mathrm{IF}}t$ and $\sin\omega_{\mathrm{IF}}t$, and the intermediate-frequency (IF) signal $I\cos\omega_{\mathrm{IF}}t + Q\sin\omega_{\mathrm{IF}}t$ is upconverted with a local signal $\cos\omega_{\mathrm{RF}}t$. Then, the quadrature-modulated signal

$$(I\cos\omega_{\mathrm{IF}}t + Q\sin\omega_{\mathrm{IF}}t)\cos\omega_{\mathrm{RF}}t \tag{7.3}$$

can be obtained. By varying the amplitude of I and Q, the amplitude and phase of the output signal, i.e., Eq. (7.3), can be controlled arbitrarily, thus achieving QAM.

In backscattering, shown at the bottom of Figure 7.2, when $\cos\omega_{\mathrm{RF}}t$ is supplied by the reader, the signal $\Gamma\cos\omega_{\mathrm{RF}}t$ is reflected. Our idea is that by changing the reflection coefficient Γ to $I\cos\omega_{\mathrm{IF}}t + Q\sin\omega_{\mathrm{IF}}t$, we can obtain the same quadrature-modulated reflection-signal as same in Eq. (7.3).

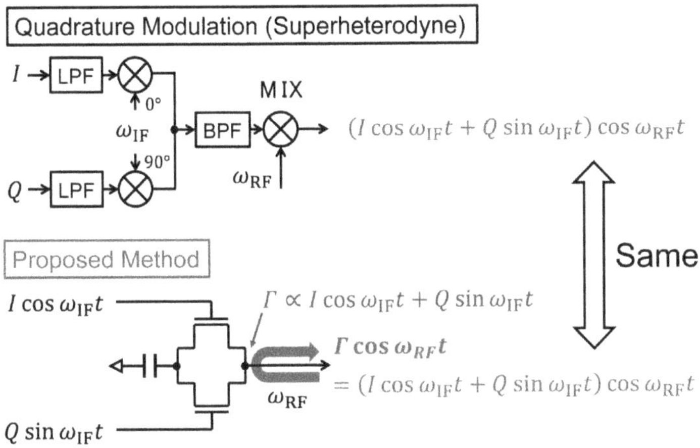

Figure 7.2 Basic idea of quadrature modulation by backscattering.

7.3.1 Method Based on MOS Transistors as Variable Resistors

This idea of quadrature modulation by backscattering has been proposed by our literature [5]. This subsection explains one of the circuit implementations of the quadrature backscattering technique and shows its limitation, which has not been described in [5].

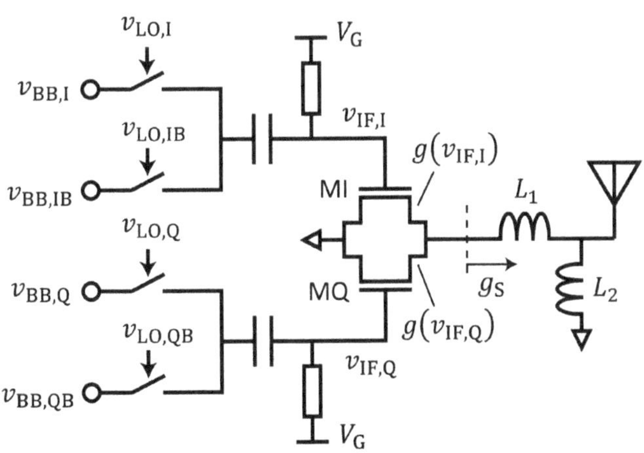

Figure 7.3 Schematic of the RF front-end circuit in the conventional quadrature backscattering transmitter [5].

Figure 7.3 shows the schematic of the RF front-end circuit in the quadrature backscattering transmitter based on using MOS transistors MI and MQ as variable resistors. Differential baseband signals $v_{BB,I}$, $v_{BB,IB}$, $v_{BB,Q}$, and $v_{BB,QB}$ are up-converted to IF signals $v_{IF,I}$ and $v_{IF,Q}$ by mixing with local signals $v_{LO,I}$, $v_{LO,IB}$, $v_{LO,Q}$, and $v_{LO,QB}$, where subscripts I and Q mean in and quadrature phases, and a subscript B means a reverse phase. The IF signals $v_{IF,I}$ and $v_{IF,Q}$ change drain-source conductance $g(v_{IF,I})$ and $g(v_{IF,Q})$ of NMOS transistors (MI and MQ), respectively, and modulate the reflection coefficient given by

$$\Gamma = \frac{g_S - \{g(v_{IF,I}) + g(v_{IF,Q})\}}{g_S + \{g(v_{IF,I}) + g(v_{IF,Q})\}} \tag{7.4}$$

$$= \Gamma_0 + \Gamma_I \cos\omega_{IF}t + \Gamma_Q \sin\omega_{IF}t, \tag{7.5}$$

where g_S is the conductance of the matching circuit as seen from the RF mixer consisting of MI and MQ. Γ_0 is the constant reflection coefficient, Γ_I and Γ_Q are the reflection coefficient controlled by IF signals $v_{IF,I}$ and $v_{IF,Q}$, respectively, and ω_{IF} is the intermediate angular frequency. The backscattered RF voltage signal can be written as

$$\begin{aligned} v_{out} &= (\Gamma_0 + \Gamma_I \cos\omega_{IF}t + \Gamma_Q \sin\omega_{IF}t)\cdot v_{in}\cos\omega_{RF}t \\ &= \Gamma_0 v_{in}\cos\omega_{RF}t + \frac{\Gamma_I v_{in}}{2}\cos(\omega_{RF} \pm \omega_{IF})t \\ &+ \frac{\Gamma_Q v_{in}}{2}\sin(\omega_{RF} \pm \omega_{IF})t, \end{aligned} \tag{7.6}$$

where $v_{in}\cos\omega_{RF}t$ is the carrier signal supplied from an external reader and received from the antenna. Again, the idea of the IF-based quadrature backscattering technique is to control Γ_I and Γ_Q separately so that arbitrary amplitude and phase changes occur in the backscattered signal v_{out}.

To simplify understanding, consider Eq. (7.4) in the vicinity of $g(v_{IF,I}) + g(v_{IF,Q}) = g_S$ as a first-order approximation as follows:

$$\Gamma = -1 + \frac{2}{1 + \frac{g(v_{\mathrm{IF,I}}) + g(v_{\mathrm{IF,Q}})}{g_{\mathrm{S}}}}$$
$$\approx \frac{1}{2g_{\mathrm{S}}}[g_{\mathrm{S}} - \{g(v_{\mathrm{IF,I}}) + g(v_{\mathrm{IF,Q}})\}]. \tag{7.7}$$

$g(v_{\mathrm{IF,I}})$ and $g(v_{\mathrm{IF,Q}})$ are given by the reciprocal of the on-resistance of NMOS transistors operating in the linear region.

$$g(v_{\mathrm{IF}}) = \mu_0 C_{\mathrm{ox}} \frac{W}{L}(V_{\mathrm{G}} + v_{\mathrm{IF}} - V_{\mathrm{th}})$$
$$= \beta(V_{\mathrm{G}} + v_{\mathrm{IF}} - V_{\mathrm{th}}) \tag{7.8}$$

where μ_0, C_{ox}, W, L, V_{G}, and V_{th} is mobility, gate capacitance per unit area, gate width, gate length, gate bias-voltage, and threshold voltage of the transistor, respectively. Assuming that the NMOS transistor sizes are equal, Eq. (7.7) becomes

$$\Gamma \approx \frac{1}{2g_{\mathrm{S}}}\{g_{\mathrm{S}} - \beta(2V_{\mathrm{G}} - 2V_{\mathrm{th}} + v_{\mathrm{IF,I}} + v_{\mathrm{IF,Q}})\}$$
$$= \frac{1}{2g_{\mathrm{S}}}\{g_{\mathrm{S}} - \beta(2V_{\mathrm{G}} - 2V_{\mathrm{th}} + V_{\mathrm{IF,I}} \cos\omega_{\mathrm{IF}}t + V_{\mathrm{IF,Q}} \sin\omega_{\mathrm{IF}}t)\} \tag{7.9}$$

where $V_{\mathrm{IF,I}}$ and $V_{\mathrm{IF,Q}}$ are AC amplitude of IF signals in I and Q path, respectively. Therefore, each reflection coefficient Γ_0, Γ_{I}, and Γ_{Q} shown in Eq. (7.5) is

$$\Gamma_0 \approx \frac{1}{2g_{\mathrm{S}}}\{g_{\mathrm{S}} - \beta(2V_{\mathrm{G}} - 2V_{\mathrm{th}})\} \tag{7.10}$$

$$\Gamma_{\mathrm{I}} \approx -\frac{\beta V_{\mathrm{IF,I}}}{2g_{\mathrm{S}}} \cos\omega_{\mathrm{IF}}t \tag{7.11}$$

$$\Gamma_{\mathrm{Q}} \approx -\frac{\beta V_{\mathrm{IF,Q}}}{2g_{\mathrm{S}}} \sin\omega_{\mathrm{IF}}t. \tag{7.12}$$

Thus, quadrature amplitude modulation can be realized by changing each AC amplitude of the IF signals $V_{IF,I}$ and $V_{IF,Q}$ in the range where both transistors MI and MQ operate in the linear region.

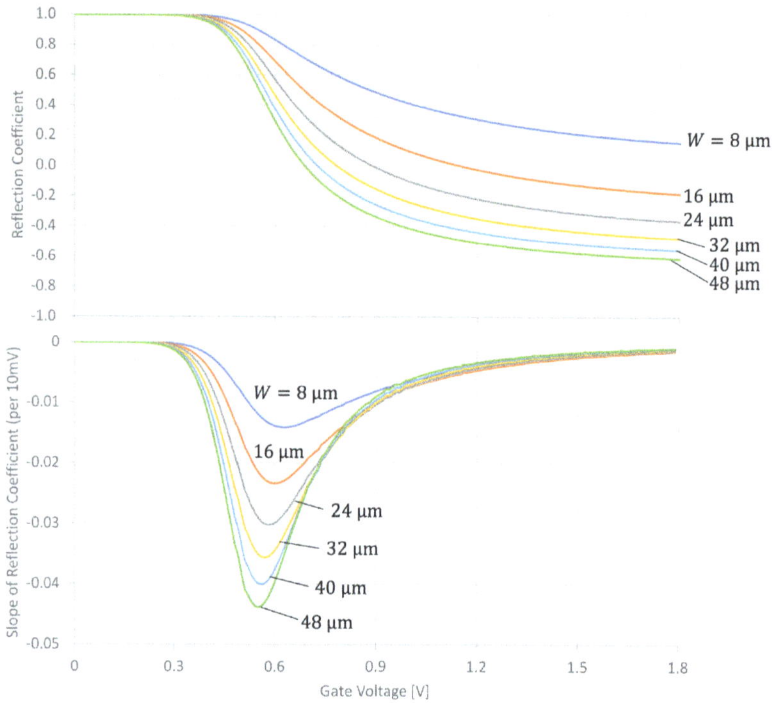

Figure 7.4 Simulated reflection coefficient of an NMOS transistor in 180 nm Si CMOS technology. Drain-Source voltage is 0 V, and gate length is 180 nm. The reference impedance is 50 Ω.

However, in reality, due to the non-linearities of Eq. (7.4) and MOS transistors, the reflection coefficient does not vary linearly with the gate voltage, i.e., IF signal amplitude, as shown in Figure 7.4. For example, even if non-linearity in the reflection coefficient up to 10% is acceptable, the range of available reflection coefficients around 0 reflection (0.9 V gate voltage, the vicinity of $g(v_{IF,I}) + g(v_{IF,Q}) = g_S$) at W = 24 μm is only about ±0.02. Thus, this method can transmit only very small power by backscattering, so there is little room for link budgets and only ultra-short-distance communication is possible. Alternatively, pre-distortion techniques could extend the linear range of the backscattering, but this would require additional calibration circuits because variations in individual chips would have to be considered, increasing energy consumption and circuit area [6].

7.3.2 Proposed Quadrature Backscattering Technique

Since the number of required symbols is finite, the idea is to realize QAM by dynamically switching the reflection coefficient. When not considering the side lobes of the modulated signal for simple discussion here, for example, 64QAM can be obtained by eight reflection coefficients, ±1, ±5/7, ±3/7, and ±1/7 on the in- and quadrature-phases, respectively.

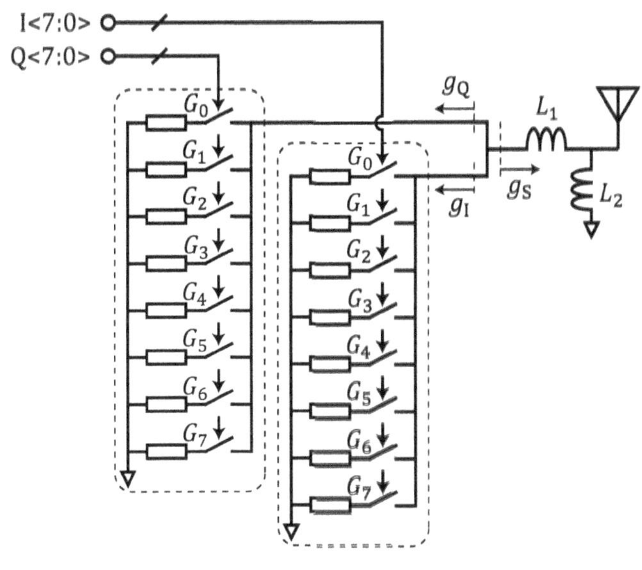

Figure 7.5 RF front-end schematic of the proposed quadrature backscattering transmitter [6].

Figure 7.5 shows the circuit diagram for realizing 64QAM by the proposed switching concept [6]. Note that this chapter reorganizes the content of the literature [6] and adds information and measurements for better understanding. The conventional switching scheme has used area-consuming inductors and capacitors for achieving QPSK [4]. Our method consists only of resistive switches that turn on and off at intermediate frequencies, which can reduce the circuit area of the modulators. The digital control signals I<7:0> and Q<7:0> for in and quadrature phases turn on only one switch of each phase at a certain time. In other words, since only two switches are on at the same time, the impedance seen from the antenna is in the form of two resistors connected in parallel. Thus, the reflection coefficient is

$$\Gamma = \frac{g_S - (g_I + g_Q)}{g_S + (g_I + g_Q)} = -1 + \frac{2}{1 + \dfrac{g_I + g_Q}{g_S}} \tag{7.13}$$

where g_S is conductance seen from switches, and g_I and g_Q are conductance of in and quadrature phases seen from the antenna side, as shown in Figure 7.5. As in the case of Eq. (7.7), a first-order approximation of Eq. (13) near $g_I + g_Q = g_S$ gives

$$\Gamma \approx \frac{1}{2g_S}\{g_S - (g_I + g_Q)\}. \tag{7.14}$$

Assuming that g_I and g_Q are rectangular waves with a phase difference of 90 degrees and change at the intermediate frequency.

$$g_I = g_{I0} + g_{I1}\cos\omega_{IF}t + g_{I3}\cos 3\omega_{IF}t + \cdots \tag{7.15}$$

$$g_O = g_{O0} + g_{O1}\sin\omega_{IF}t + g_{O3}\sin 3\omega_{IF}t + \cdots \tag{7.16}$$

Thus, the reflection coefficient is

$$\Gamma \approx \frac{1}{2g_S}\{g_S - (g_{I0} + g_{Q0} + g_{I1}\cos\omega_{IF}t + g_{Q1}\sin\omega_{IF}t + \cdots)\}. \tag{7.17}$$

Thus, QAM can be realized by controlling the magnitude of g_I and g_Q respectively through switching arbitrary conductance $G_7 - G_0$ with digital signals I<7:0> and Q<7:0>.

The specific implementation of this technique is described below. To achieve a reflection coefficient of −1, a very small resistance in the order of single-digit ohms, including the on-resistance of the MOS switch, is required, which is not easy to achieve in the CMOS process. Thus, for mitigating this requirement, the reflection coefficient range is set to ±0.9 in the design. To achieve 64QAM, reflection coefficients of ±0.9, ±0.9 × 5/7, ±0.9 × 3/7, and ±0.9 × 1/7 need to be provided in I and Q. The conductance of each switch normalized by a reference conductance is determined as shown in Figure 7.6. The actual output conductance $g_I + g_Q$ is affected by the parasitic capacitance and parasitic resistance of PADs, wirings, and MOS transistors, so the gate width of the MOS switches and the values of the inductors L_1 and L_2 for impedance matching are designed considering them while also performing post-layout simulations. In our design using 180 nm CMOS technology, the resistor values of I/G_0 to I/G_7 were 0 Ω, 19 Ω, 29 Ω, 42 Ω, 60 Ω, 87 Ω, 132 Ω, and 220 Ω, and the gate width and length of the NMOS transistor switch was 1.5 μm × 52 and 180 nm, respectively [6]. The values of L_1 and L_2 were 500 pH and 3 nH when designed for 920 MHz band operation. However, note that the better policy for increasing G_0/g_S, i.e., obtaining conductance close to a short circuit, is not to increase the transistor gate width, which carries a high risk of increasing parasitic capacitance, but to increase the reference impedance $1/g_S$ as much as possible.

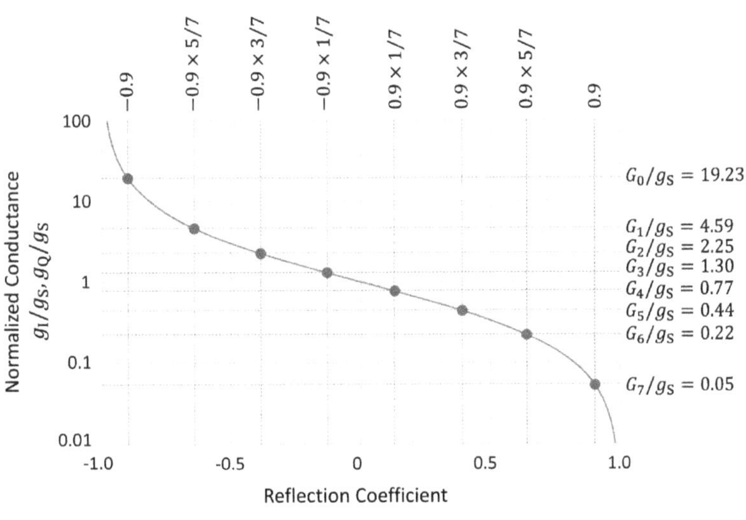

Figure 7.6 Examples of G_7 to G_0 values to achieve 64QAM. The maximum reflection coefficient is determined to be |0.9| in this design.

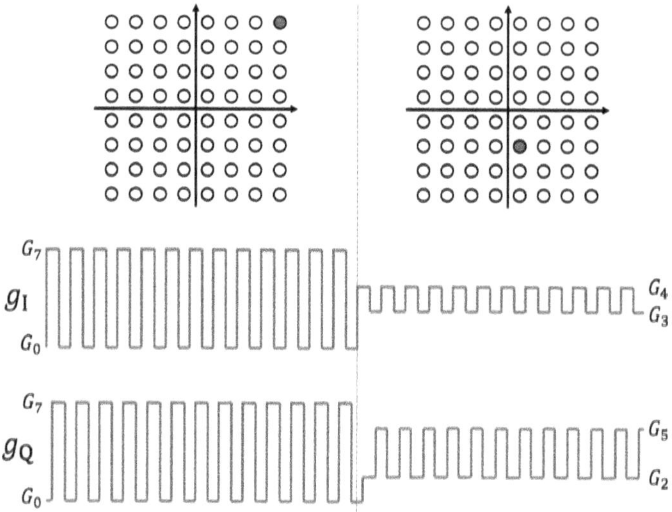

Figure 7.7 Example of a constellation and the conductance time-domain waveform to obtain it.

A 64QAM signal can be realized by switching from G_7 to G_0 at the IF frequency according to the symbols. Figure 7.7 shows an example of the relationship between the constellations and the time-domain waveforms of the I and Q conductance. For example, to obtain the upper right symbol on the constellation as shown on the left side of the figure, the reflection coefficient should be

$$\begin{aligned}\Gamma &= \Gamma_I \cos\omega_{IF}t + \Gamma_Q \sin\omega_{IF}t \\ &= 0.9\cos\omega_{IF}t + 0.9\sin\omega_{IF}t.\end{aligned} \tag{7.18}$$

In this case, the maximum and minimum values of the I and Q reflection coefficients are 0.9 and –0.9, respectively, so the conductance at which this reflection coefficient is obtained, that is, G_7 to G_0, should be switched alternately at the IF frequency In the example on the right of the figure, the reflection coefficient should be

$$\Gamma = (0.9\times 1/7)\cos\omega_{IF}t - \left(0.9\times\frac{3}{7}\right)\sin\omega_{IF}t. \tag{7.19}$$

To obtain a reflection coefficient Γ_I = $(0.9 \times 1/7)\cos\omega_{IF}t$, switch the conductance of G_4 and G_3 at the IF frequency. In the case of $\Gamma_Q = -(0.9 \times 3/7)\sin\omega_{IF}t$, start with G_2 and switch between G_2 and G_5 because the phase is inverted. Note that, in this article, the reflection coefficient, i.e., conductance, is switched in a square-wave shape to demonstrate the concept simply, and this will increase the sidelobe level of the reflected signal. To lower the sidelobes, we can use the technique of gradually varying the conductance in a staircase-like shape in order to approximate a sinusoidal reflection coefficient, as shown in Figure 7.8 [6].

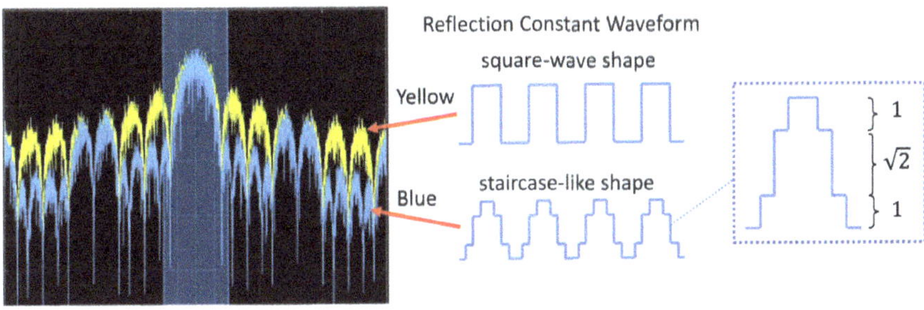

Figure 7.8 One idea to suppress sidelobe level of the reflected signal [6].

①	Carrier frequency	920 MHz	
②	Communication distance	1 m	
③	Modulation order (QAM)	64	
④	Input power	-4.7 dBm	Reader output EIRP 24dBm.
⑤	Losses until input/output to antenna	-6.0 dB	
⑥	Maximum reflection power	-10.7 dBm	④ + ⑤
⑦	Minimum reflection power	-27.6 dBm	④ + ⑤ - 20log(sqrt(③) - 1)
⑧	Antenna gain	3.0 dBi	
⑨	Propagation loss	-31.7 dB	147.56 - 20log(① × ②)
⑩	Reader's antenna gain	2.1 dBi	
⑪	Maximum received power	-37.3 dBm	⑥ + ⑧ + ⑨ + ⑩
⑫	Minimum received power	-54.2 dBm	⑦ + ⑧ + ⑨ + ⑩
⑬	Noise floor	-174.0 dBm/Hz	
⑭	Symbol rate	200 ks/sec.	
⑮	Noise margin	40.0 dB	
⑯	Total noise	-81.1 dBm	⑬ + 10log(⑭)+⑮
⑰	Target SNR	25.0 dB	BER = 0.001 @ 64QAM
⑱	Required received power	-56.0 dBm	⑯ + ⑰ < ⑫ => OK

Figure 7.9 Rough estimation of link budget [6].

Figure 7.9 shows the approximate link budget when a reflection coefficient of up to 0.9 is obtained by the proposed method. Even if the sum of the losses due to reflection by the RF-FE and implementation is 6.0 dB, it can be seen that the SNR required for 64QAM can be maintained in principle at a communication distance of 1 m.

7.4 Block Diagram and Circuit Implementation

A block diagram for realizing the proposed method is shown in Figure 7.10. First, 6-bit serial data, i.e., baseband signals, synchronized with the baseband clock are converted to parallel signals by the serial-to-parallel (S2P) circuit. The decoder determines the switches to be ON in the RF front-end (RF-FE) corresponding to a symbol according to the parallel signal. The upper 3 bits determine I and the lower 3 bits determine Q. The mixer is essentially a MUX circuit that selects the output of the decoder according to the high/low level of the local signal. This upconverts the baseband signal to the IF frequency and outputs I<7:0> and Q<7:0> to switch in the RF-FE.

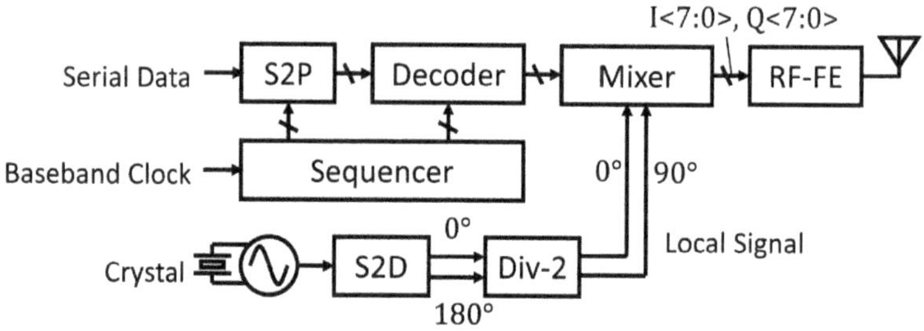

S2P: Serial to Parallel Converter, RF-FE: RF front-end,
S2D: Single to Differential Converter, Div-2: Frequency Divider

Figure 7.10 Block diagram of the transmitter [6].

The local signal is generated by dividing a crystal oscillator with a 10 MHz inverter-type Pierce topology. The single-to-differential converted oscillator-output signal is input to a divider with D-flip-flops to generate 0° and 90° IF local signals.

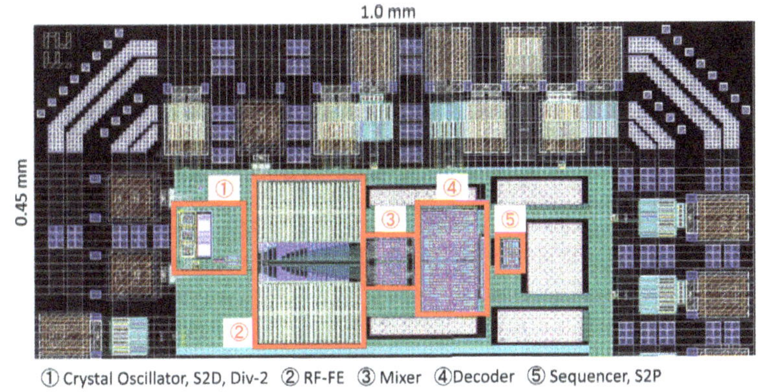

Figure 7.11 Chip layout of the transmitter in 180 nm Si CMOS technology [6].

Figure 7.11 shows the chip layout of the entire transmitter, which has an area of 1.0 mm × 0.45 mm including IOs. Off-chip inductors are used for L_1 and L_2. The total power consumption is 82 μW, 90% of which is dominated by the mixer (53 μW) and the crystal oscillator (21 μW). Simulations using the envelope transient showed that the reflected wave power of our circuit for CW power input from −15 dBm to 0 dBm was more than 10 dB better than that of the conventional circuit [5], suggesting the effectiveness of the proposed technique.

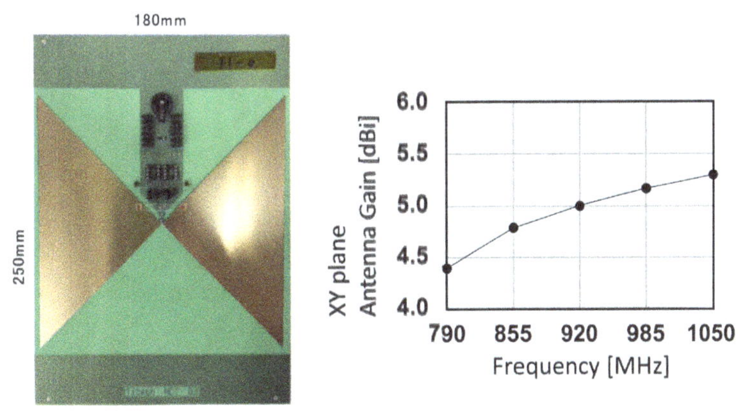

Figure 7.12 Picture of the transmitter board and simulated antenna gain [6].

Figure 7.12 shows a picture of a transmitter board, which consists of the prototype backscattering transmitter, bow-tie antenna, balun, connectors, crystal resonator, capacitive sensor circuit, reset circuit, LDO, button battery, and so on. When 3.0 V is supplied, the LDO provides the 2.5 V and 1.0 V supply voltages. The XY-plane antenna gain of the bow-tie antenna is shown on the right side of Figure 7.12. The antenna gain exceeds 5 dBi, and even allowing the 1-dB insertion loss of the balun, the antenna gain of over 3 dBi is expected. Thus, this meets the 3-dBi antenna gain used to estimate the link budget and a communication distance of 1 m is expected.

7.5 Measurement Results

Figure 7.13 shows a 1-meter wireless communication measurement. A 920 MHz sine wave with 18 dBm power is output from the signal generator (Agilent, E8257D) through the antenna, and the backscattered signal is received by the same antenna and evaluated by a vector signal analyzer (Agilent, 89600S). Transmit and receive signals are separated by a circulator. The backscattering transmitter is fed with a pseudo-random bit stream and a clock externally.

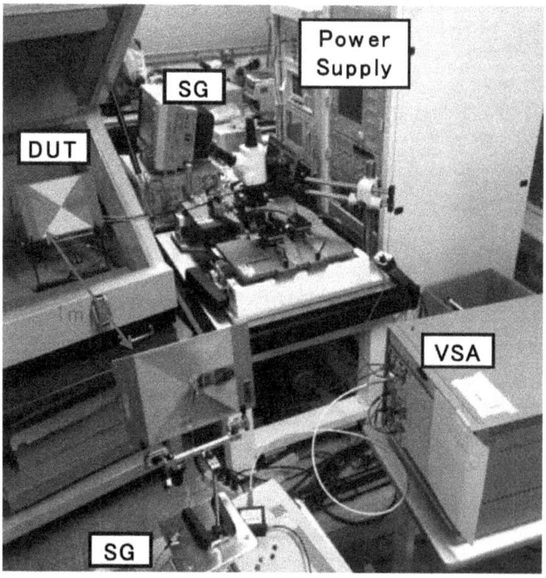

Figure 7.13 Measurement equipment.

Our backscattering transmitter also allows QPSK and 16QAM by specifying the input bits to be limited to specific reflection coefficients. Figure 7.14 shows the QPSK measurement results. EVM at 400 kbps and 4 Mbps were 6.9% and 9.4%, and current consumption from the 3 V supply was 45.35 μA and 59.76 μA, respectively. The EVMs of 800 kbps and 8 Mbps for 16QAM shown in Figure 7.15 were 9.1% and 11.4%, and the current consumption was 43.46 μA and 58.25 μA, respectively. 64QAM 1.2 Mbps is shown in Figure 7.16, and the constellation is distorted. These results show that only QPSK has succeeded in 1-meter wireless communication with low BER. However, it was shown that QAM can be achieved by the proposed method. The presence of deterministic distortion in the constellation suggests that process variations in resistors and switch-on resistance are the main cause of BER degradation in multi-level modulation. The next development step is to take this measure.

7.6 Summary

This chapter introduced quadrature backscattering technology that can achieve both low power consumption and Mbps-class data rates. After showing the challenges of using MOS transistors as variable resistors, the principle and implementation of a method to control the amplitude and phase of the reflection coefficient by switching the resistor were introduced. The prototype with the silicon CMOS integrated circuit and the board is presented, and its actual measurements showed that QAM is possible as proposed, and future issues are also discussed.

Acknowledgments

This work was partially supported by SCOPE (165003004) and the activities of VDEC, The University of Tokyo, in collaboration with Cadence Design Systems, Mentor Graphics, Keysight Technologies Japan, and NIHON SYNOPSYS G.K. The author thanks K. Miyauchi, N. Ishihara at Tokyo Institute of Technology, A. Kasamatsu at NICT for their kind supports.

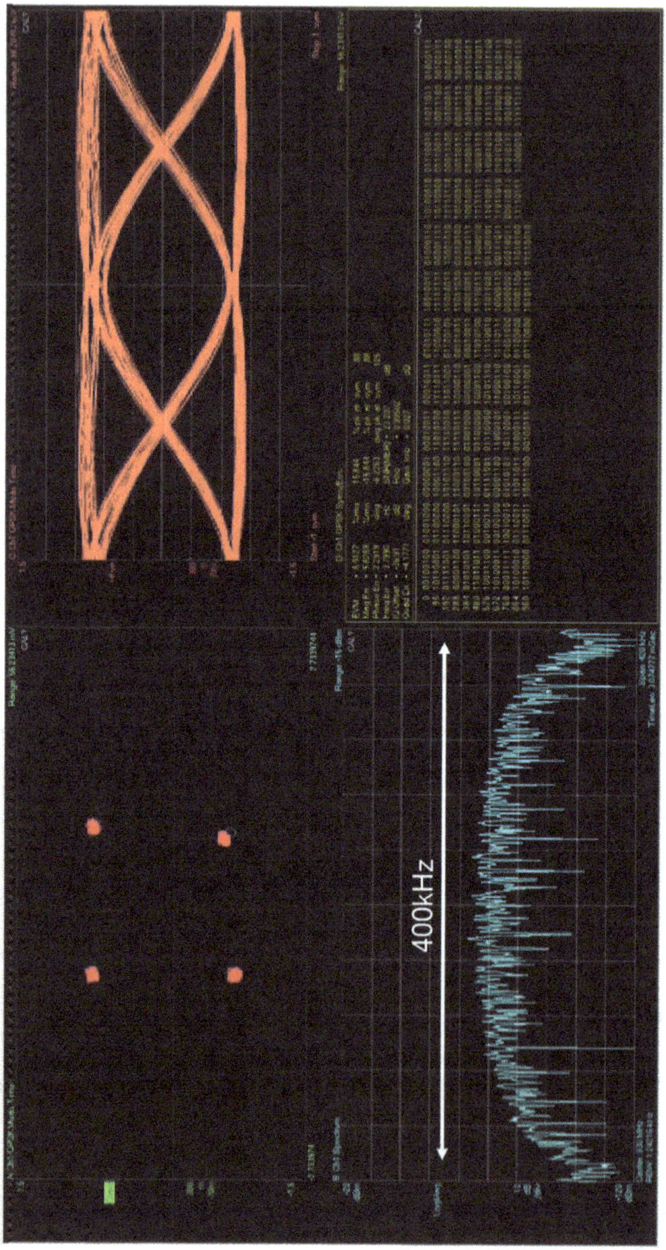

(a) 400 kbps

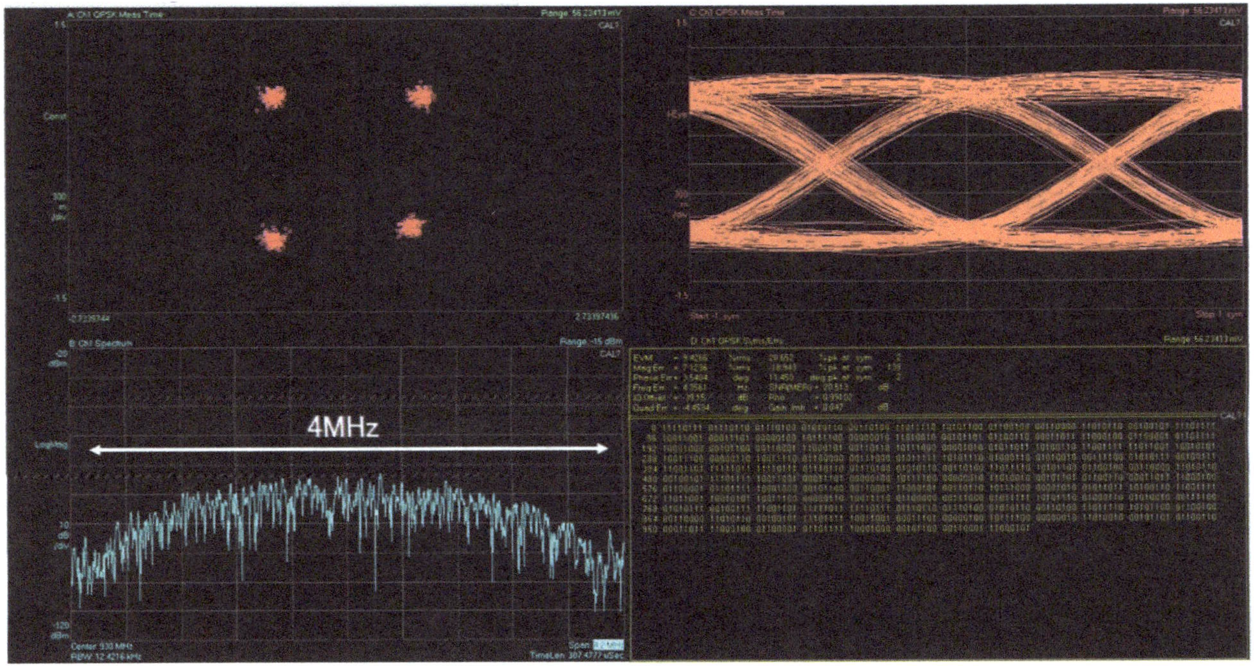

(b) 4 Mbps

Figure 7.14 Measurements of QPSK.

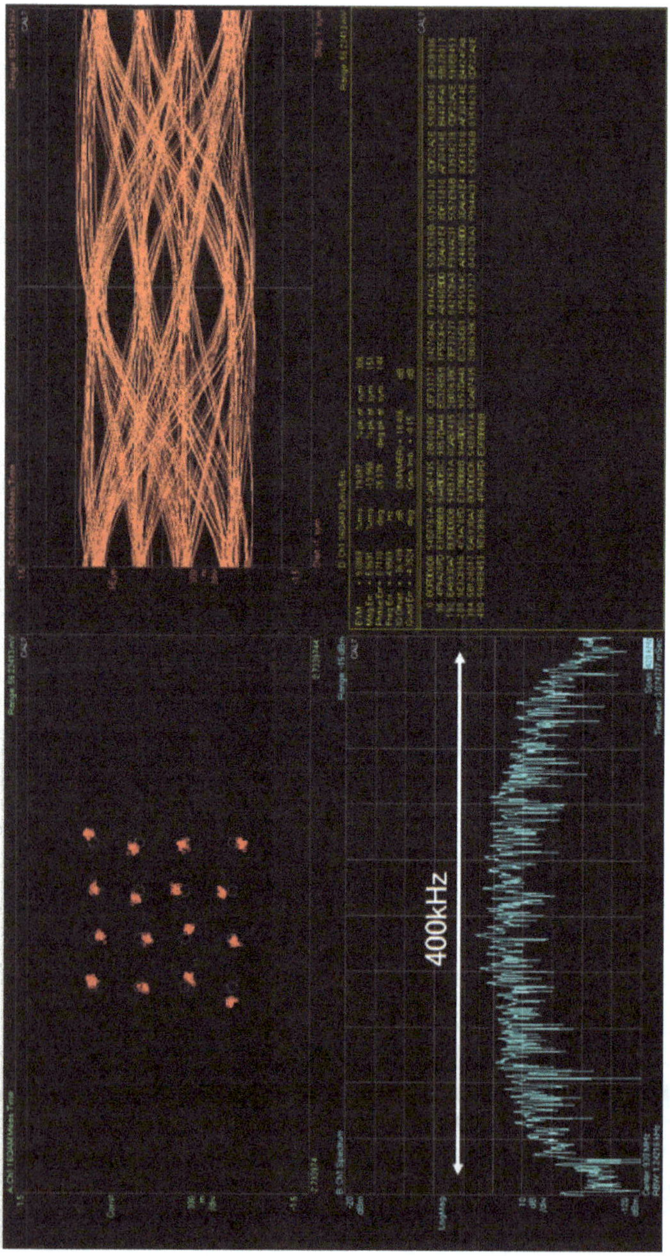

(a) 800 kbps

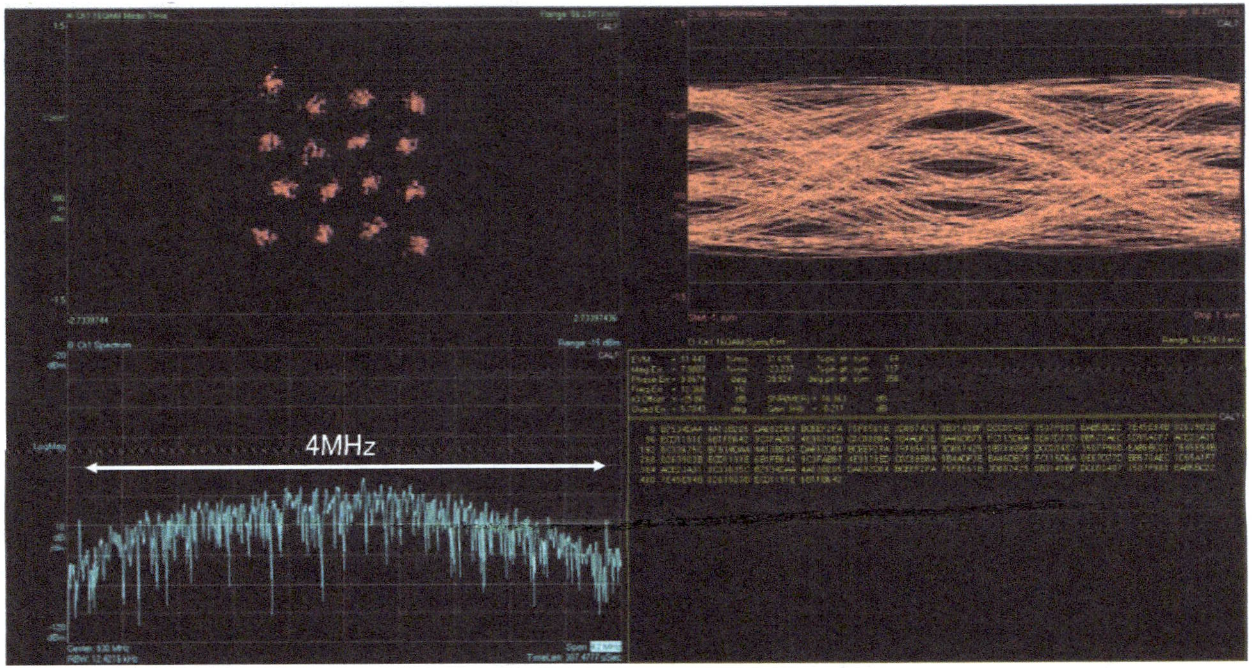

(b) 8 Mbps

Figure 7.15 Measurements of 16QAM.

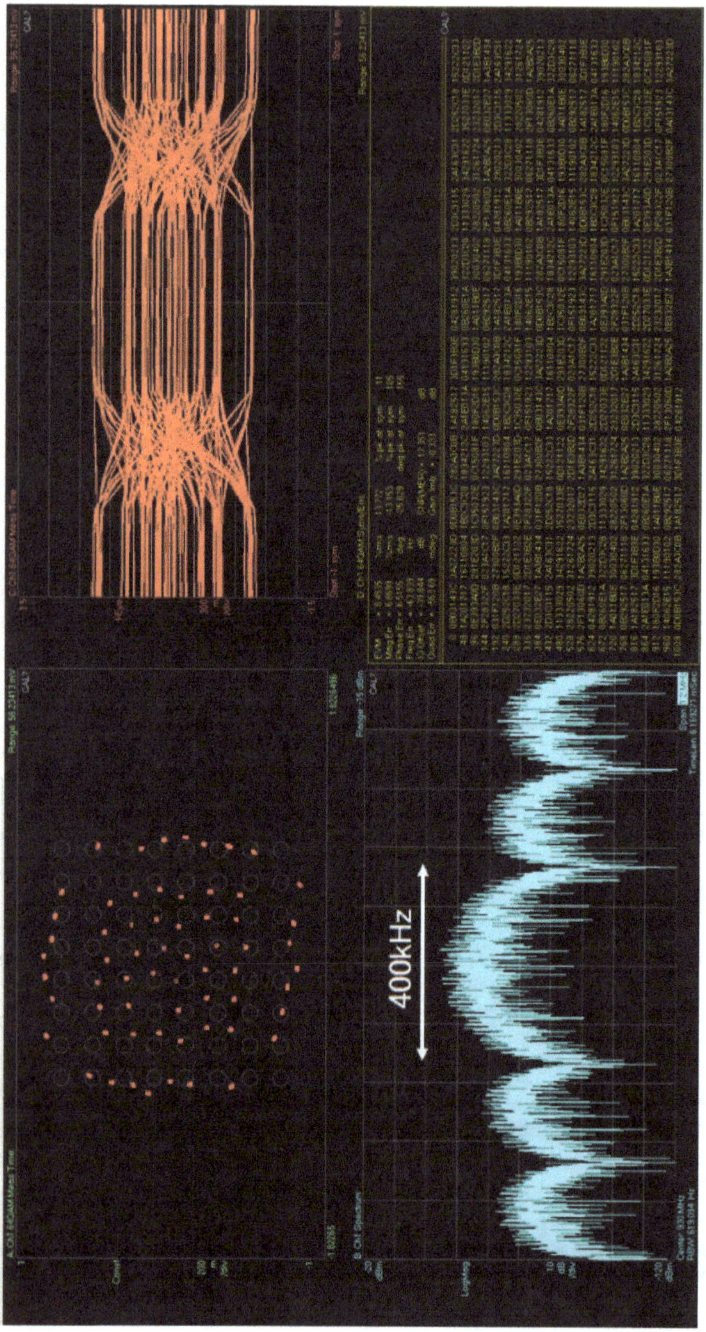

Figure 7.16 Measurements of 64QAM. The data rate is 1.2 Mbps.

References

1. Song, M., Yu Huang, Y., Shen, Y., Shi, C., Breeschoten, A., Konijnenburg, M., Visser, H., Romme, J., Dutta, B., Alavi, M. S., Bachmann, C. and Liu, Y.-H. (2022). A 1.66Gb/s and 5.8pJ/b Transcutaneous IR-UWB Telemetry System with Hybrid Impulse Modulation for Intracortical Brain-Computer Interfaces, *Proc. IEEE International Solid-State Circuits Conference*, pp. 394–395.
2. Lo, Y.-K., Chang, C.-W., Kuan, Y.-C., Culaclii, S., Kim, B., Chen, K., Gad, P., Edgerton, V. R. and Liu, W. (2016). A 176-Channel 0.5 cm^3 0.7g Wireless Implant for Motor Function Recovery after Spinal Cord Injury, *Proc. IEEE International Solid-State Circuits Conference*, pp. 382–383.
3. Nakamoto, H., Yamazaki, D., Yamamoto, T., Kurata, H., Yamada, S., Mukaida, K., Ninomiya, T., Ohkawa, T., Masui, S. and Gotoh, K. (2006). A Passive UHF RFID Tag LSI with 36.6% Efficiency CMOS-Only Rectifier and Current-Mode Demodulator in 0.35 um FeRAM Technology, *Proc. IEEE International Solid-State Circuits Conference.*
4. Thomas, S. J., Wheeler, E., Teizer, J. and Reynolds, M. S. (2012). Quadrature Amplitude Modulated Backscatter in Passive and Semipassive UHF RFID Systems, *IEEE Transactions on Microwave Theory and Techniques*, **60**, 4, pp. 1175–1182.
5. Shirane, A., Fang, Y., Tan, H., Ibe, T., Ito, H., Ishihara, N. and Masu, K. (2015). RF-Powered Transceiver with an Energy- and Spectral-Efficient IF-Based Quadrature Backscattering Transmitter, *IEEE Journal of Solid-State Circuits*, **50**, 12, pp. 2975–2987.
6. Miyauchi, K. (2019). Master Thesis (Tokyo Institute of Technology) (in Japanese).

Chapter 8

Representation by Extended Reality in X-Ray Three-Dimensional Imaging

Hiroki Kase, Kento Tabata, Katsuyuki Takagi, and Toru Aoki

Research Institute of Electronics, Shizuoka University
3-5-1 Johoku, Naka-ku, Hamamatsu 432-8011, Japan

aoki.toru@shizuoka.ac.jp

This chapter discusses the three-dimensional representation of complete voxel data including internal structures obtained from invisible information, X-ray computed tomography (CT). Since humans are always aware of three dimensions but use surface information of objects, three dimensions including internal structures such as X-ray CT are difficult to understand. In this chapter, we introduce the use of extended reality (XR) to achieve a representation that is easy for humans to understand, as well as a method to facilitate pointing of the desired location of 3D information. In addition, examples of these applications in the medical field are presented, showing that xR can be used not only for X-ray CT but also for magnetic resonance imaging (MRI) and other types of information that can provide 3D information including internal structures.

Biomedical Engineering: Imaging Systems, Electric Devices, and Medical Materials
Edited by Akihiro Miyauchi and Hiroyuki Kagechika

ISBN 978-981-5129-16-8 (Hardcover), 978-1-003-46404-4 (eBook)
www.jennystanford.com

8.1 Introduction

In recent years, extended reality (xR) technologies such as virtual reality (VR), augmented reality (AR), and mixed reality (MR) have been used in a wide range of fields. Their primary applications are in the representation of VR spaces, for example, in games and metaverse, and in entertainment using moving images and computer graphics. However, their use is also expanding into practical fields, such as inspection and security, because these technologies can directly represent three dimensions.

Meanwhile, computed tomography (CT) technology has become common in the world of X-ray imaging and is widely used not only in medicine but also in fields such as nondestructive testing and security. This is because CT provides three-dimensional (3D) data that can be analyzed, thus offering various advantages in terms of applications.

It is, therefore, natural to want to use 3D data captured by 3D X-ray CT for 3D representation in VR, AR, and other applications. Until now, data captured by 3D X-ray CT are generally represented as a two-dimensional tomographic image, and if necessary, the three directions of sagittal, axial, and coronal sections are displayed to understand the 3D image of a human brain. Although this method allows human beings to understand positional information accurately, the three axial directions of sagittal, axial, and coronal sections do not always coincide with the viewing position to be observed, and this has been handled by performing axis rotation operations as necessary. Generally, 3D X-ray CT outputs voxel data (pixel data in two dimensions) in the standard called digital imaging and communications in medicine (DICOM) [1]. The three directions (sagittal, axial, and coronal) are determined according to the slice at the time of X-ray CT imaging. Therefore, the voxels are calculated and the sagittal, axial, and coronal sections are reconstructed as axes according to the line of sight, instead of these three directions according to the viewpoint.

Humans normally recognize three dimensions through visual information that they receive as a two-dimensional light pattern. When human vision perceives a 3D object, the object is recognized as a 3D volume or configuration of parts and as a set of viewpoint-specific local features [2]. In addition, as the information is naturally obtained from visible light, the light on the surface of the object, in most cases reflected light, is seen and recognized. Therefore, most of the time we recognize only surface information, even if it is a 3D object, and when the volume of this information is exceeded, recognition suddenly becomes difficult for humans. Because we recognize limited 3D information, including internal information (for example, a model of the human body made of transparent acrylic of multiple colors), we have little experience and an excessive amount of information. This makes it difficult to recognize not only the internal 3D information of a 3D object but also the surface 3D information. Therefore, to capture the internal information of an object accurately, for example, when one wants to obtain accurate information about the inside of a body for surgery, it is often necessary to make a judgment by looking at a two-dimensional tomographic image. The reason is that the 3D DICOM data from a 3D X-ray CT lack comprehensibility even if the data are represented as a 3D image by xR or holograms. Furthermore, as mentioned above, although the axial direction of the gaze axis and the axial direction of the two-dimensional tomogram should be aligned and represented, it is not easy to point to the gaze position or the display position of the necessary tomogram. Currently, the gaze axis and tomogram axis are not aligned. Thus, the cross points of the three axes (sagittal, axial, and coronal) are manipulated with the help of the physician and technician using a mouse or other device to point to the tomogram position they wish to see.

Therefore, it is difficult to understand the internal information spatially with a simple 3D representation, and it is not easy to indicate the position accurately. In this paper, we describe a composite type of 3D representation that considers the 3D recognition characteristics of humans and examines the information that humans need to know by combining voxel data from 3D X-ray CT and two-dimensional tomographic images. We also discuss the recent advances in the use of wavelength information, such as dual-energy X-ray CT, to further increase the amount of information. In addition, surgical assistance using

AR technology and alignment adjustment of X-ray CT using these technologies are briefly introduced. These issues are not limited to X-ray CT but are common to magnetic resonance imaging (MRI), terahertz wave CT, visible light CT, and other 3D representations with internal information, but the discussion in this paper is limited to X-ray CT.

8.2 Three-Dimensional Representation of X-Ray CT Using Two-Dimensional Tomograms (Three-Plane Display)

The general 3D representation in the current X-ray CT and MRI systems consists of three two-dimensional tomographic images (sagittal, axial, and coronal sections) plus a pseudo-3D image (displayed in two dimensions) that assists in specifying the observation position, and these four images are displayed on a single large display or four displays. The images are displayed indicating a single point to be observed, i.e., the cross points of the sagittal, axial, and coronal sections (Figure 8.1). These tomographic images are an excellent method of presentation that allows the surgeon to determine the location of the surgery accurately and to understand it rapidly and easily. The challenges are that it is not easy to specify the observation points to be viewed (pointing), and the axis of the physician's viewpoint during surgery does not necessarily coincide with the axis presented by the DICOM data. This is because the DICOM data returns sagittal, axial, and coronal sections of three orthogonal axes in the patient's height, width, and vertical width directions, while the physician's line of sight is from an oblique direction when viewed from these axes. Although it is not difficult to convert DICOM data to the physician's gaze axis on a computer and recalculate the data, it is not easy to specify the point to be observed, and pointing movements that take the physician's gaze axis into consideration become necessary (Figure 8.2). Therefore, the three tomographic images of sagittal, axial, and coronal sections provide important and accurate information that the operating physician can understand immediately. However, the axes of the sagittal, axial, and coronal sections from DICOM data are different from those of the physician's line of sight during surgery and need to be converted in the mind of the physician. It is possible to align the axes from DICOM data with the gaze axis of the physician, but pointing becomes difficult in this case.

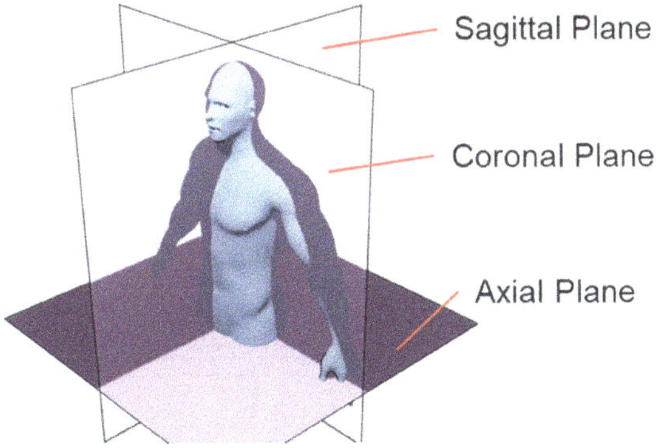

Figure 8.1 Axes of three-dimensional (3D) X-ray computed tomography (CT).

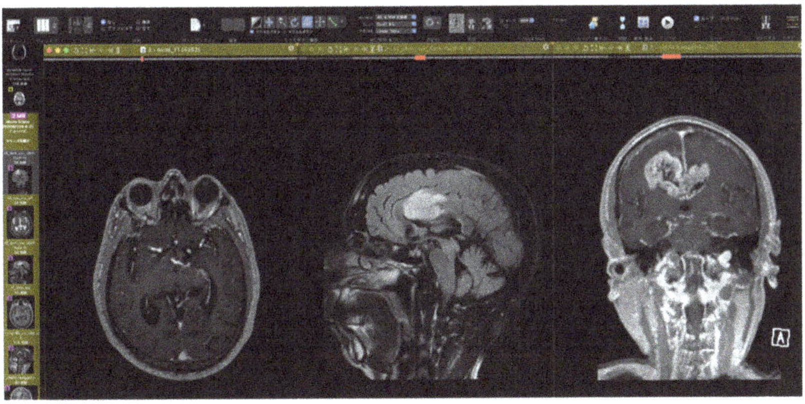

Figure 8.2 Human head image from each axis.

8.3 Three-Dimensional Representation of X-Ray Computed Tomography Data Using Extended Reality

This section describes the 3D representation of X-ray CT data using xR with the goal of clearly representing the internal structure of invisible objects imaged by 3D X-ray CT. This approach does not aim to replace the representation using the previously described three-plane tomogram but provides a distinct representation or specifies a clear position and axis angle of the observation point.

When an object imaged by 3D X-ray CT is represented as a 3D object in a virtual space, the observer can confirm the object spatially. The displayed object is represented as meshed 3D data in the virtual space and can be confirmed from any direction by moving or rotating the position of the object's cross section. The objective is to allow verifying the object from any direction by moving and rotating the position of the object's cross section.

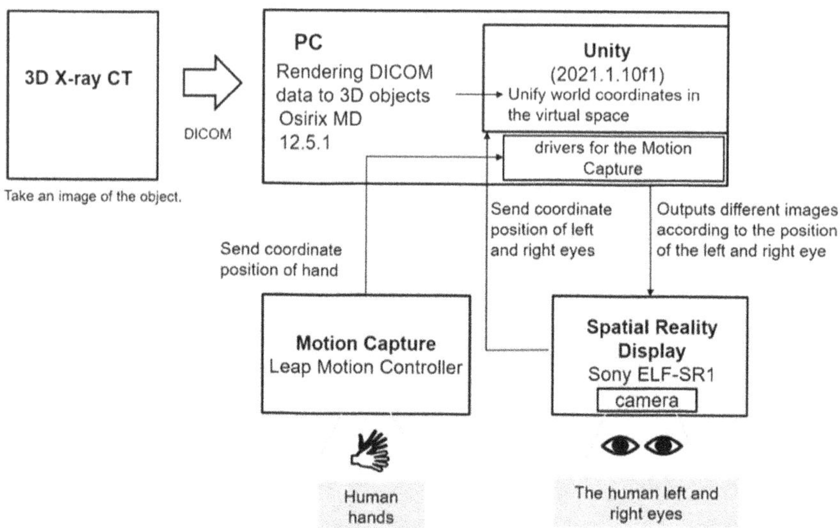

Figure 8.3 Actual configuration of the device.

The actual configuration of the device is shown in Figure 8.3. This figure also includes a system for pointing operations (viewpoint position and viewpoint axis specification) using motion capture, which will be explained in the next section. The DICOM data captured by the 3D X-ray CT are sent to a PC and meshed by surface rendering. Using the Unity (2021.1.10f1) [3] gaming engine, the meshed data are represented in a virtual space, and the object data are represented in 3D by a spatial reality display (SONY ELF-SR1) [4] connected to the PC. The spatial reality display has a camera mounted on top of the front display and is equipped with gaze recognition technology that detects the position of the observer's left and right eyes in real-time in horizontal, vertical, and depth directions and transmits this information to Unity. When different images are output according to the positions of the left and right eyes, the spatial reality display outputs separate images for the left and right fields of vision (naked-eye 3D display), which makes the observer feel as if the object is being represented in three dimensions.

We have developed a system in which a two-dimensional image consisting of DICOM data is superimposed on the cross section of a surface-rendered object, as shown in Figure 8.4. This is described in detail below regarding the cross-sectional representation. The system adds a function that allows the observer to move freely and rotate the cross section in MR, rather than displaying the cross section as a 3D view from a specific direction. First, when an observer determines the position and rotation direction of a cross section on a surface-rendered object model, a two-dimensional cross section in the same position and rotation direction is generated on the DICOM voxel data. The cross section is then overlaid on the surface-rendered object model. The most important feature of this method is that the cross-sectional orientation can be arbitrarily determined when displaying the cross section, rather than in a specific direction (X, Y, or Z direction). For example, in full-body X-ray CT, in the direction of the body width axis relative to the body length axis or the front-back axis of the body. Rotating the object and displaying the cross section on the boundary plane is synonymous with fixing the object and determining the position and angle of the cross section. This means that when the object touches the boundary surface in the world coordinates in the virtual space, it is converted to a specific point on the boundary surface as a point (x, y, z) in the plane of the axes (X, Y, Z) with respect to the boundary surface, as shown in Figure 8.5. It is further converted to a point (x′, y, z) in the plane of the axes (X′, Y′, Z) with respect to the object axes (X′, Y′, Z′ axes) and then converted to a specific point (x′, y′, z′) in the axes (X′, Y′, Z′ axes) with respect to the object as reference.

This allows us to calculate the position on the voxel data of the cross section that the observer wants to see.

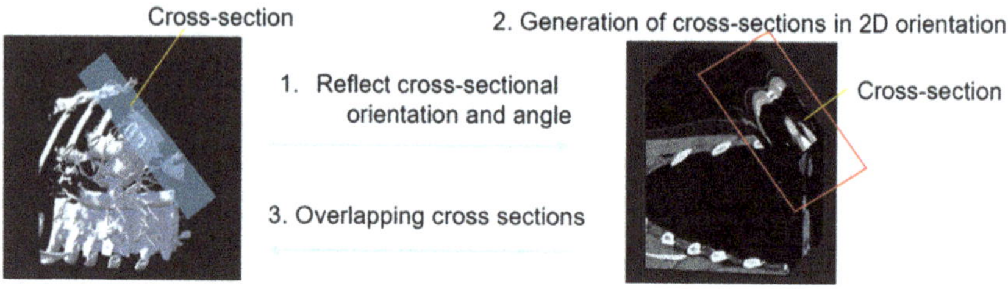

Figure 8.4 Representation of cross section from DICOM 2D image.

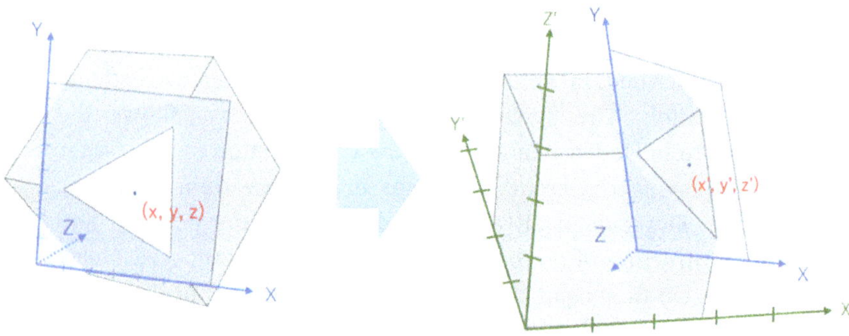

Figure 8.5 Transformation of world coordinates and axes in virtual space.

In this paper, sample data of the heart from Pixmeo's DICOM Image Library [5] were used. Figure 8.6 (0) is an illustration of surfaces and axes, (A) is a cross section of a surface rendering of an object, (B) is a cross section of a volume rendering, (C) is a cross section in the two-dimensional direction using DICOM, and (D) is a cross section of a surface rendering of an object. (D) shows a two-dimensional cross section from DICOM superimposed on a surface-rendered object cross section. In (A), the surface layer of the object is meshed to express a 3D effect and shading, making it easy to understand the spatial structure in the depth direction, but there are no data in the cross section. Thus, the object is generally expressed in white, and no internal information is expressed. In (B), the transparency is reflected according to the density information of the CT values, and the internal structure can be observed, but it is difficult to determine where the cross section is located because the density information in the depth direction is expressed at the same time. (C) shows a two-dimensional image generated from DICOM voxel data, but because it is an image, it does not provide a 3D representation. Therefore, a new representation method, (D), superimposes a two-dimensional cross section from DICOM on a surface-rendered cross section. By incorporating a process (stencil buffer [6]) that determines whether or not to draw a two-dimensional cross-sectional image on the far side by referring to the cross-sectional shape of the 3D data, a surface-rendered model is depicted if it exists in the depth direction based on the viewpoint. If it does not exist, it is not depicted. This prevents the 3D data in the depth direction from being obscured by the cross-sectional image. This method of representation complements the advantages and disadvantages of both surface rendering and volume rendering and allows us to understand the internal structure and the depth direction.

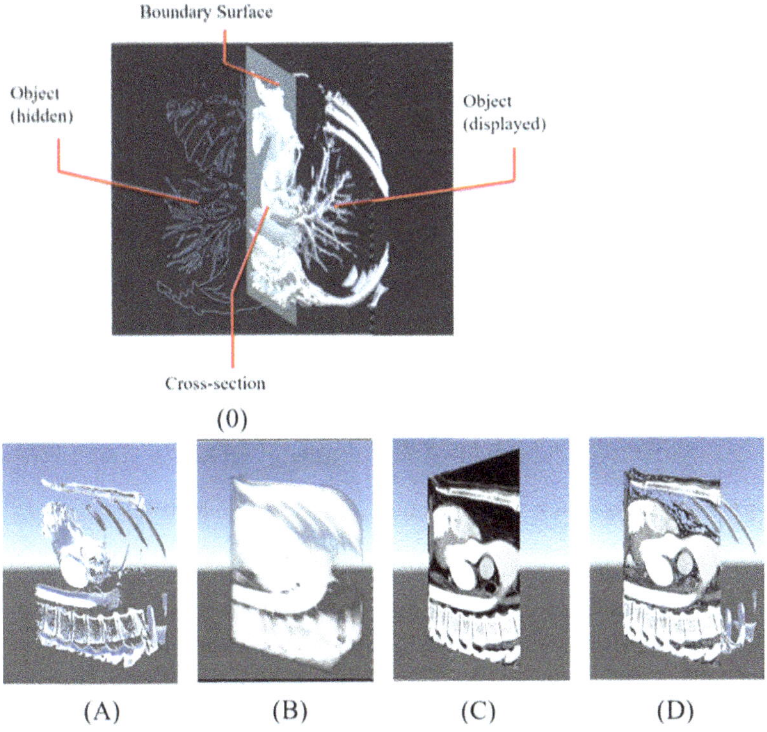

Figure 8.6 Comparison of expression methods.

8.4 Three-Dimensional Pointing Using Extended Reality and Motion Capture

As described in the previous section, xR enables the simultaneous representation of internal structures using cross-sectional views and 3D displays that are easy for humans to recognize. However, the information provided by the operator also increases and pointing becomes even more difficult with the addition of the specification of the viewing axis with a degree of freedom in the entire 3D region along with the specification of the position where the tomogram is to be displayed in the 3D voxel data. This is not easy even for a conventional pointing device such as a mouse. In fact, in first-person games, these two axes are manipulated by superhuman manipulation of the mouse and keyboard, which creates a game-like effect. Here, the position of the cross section is rotated and moved not by keyboard or mouse operation, but by intuitive operation as if the observer were actually grasping, moving, and rotating the 3D data of the object with their hands. We propose and demonstrate a system that allows users to observe the cross section freely.

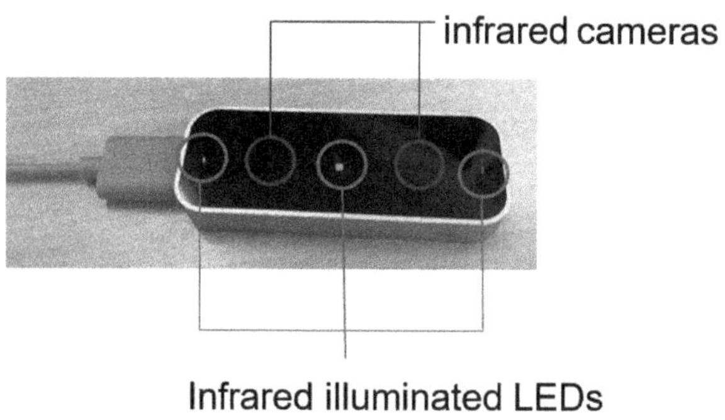

Figure 8.7 Motion capture (leap motion controller).

The motion capture shown in Figure 8.7 can be operated intuitively only by gestures; the Leap Motion Controller [7] is equipped with two infrared cameras and three LED lights to acquire hand and finger movement and angle information. It is capable of recognizing specific gestures such as grasping, picking, and rotating objects. Hand and finger information is also transmitted to Unity. In this study, the motion capture camera is attached to the observer's neck so that it can recognize the entire hand movement.

Here, the use of a spatial reality display and motion capture enables the observer to rotate and move the object by hand gestures to observe the cross section in any direction. Figure 8.8 shows an actual observer wearing the motion capture camera and performing a grasping gesture in front of the spatial reality display. The observer's hand is represented as a virtual hand on the spatial reality display, as shown in Figure 8.9, and can move and rotate in all 3D angles in the 4π direction. The virtual hand, object, and cross section are displayed on the same screen, and the virtual hand and object are designed to interact with each other in the same way as in the real world, that is, making contact, grasping, and holding.

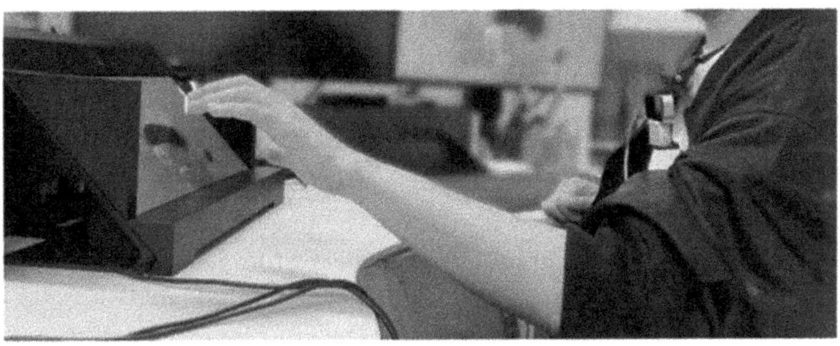

Figure 8.8 Performing a grasping gesture in front of the spatial reality display.

The above system provides a representation that allows the observer to perceive freely the cross section of an object in MR, including density information. Issues of the system include the lack of feedback to the hand and the fact that it does not provide the sensation of actually grasping the object. In addition, questions arise such as whether it is appropriate to lift up a person in VR to match their viewpoint in actual surgery, even if it is good for educational purposes in the medical field, and whether AR can be used by doctors for surgery in the future. A method has been demonstrated to display 3D data including internal information in an easy-to-understand manner for humans and to specify the position of the data easily.

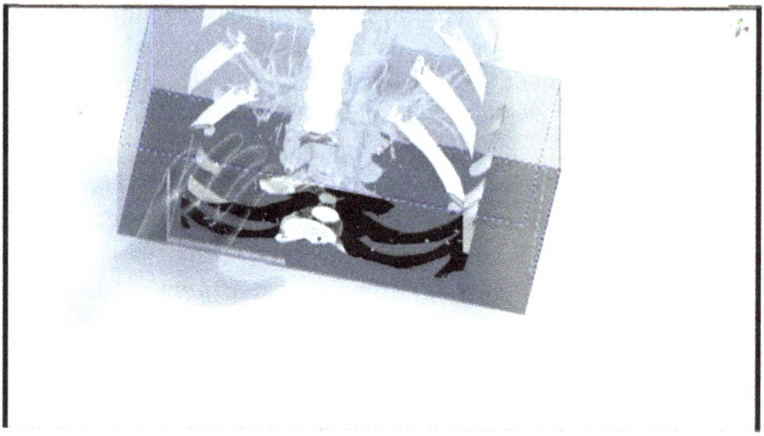

Figure 8.9 Virtual hand on the spatial reality display.

8.5 Application of Extended Reality Technology in the Medical Field

The use of 3D data captured by 3D X-ray CT and MRI to fabricate jigs and other components necessary for surgery and treatment or to assist in surgery and treatment has begun. The technology is being utilized, for example, to fabricate prototypes of parts using a 3D printer or to fabricate components based on prototyped parts when they are to be placed inside the body [8]. However, although improvements have been made, prototypes made with 3D printers are not always sufficiently strong or biocompatible. In addition, the use of 3D printed parts requires further research, because plastic materials are mainly used, heat treatment is difficult, and 3D printing of sterilized metal parts still requires a long manufacturing process and is expensive. Meanwhile, prototyping a component by simulating a mold made by 3D printing is used to create the shape of catheters and other elements [9]. In this method, sterilized components can be used as they are, and there is no biocompatibility issue. However, if a 3D printed component is touched even slightly, it cannot be used for a jig to be introduced into the body, and the precise printing and fabrication with a 3D printer takes time in the order of days, making it difficult to apply in urgent cases.

Therefore, we attempted to deform and process the wire by overlaying the 3D display on the aforementioned spatial reality display. In this system, the 3D image is composed from 3D DICOM data, and the 3D face is checked while it is moved or the object is moved as described in the previous section, and the position of the object is adjusted while being expressed. The problem in this case is that voxels in DICOM are not always manufactured in the same way (the distance between pixels in the three axes is not constant). Voxels must be square to avoid stretching in images from arbitrary viewpoint axes and to ensure that the image is represented at equal magnification (not only in the horizontal direction but also in the depth direction of the screen). However, voxels are not always square. Therefore, calibration including adjustment operations with drivers and displays is necessary. To confirm the results of these calculations, a ruler is displayed on the spatial reality display with the display axis after the calculations, and the "scale of the ruler in virtual space" is measured with a "real caliper" to confirm that the error is within the minimum scale or less. Because there is no real object in this measurement, it is not easy to fix the real caliper and it is difficult to verify the accuracy of the caliper.

In addition, the X-ray beam must be carefully aligned for the correct and safe use of various X-ray devices. While many medical devices are always aligned by the manufacturer's technicians, there are occasional cases where alignment of the X-ray source and detector (including the imaging plates) must be performed by a physician or radiologist, for example, in dental applications. Currently, physicians and technologists work together to confirm that the positions of the X-ray tube beam, collimator, and detector are in a linear relationship, and then the image is taken. By measuring the collimated X-ray beam in three dimensions using an X-ray imaging device and converting it into 3D data, it is possible to visualize the X-ray beam and represent it in real 3D space. This is performed by displaying the X-ray beam data in AR using the equipment and landmarks in the examination room as markers. Some issues should still be solved, such as the need to set up an X-ray FPD and its driving axis to acquire 3D X-ray beam data in the real world and to set up and identify markers to ensure consistency between the virtual and real spaces in a wide range of locations with high accuracy. In the future, however, xR will be used to display scattered radiation by combining a Monte Carlo simulation of radiation and energy-differentiated X-ray 3D data. In addition, xR will make it possible to display appropriately an increased amount of information, such as reduced exposure and scattered noise, by combining it with 3D measurement data of the examination room structure and equipment. This will facilitate human understanding and make X-ray useful and safe in the medical field. Additionally, the visualization of invisible light using xR has great potential for making X-rays useful and safe in the medical field.

References

1. Tomonori Yamauchi, Masashi Yamazaki, Akihiko Okawa, Takeo Furuya, Koichi Hayashi, Tsuyoshi Sakuma, Hiroshi Takahashi, Noriyuki Yanagawa, Masao Koda, Efficacy and reliability of highly functional open source DICOM software (OsiriX) in spine surgery, *Journal of Clinical Neuroscience*, Vol. 17, Issue 6, pp. 756–759, 2010.
2. Michael J Tarr, Heinrich H Bülthoff, Image-based object recognition in man, monkey and machine, *Cognition*, Vol. 67, Issues 1–2, pp. 1–20, 1998.
3. Unity, https://unity.com/ (14 November 2022).
4. Sony, Spatial Reality Display, https://www.sony.net/Products/Developer-Spatial-Reality-display/jp/ (14 November 2022).
5. Pixmeo, DICOM Image Library, https://www.osirix-viewer.com/resources/dicom-image-library/ (accessed Oct. 12, 2022).
6. Kilgard, Mark J, Improving shadows and reflections via the stencil buffer, *Advanced OpenGL Game Development*, pp. 204–253, 1999.
7. Ultraleap, Leap Motion Controller, https://www.ultraleap.com/product/leap-motion-controller/ (14 November 2022).
8. Ventola CL, Medical applications for 3d printing: Current and projected uses, P T. 2014 Oct, Vol. 39(10), pp. 704–11. PMID: 25336867; PMCID: PMC4189697.
9. M. Błaszczyk, R. Jabbar, B. Szmyd, M. Radek, 3D printing of rapid, low-cost and patient-specific models of brain vasculature for use in preoperative planning in clipping of intracranial aneurysms, *Journal of Clinical Medicine*, Vol. 10, No. 6, p. 1201, 2021.

Chapter 9

Refractive Index Measurement by Photodiode with Surface Plasmon Antenna and Its Application to Biosensing

Hiroaki Satoh and Hiroshi Inokawa

Research Institute of Electronics, Shizuoka University, 3-5-1 Johoku, Naka-ku, Hamamatsu, Shizuoka 432-8011, Japan

satoh.hiroaki@shizuoka.ac.jp

Gold line-and-space (L/S) surface plasmon antenna is introduced to enhance the sensitivity of silicon-on-insulator photodiode (PD), which also realizes sensitive refractive index (RI) measurement of the medium around the antenna, providing a new opportunity in optical biosensing for unlabeled analytes. Unlike the conventional device such as the surface plasmon resonance (SPR) sensor, it has a built-in photodetector, features a small footprint, and can be integrated in large numbers for high-throughput analysis. A chip and a flow system compatible with aqueous solutions are fabricated and tested with sucrose solutions. Thanks to the two-PD configuration with different L/S periods, a minimum detectable RI of 1.11×10^{-5} is attained, which is comparable to that of the

Biomedical Engineering: Imaging Systems, Electric Devices, and Medical Materials
Edited by Akihiro Miyauchi and Hiroyuki Kagechika

ISBN 978-981-5129-16-8 (Hardcover), 978-1-003-46404-4 (eBook)
www.jennystanford.com

SPR sensor. Furthermore, the change in the quantum efficiency of the PD with respect to the thickness of the analyte covering the Au line is simulated, and it is found that a few-nanometer-thick analyte such as avidin-biotin complex could be detected.

9.1 Introduction

A method of detecting the target analyte such as DNA, virus, bacteria, and disease marker molecules by utilizing the specific affinity or reactivity of biological receptors such as DNA, antibody, and enzyme is called biosensing, and the device to embody such a method is called a biosensor [1, 2].

Among various biosensors, one based on refractive index (RI) measurement can directly detect the capture of analyte by the receptor via the change in RI at the sensor surface [2], as shown in Figure 9.1. In contrast to other methods, such as enzyme-linked immunosorbent assay (ELISA) [3] that requires the modification (labeling) of the receptor or analyte with enzyme or fluorescent material to detect the capture via the change in the color density of a by-product or fluorescence intensity, the RI-based sensor does not require the labeling, which simplifies the experimental procedure and prevents the undesirable change of receptor/analyte properties by the modification process.

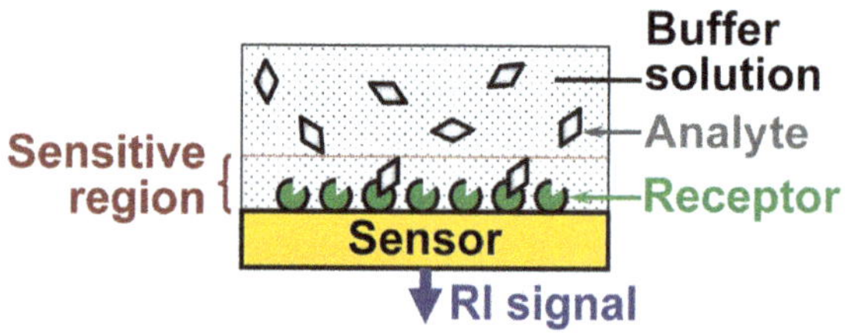

Figure 9.1 Schematic illustration of biosensor based on refractive index (RI) measurement.

As a representative of the existing RI-based biosensors, the surface plasmon resonance (SPR) sensor based on the prism coupling [2] is depicted in Figure 9.2(a). The resonant incident angle, at which the surface plasmon (SP) wave is induced and the reflectance is largely decreased, is sensitively shifted when a material with a different RI is attached to the metal surface, as shown in Figure 9.2(b). The detection limit of the SPR sensor is summarized in Table 9.1. Note that an extremely small amount of the deposited molecules in the order from nano to picogram per square centimeter can be detected, due to the short range of the near-field light generated by the SP wave in the order of the wavelength of the incident light. Since the SPR sensor can sensitively detect biomedical substances by the simple principle of RI measurement, it has been widely used in drug development, clinical diagnosis, agricultural and environmental monitoring, and so on. However, the number of samples that can be analyzed simultaneously is limited. Additionally, the optical system is bulky and requires a separate light source and detector, and the sensor size is large in the order of centimeters. As a result, there are difficulties in integrating a large number of sensors and improving the throughput of analysis. In order to address the above issues of the SPR sensor and to realize the high-throughput biosensing, we have investigated the photodiode (PD) with an SP antenna [4–6].

Table 9.1 Performance of the conventional SPR sensor

Detection limit of RI	$10^{-5} \sim 10^{-8}$	RIU
Detection limit of deposited molecules	$5 \times 10^{-9} \sim 5 \times 10^{-12}$	g/cm^2

RIU: refractive index unit

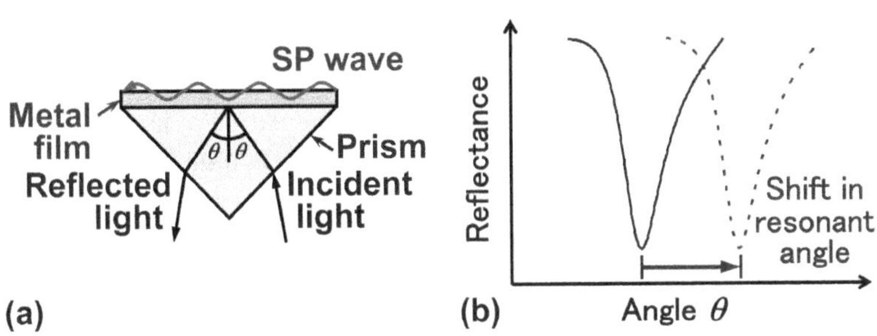

Figure 9.2 Conventional surface plasmon resonance (SPR) sensor. (a) Schematics and (b) response to the RI change at the metal surface.

9.2 PD with SP Antenna

Figure 9.3 shows the device structure of the PD with an SP antenna [6, 14, 15]. The lateral p-n junction PD is fabricated in the silicon-on-insulator (SOI) substrate. Line-and-space (L/S) grating-type SP antenna is placed on the thin silicon dioxide (SiO_2) layer that covers the PD. The grating is made of gold (Au) with titanium (Ti) adhesion layer beneath. The period p of the grating is varied from 260 nm to 340 nm. The photocurrent is taken from the positively biased (V_c) cathode terminal. The SP antenna also works as a gate electrode, and the volume of the depletion layer in the silicon (Si) layer, which is related to the PD sensitivity, is maximized by adjusting the gate voltage V_g and the substrate voltage V_{sub}.

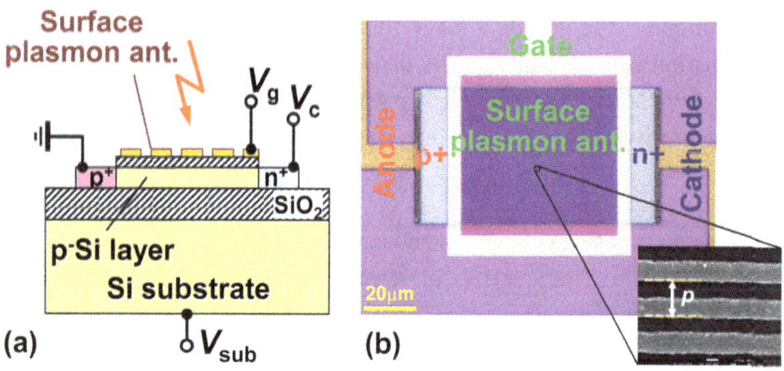

Figure 9.3 (a) Cross-sectional structure of the SOI photodiode with surface plasmon antenna. (b) Optical and scanning electron micrographs of the fabricated photodiode. The antenna consists of Au/Ti grating with a period p from 260 nm to 340 nm.

Figure 9.4 shows the spectroscopic sensitivity, i.e., external quantum efficiency (QE), for various p's with illumination by a TM-polarized light [4]. There are peaks of QE depending on p. Compared to the case without an SP antenna, 8.2 times larger QE (25%) is obtained at the wavelength of 680 nm even if the Si thickness is only 95 nm.

Figure 9.5 plots the experimental relationship between the peak wavelength and the grating period p [4]. Since the Si layer of PD is sandwiched by SiO_2 layers with smaller RI, the Si layer works

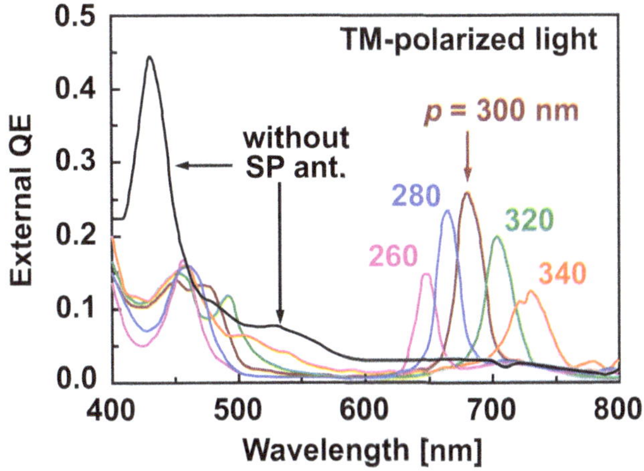

Figure 9.4 External quantum efficiency (QE) of photodiodes with various grating periods p and a Si thickness of 95 nm for TM-polarized light, i.e., the magnetic field parallel to the grating lines.

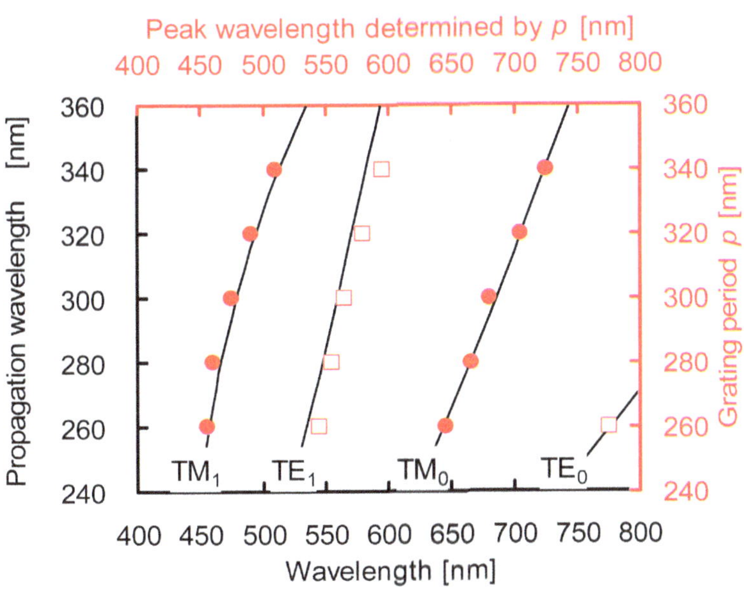

Figure 9.5 Experimental wavelength at QE peaks plotted against the grating period p (symbols), and theoretical dispersion relationship of various modes in the Si slab waveguide (solid lines). Note that the QE is enhanced at the wavelength where the propagation wavelength in Si coincides with the grating period (the phase matching is attained).

as a slab waveguide whose theoretical dispersion relationship (propagation wavelength λ_g in Si vs. free space wavelength λ) is also plotted as solid lines [7]. The experimental data points and the theoretical lines coincide well, indicating that the light absorption (QE) is enhanced when the λ_g and p are matched. Under the phase matching condition ($\lambda_g = p$), the diffracted light by the SP antenna grating is coupled to the waveguiding mode in the Si, and the incident light is efficiently converted to the laterally propagating light in the Si PD to generate a large photocurrent [4–6, 8–10].

9.3 Refractive Index Measurement

When the light enters the grating in an oblique direction, there is a phase difference between lights entering the adjacent grating lines, as shown in Figure 9.6, and the phase matching condition is modified [11]. The diffracted light generates forward and backward waves in the Si waveguide with propagation wavelengths expressed by the following equations.

$$\lambda_{gf} = 1/\{(1/p) + (n/\lambda)\sin\theta\} \text{ for forward wave} \tag{9.1}$$

$$\lambda_{gb} = 1/\{(1/p) - (n/\lambda)\sin\theta\} \text{ for backward wave} \tag{9.2}$$

These waves are coupled to the waveguiding mode at different wavelengths. The RI of the medium around the SP antenna n affects the λ_{gf} and λ_{gb} as long as the incident light is tilted ($\theta \neq 0$).

In Figure 9.7, λ_{gf} and λ_{gb} for $n = 1.0, 1.5$, $\theta = 0, 20°$, and $p = 300$ nm are plotted with respect to λ based on Eqs. (9.1) and (9.2), respectively, and the dispersion curve for the TM_0 mode in 100-nm-thick Si waveguide is also shown. The absorption (QE) peaks are expected at the crossing points (open circles) of these curves.

The prediction is experimentally verified as spectroscopic photocurrents shown in Figure 9.8 for $n = 1, 1.493$, $\theta = 0, 10, 20°$, $p = 300$ nm, and the Si thickness of 100 nm [11]. The photocurrent peak for the normal light incidence ($\theta = 0$) is split into two when the light enters obliquely. The peak split becomes larger for a larger incident angle and larger RI as predicted by the theory explained above. The RI measurement by the PD with SP antenna is successfully demonstrated.

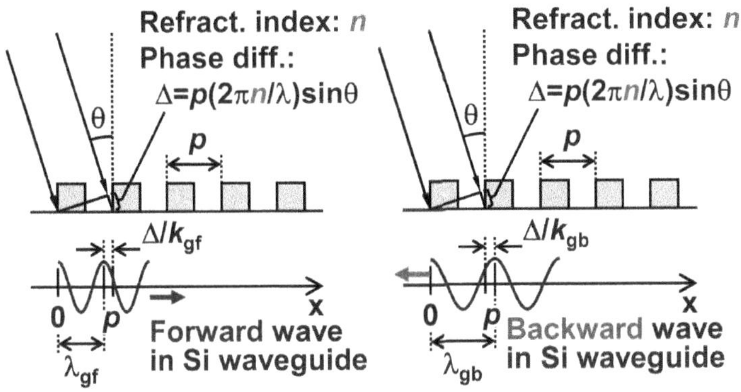

Figure 9.6 Phase matching conditions for oblique incident light with an effect of the refractive index of the medium around the surface plasmon antenna. For oblique incidence, the diffracted light generates forward and backward waves in the Si layer, which are coupled to the waveguiding mode at different wavelengths.

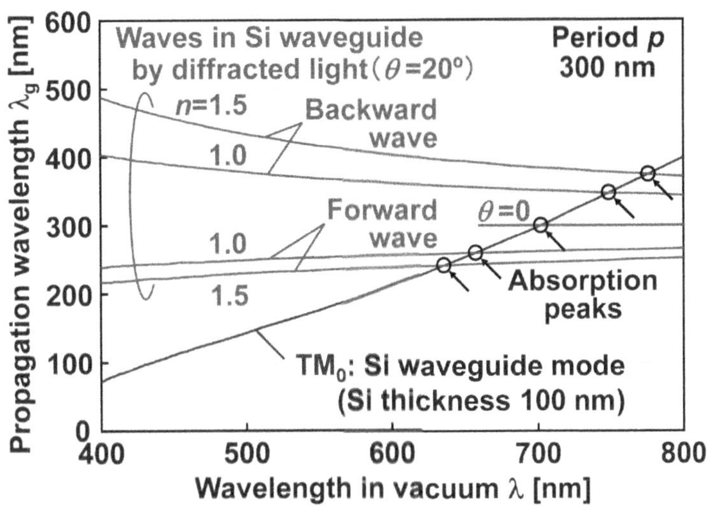

Figure 9.7 Theoretically expected peak wavelengths (open circles) where the light absorption (photodiode QE) is maximized for light incident angle θ of 0 and 20°, and refractive index n of 1.0 and 1.5.

9.4 Two-PD Method

To obtain the RI information by the spectroscopic measurement in Figure 9.8, the wavelength needs to be swept, which takes a long time and is not desirable for high-throughput analysis. In order to perform real-time measurement, the two-photodiode (2PD) method is invented [11–13]. As shown in Figure 9.9(a), two PDs with different grating periods and a monochromatic light source such as a laser diode are employed. In the initial condition, where $n = n_0$, the grating periods p_1 and p_2, the wavelength λ, and the incident angle θ are adjusted so that the photocurrent difference is nullified. As the n changes from n_0 to $n_0 + \Delta n$, the peak profiles of the two PDs are shifted, and the differential photocurrent that reflects the RI change Δn appears. This method allows sensitively detect Δn and can cancel a part of the drift or noise that is common to both PDs.

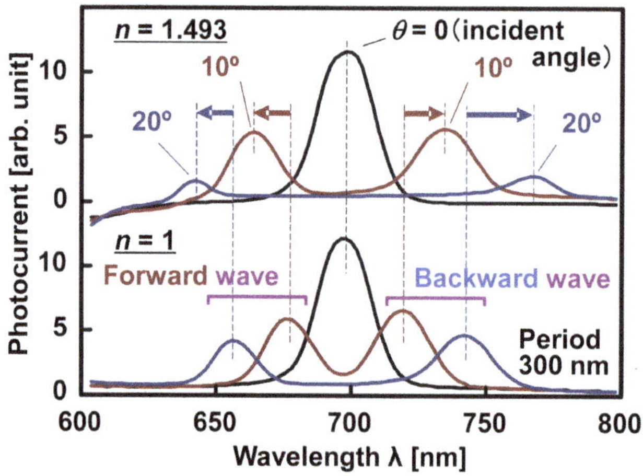

Figure 9.8 Measured photocurrent vs. wavelength for light incident angle θ of 0, 10, and 20°, and refractive index n of 1 and 1.493.

Figure 9.9(b) shows the measurement circuit diagram for the 2PD method. The amplitude of the light intensity is modulated, and the differential photocurrent is detected by the lock-in amplifier to further improve the signal-to-noise ratio and the detection limit of the Δn. As shown in Figure 9.9(c), multiple PDs are fabricated in a chip, and contained in the liquid-tight package (flow system) to realize the continuous monitoring of the RI change of the sample liquid or the process of depositing molecules on the surface of the Au grating lines. As 32 PDs are integrated in a small chip, the throughput of the analysis could be appreciably improved by the parallel operation if different receptors were attached to PDs.

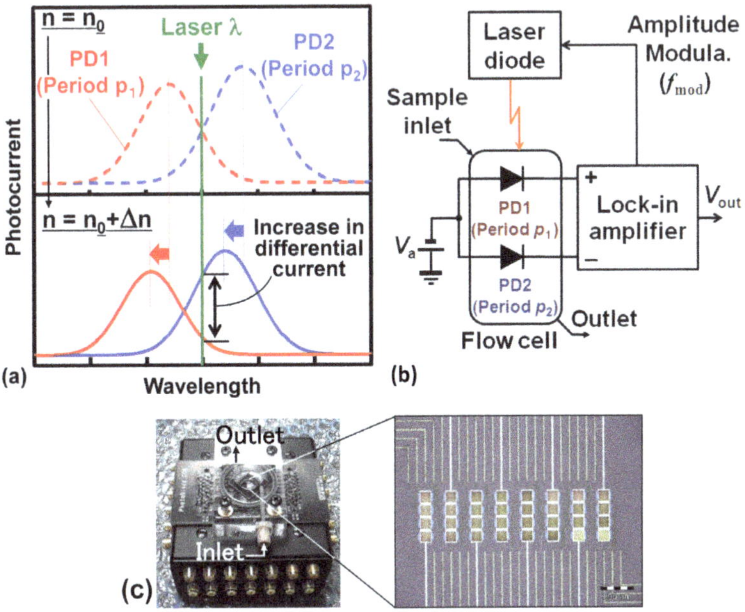

Figure 9.9 (a) Operation principle of two-photodiode (2PD) method for real-time refractive index measurement and improved signal-to-noise ratio. (b) Measurement circuit for 2PD method. Two PDs are set in a liquid-tight package to allow the flow of sample liquid from the inlet to the outlet. (c) Photograph of the package (flow system) and micrograph of the chip including multiple PDs for high-throughput parallel analysis.

Figure 9.10(a) shows the time series graph of the output signal (sensorgram) while the sucrose solutions with concentrations of 0.4, 0.6, 0.8, and 1.0 wt.% are sequentially injected in the flow of water [14, 15]. The p_1, p_2, λ, θ, light intensity, modulation frequency, and current sensitivity of the amplifier are 330 nm, 340 nm, 685 nm, 16.8°, 48 mW/cm^2, 500 Hz, and 10 MV/A, respectively.

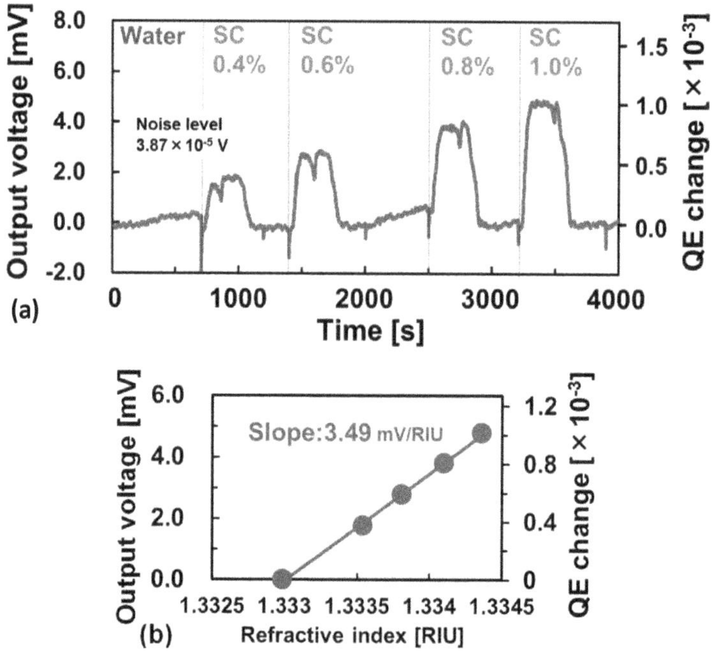

Figure 9.10 (a) Sensorgram of the sequentially injected sucrose solution with various concentrations in the flow of water. Photodiodes with the grating periods of 330 and 340 nm are illuminated by a 685-nm light at an incident angle of 16.8°. (b) Output voltage as a function of the refractive index calculated from the sucrose concentration. By dividing the baseline noise voltage by the slope, the detection limit of the refractive index is found to be 1.11×10^{-5} RIU.

From the slope of the regression line of the output voltage vs. RI in Figure 9.10(b) and the noise level of the baseline in Figure 9.10(a), the detection limit is calculated to be 1.11×10^{-5} RIU, which is comparable to that of the SPR sensor. Note that the main feature of the PD with SP antenna is the capability of integrating a large number of sensors, thereby increasing the throughput of the analysis although the attained detection limit is not strikingly low.

9.5 Sensing of Biomolecules

Avidin, which is a protein found in egg white and has a strong affinity to biotin (also known as Vitamin B_7) [16, 17] is selected as a model biomolecule to test the sensor. The procedure to attach the molecules at the Au surface is as follows.

1. Clean the Au surface with the 1:3 mixture of hydrogen peroxide solution and sulfuric acid for 30 s.
2. Dip the sample in 1 mM cysteamine water solution for 30 min. Cysteamine [Figure 9.11(a)] is a kind of thiol having an affinity to Au and provides an amino end group to facilitate the biotinylation reagent in the next step.
3. 50 mM biotin N-hydroxy-sulfosuccinimide ester (Biotin Sulfo-OSu) water solution is first prepared, and then diluted by 10 with phosphate-buffered saline (PBS) having a pH of about 7.4. The sample is dipped in the solution for 30 min to make a cysteamine-biotin complex [Figure 9.11(b)].
4. 100 μg/mL water solution of avidin [Figure 9.11(c)] is first prepared, and then diluted by 10 with PBS. The sample is dipped in the solution for 30 min.

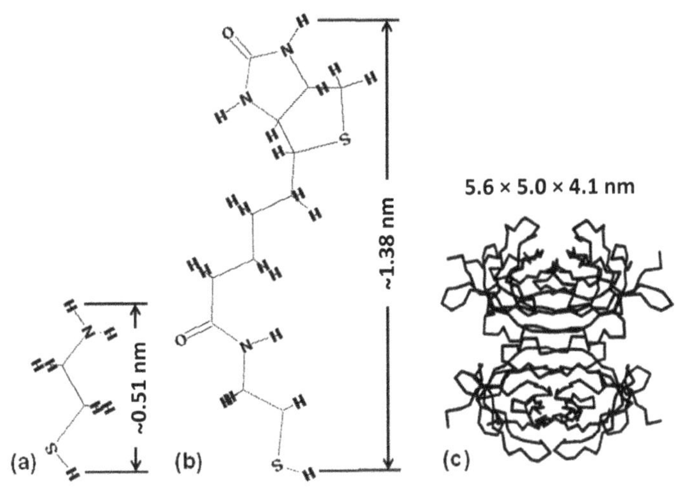

Figure 9.11 Model molecules to test the capability as a biosensor. (a) Cysteamine [18], (b) biotin-cysteamine complex [18], and (c) avidin tetramer [17].

At the end of each step, the sample is washed with pure water, dried by blowing nitrogen, and measured by ellipsometry for thickness. The results are shown in Figure 9.12. Sequential attachment of the nanometer-scale molecules is reproducibly observed. The thickness of the deposited film is about half of the molecular sizes, as given in Figure 9.11, probably due to the inclined alignment of the molecule [19, 20] or insufficient coverage.

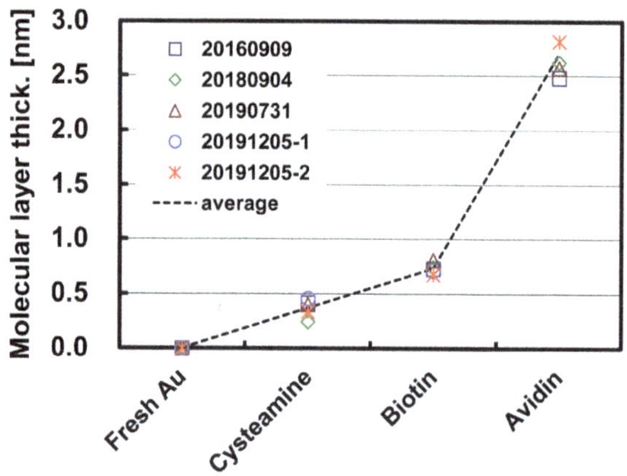

Figure 9.12 Molecular layer thickness at Au surface as a course of sequential attachment of molecules measured by ellipsometry with 632.7 nm light and the assumed layer refractive index of 1.5.

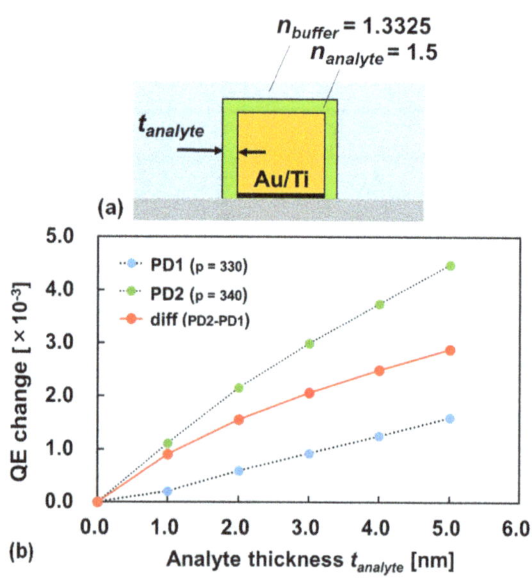

Figure 9.13 (a) Assumed cross-sectional structure of the grating line covered with a molecular layer (analyte) for finite-difference time-domain (FDTD) simulation. (b) Simulated QE change with respect to the analyte thickness. The difference between those for PD1 and PD2 corresponds to the output signal V_{out} of the 2PD method [Figure 9.9(b)].

In order to assess the possibility of detecting the nanometer-scale molecules deposited on the Au lines in the SP antenna, a finite-difference time-domain (FDTD) simulation is performed [14, 15] by assuming the cross-sectional structure shown in Figure 9.13(a). Based on the idea of the 2PD method, QE change (change in absorption efficiency) with respect to analyte (molecular) thickness from 1 to 5 nm is simulated for p_1, p_2, λ, and θ of 330 nm, 340 nm, 685 nm, and 16.4°, respectively, and shown in Figure 9.13(b). The differential QE change (PD2–PD1) up to 3×10^{-3} is attained, which is sufficiently larger than the experimentally detectable QE change demonstrated in Figure 9.10.

9.6 Conclusion

The capability of the PD with Au SP antenna for RI measurement was accessed, and the significant shift in the QE peak was observed due to the modification of the phase matching condition between the diffracted light from the SP antenna grating and the waveguiding mode in the Si layer when the incident light is tilted. Based on the 2PD method with differential lock-in detection of the modulated laser light, the detection limit of RI for sucrose aqueous solution was found to be 1.11×10^{-5} RIU, which is comparable to that of the SPR sensor. Taking the avidin-biotin complex as an example of the biomolecule, the effect of the nanometer scale deposition on the Au lines of the SP antenna is estimated by FDTD simulation. Sufficient change in QE, judging from the experimentally detectable QE change, was obtained, and the prospect of a biosensor was clarified. Featuring the small footprint and the high RI sensitivity, the proposed PD may open up a new opportunity in biosensing techniques in terms of high throughput analysis.

Acknowledgments

Authors are indebted to the Solid State Division of Hamamatsu Photonics K.K. for providing the SOI photodiodes before the fabrication of the surface plasmon antenna, and Yamaha Motor Co., Ltd. for financial and technical support. This research was also supported by the Japan Society for the Promotion of Science

(JSPS) Grant-in-Aid for Scientific Research 25286068, 25630143, 18K04261, and 22K04241, the Cooperative Research Project of the Research Center for Biomedical Engineering with RIE, Shizuoka University, and the Cooperative Research Project Program of RIEC, Tohoku University.

References

1. Castillo, J. Gáspár, S. Leth, S. Niculescu, M. Mortari, A. Bontidean, I. Soukharev, V.. Dorneanu, S.A Ryabov, A.D. Csöregi, E. (2004). Biosensors for life quality Design, development and applications, *Sensors and Actuators B* **102**, pp. 179–194.
2. Fan, X. White, I. M. Shopova, S. I. Zhu, H. Suter, J. D. and Sun Y. (2008). Sensitive optical biosensors for unlabeled targets: A review, *Analytica Chimica Acta*, **620**, pp. 8–26.
3. Engvall E. and Perlmann P. (1971). Enzyme-linked immunosorbent assay (ELISA) quantitative assay of immunoglobulin G, *Immunochemistry*, **8**, pp. 871–874.
4. Satoh, H. Ono, A. and Inokawa H. (2013). Enhanced Visible Light Sensitivity by Gold Line-and-Space Grating Gate Electrode in Thin Silicon-On-Insulator p-n Junction Photodiode, *IEEE Trans. Electron Devices*, **60**, pp. 812–818.
5. Satoh, H. Kawakubo, K. Ono, A. and Inokawa H. (2013). Material Dependence of Metal Grating on SOI Photodiode for Enhanced Quantum Efficiency, *IEEE Photonics Technology Letters*, **25**, pp. 1133–1136.
6. Inokawa, H. Satoh, H. Kawakubo, K. and Ono, A. (2013). Enhancement of SOI Photodiode Sensitivity by Aluminum Grating, *ECS Trans.*, **53**, pp. 127–130.
7. Liu, J. M. (2005). *Photonic Devices* (Cambridge University Press, Cambridge, UK) pp. 95–99.
8. Satoh, H., Kawakubo, K., Ono, A., and Inokawa, H., (2022). Angle-sensitive pixel based on silicon-on-insulator p-n junction photodiode with aluminum grating gate electrode, *IEICE Electronics Express*, **19**, pp. 20220428_1–5.
9. Nagarajan, A. Hara, S. Satoh, H. Panchanathan, A. P. and Inokawa, H. (2020). Angular selectivity of SOI photodiode with surface plasmon antenna, *IEICE Electronics Express*, **17**, pp. 20200187_1–6.

10. Nagarajan, A. Hara, S. Satoh, H. Panchanathan, A. P. and Inokawa, H. (2020). Angle-Sensitive Detector Based on Silicon-On-Insulator Photodiode Stacked with Surface Plasmon Antenna, *Sensors*, **20**, pp. 5543_1–14.

11. Satoh, H., Aso, T., Iwata, S., Ono, A., and Inokawa, H. (2016). Refractive index measurement of aqueous solution using silicon-on-insulator photodiode with surface plasmon antenna. In *Proc. Asia-Pacific Workshop on Fundamentals and Applications of Advanced Semiconductor Devices* (Hakodate, Japan (pp. 70–73).

12. Inokawa, H. Satoh, H. and Ono, A. (2016). Refractive index measurement device, Japanese Patent JP2016151421 A.

13. Inokawa, H. Satoh, H. and Ono, A. (2018). Refractive-index measuring method, Japanese Patent JP6260950 B2.

14. Satoh, H. Isogai, K. and Inokawa, H. (2019). Optical Response of SOI Photodiode with Gold Line-and-space Grating to Biomolecular Interactions, In *Photonics & Electromagnetics Research Symposium Abstracts*, Xiamen, China.

15. Satoh, H., Isogai, K., Iwata, S., Aso, T., Hayashi, R., Takeuchi, S., and Inokawa, H., (2023). Refractive index measurement using SOI photodiode with SP antenna toward SOI-CMOS-compatible optical biosensor, *Sensors*, **23**, pp. 568_1–17.

16. Livnah, O. Bayert, E. A. Wilchekt, M. and Sussman, J. L. (1993). Three-dimensional structures of avidin and the avidin-biotin complex, *Proc. Natl. Acad. Sci. USA*, **90**. pp. 5076–5080.

17. Rosano, C. Arosio, P. and Bolognesi, M. (1999). The X-ray three-dimensional structure of avidin, *Biomolecular Engineering*, **16**, pp. 5–12.

18. ChemSketch Version 5.0 (2001). Advanced Chemistry Development, Inc., Toronto, Ontario M5C 1B5 Canada.

19. Bain, C. D. Troughton, E. B. Tao, Y. T. Evall, J. Whitesides, G. M. and Nuzzo, R. G. (1989). Formation of monolayer films by the spontaneous assembly of organic thiols from solution onto gold, *J. Am. Chem. Soc.*, **111**, pp. 321–335.

20. Tour, J. M. Jones II, L. Pearson, D. L. Lamba, J. J. S. Burgin, T. P. Whitesides, G. M. Allara, D. L. Parikh, A. N. and Atre S. (1995). Self-Assembled Monolayers and Multilayers of Conjugated Thiols, alpha, omega. Dithiols, and Thioacetyl-Containing Adsorbates. Understanding Attachments between Potential Molecular Wires and Gold Surfaces, *J. Am. Chem. Soc.* **117**, pp. 9529–9534.

Chapter 10

Application of THz Spectroscopy for Crystal-Structure Refinement of Bio-Related Molecules and Functional Materials

Feng Zhang,[a,b,c] Izuru Karimata,[d] Houng-Wei Wang,[e] Takashi Tachikawa,[a,d] Takashi Nishin,[f] Keisuke Tominaga,[a,d] Michitoshi Hayashi,[e] and Tetsuo Sasaki[g]

[a]*CAS Key Laboratory of Functional Materials and Devices for Special Environments, Xinjiang Technical Institute of Physics & Chemistry, CAS, and Xinjiang Key Laboratory of Electronic Information Materials and Devices, 40-1 South Beijing Road, Urumqi 830011, China*
[b]*Research Center for Crystal Materials, University of Chinese Academy of Sciences, Beijing 100049, China*
[c]*Molecular Photoscience Research Center, Kobe University, Nada, Kobe 657-8501, Japan*
[d]*Department of Chemistry, Graduate School of Science, Kobe University, Nada, Kobe 657-8501, Japan*
[e]*Center for Condensed Matter Sciences, National Taiwan University, 1 Roosevelt Rd., Sec. 4, Taipei 10617, Taiwan*
[f]*Department of Chemical Science and Engineering, Graduate School of Engineering, Kobe University, Kobe 657-8501, Japan*
[g]*Research Institute of Electronics, Shizuoka University, Hamamatsu 432-8011, Japan*

zhangfeng@ms.xjb.ac.cn

Biomedical Engineering: Imaging Systems, Electric Devices, and Medical Materials
Edited by Akihiro Miyauchi and Hiroyuki Kagechika

ISBN 978-981-5129-16-8 (Hardcover), 978-1-003-46404-4 (eBook)
www.jennystanford.com

In the past decade, remarkable advances have been made toward establishing terahertz (THz) spectroscopic techniques in terms of experimentation and theory. Terahertz spectroscopy has proven to be a powerful tool in analytical chemistry for identifying molecules, distinguishing polymorphs, and detecting impurities. With the accumulation of large amounts of spectroscopic data, researchers have recognized another potential application of THz spectroscopy, i.e., refining the structures of crystalline matter. Here, we review the applications of THz spectroscopy to shed light on two crucial problems in crystallography: resolving hydrogen atoms and analyzing disorder. We discuss the first problem using the example of poly(lactic acid) stereocomplex (scPLA). We determined that the derivations of hydrogen atoms from their ideal symmetry sites in the poly(L-lactic acid) (PLLA) and poly(D-lactic acid) (PDLA) break the *R3c* space group symmetry. We discuss the second problem using two prototype case studies, occupational and orientational disorders, where Form I of diflunisal and the low-temperature orthorhombic phase of the $MAPbBr_3$ perovskite are used as examples, respectively. We found that THz spectroscopy reflects the fingerprint information of the local domains induced by short-range order (SRO). Finally, we report that the disordered domains in a highly oriented film of poly(glycolic acid) (PGA) show an abundance of features in THz spectroscopy that can be used to retrieve microscopic structural information.

10.1 Introduction

Terahertz (THz) radiation interacts with phonon modes at the long wavelength limit, generating the spectroscopic fingerprints of crystals [1]. By exploiting this property, the research community has made significant progress in terms of applying THz spectroscopy to molecular identification [1, 2], impurity detection [3], and phase-transition monitoring [4, 5]. Recently, the Sasaki group at Shizuoka University released a THz spectroscopic database containing 600+ broadband and high-resolution THz spectra of pharmaceuticals [6]. In parallel, the advances in the solid-state density functional theory have enabled relatively reliable representations of intermolecular interactions. Many research groups have achieved good theoretical reproductions of the experimental THz peaks, and calculating THz modes has become a routine practice [7–13]. Moreover, an analysis method has been developed to reveal the presence of different vibrational components in any THz mode, making rigorous mode assignment possible [14–16]. These advancements have deepened our understanding of the interactions between THz radiation and solid matter. Several recent studies have identified another promising application of THz spectroscopy, which could provide crucial complementary information to X-ray diffraction (XRD) when its limits are met.

X-ray crystallography is the main technique used to determine crystal structures. Despite the advances that have been made, two challenging problems remain. One is that hydrogen atoms are invisible due to their weak interactions with X-rays [17]. The other is that determining the distribution of disordered atoms is not yet a routine task. The first problem is limited to X-rays and electron beams because hydrogen atoms can be seen in association with neutron scattering. However, the second problem is inherent to any diffraction methodology. The central issue of structural analysis of disorder is determining the correlations of disordered atoms. Because diffraction methods collect signals as a spatial average, correlated disorders do not contribute to Bragg diffractions but do give rise to the diffuse scattering of X-rays. The spatial distribution information of the disordered atoms is washed out in diffuse scattering [18, 19]. Therefore, revealing the disorder in other experimental dimensions is always useful.

Terahertz radiation excites collective vibrations, typically in the 0.1–10 THz region [8, 20–22]. Collective excitations have two characteristics that can be exploited to tackle the preceding two problems. First, the structural information of all atoms, including hydrogen, is reflected in its entirety by the collective nature of the excitation. In a previous study, we revealed the capability of THz spectroscopy to determine the positions of hydrogen atoms that play a crucial role in breaking the helical symmetry of a polymer crystal [23]. Second, the collective nature of the THz modes is closely related to the dimension of order that defines the extent to which the atoms vibrate coherently [21, 24–28]. Many molecular crystals have inherent disorders, such as occupational or orientational disorders. In many cases, such disorders break long-range periodicity and lead to a short-range order (SRO). In a previous study, we found that different SRO domains in disordered crystals display fingerprint THz peaks. Terahertz spectroscopy can potentially reveal the microscopic structural information of crystals. In comparison, Fourier transform infrared spectroscopy (FT-IR) and Raman spectroscopy measurements probe the vibrations localized in functional groups or structural segments. Nuclear magnetic resonance (NMR) spectroscopy is another established approach for studying disorders in solids [29–31]. Note that NMR measures the chemical shifts of atom probes sensitive to the local environment. In summary, the THz method detects structural information on a larger scale than FTIR, Raman, and NMR spectroscopy.

In this chapter, we review several studies that used a low-frequency spectroscopic technique to refine the crystal structures of a few bio-related molecules and a light-electron conversion functional material. These samples were scPLA, PGA, Form I of diflunisal, and hybrid organic-inorganic (HOI) perovskite $MAPbBr_3$. Both ScPLA and PGA represent new-generation bio-related polymers with promising properties. ScPLA is superior in terms of mechanics, thermal resistance, and hydrolysis resistance to its chiral counterparts PLLA and PDLA. The hydrogen atoms account for 44% of the atoms in scPLA. Because the hydrogen atoms are invisible to X-rays, the coordinates of hydrogen atoms are missing in the resolved crystal structure [32, 33]. PGA is a semi-crystalline polyester with good mechanical, biocompatible, and degradative properties [34–36]. A few studies have been conducted to investigate molecular packing in the amorphous zones. Many pharmaceuticals exist in polymorphic forms [37]. Polymorphs result in remarkable changes in physicochemical properties, such as the melting point, solubility, and mechanics, which significantly impact solubility, bioactivity, and stability [38]. The determination of crystal structure, therefore, plays a central role in drug production. Diflunisal, an anti-inflammatory drug, has at least six polymorphs [39, 40]. Among them, Form I has a disordered nature with respect to the occupations of F and H at the two 2, 6-ortho sites of the fluorine-containing ring. The exact molecular configurations associated with the F/H occupation disorder have not yet been reported for this polymorph. Similar to the case of Form I of diflunisal, the crystal structure of the HOI perovskite material $MAPbBr_3$ is ambiguous concerning the orientations of the methylammonium (MA) cations in the lattice.

We used the THz spectroscopic method to retrieve quantitative information on scPLA, Form I of diflunisal, and $MAPbBr_3$. We also considered an example where the disordered zones in a highly oriented PGA film displayed an abundance of absorption bands in the far-IR spectra, providing a new perspective for characterizing disorder.

10.2 Methods

10.2.1 Gallium Phosphide (GAP)-Continuous Wave (CW)-THz, THz-Time-Domain Spectroscopy (TDS), and Far-IR Measurements

A GaP-CW-THz spectrometer characterized by broad band, high frequency accuracy, and high frequency resolution was utilized as the analytical method [41, 42]. The light source was a THz signal generator (SG) based on the difference frequency generation (DFG) method in GaP crystals. This light source had a wide bandwidth (0.1–7.5 THz) mainly due to the high transmittance of the GaP crystal for THz waves. Two pump beams were fed from a mode-hop free wavelength-tunable external cavity diode laser (ECDL) and distributed feedback (DFB) laser. These two beams were amplified by ytterbium (Yb)-doped fiber amplifiers (YbFA) with a constant value (typically 3 W). The THz wave was detected using a niobium (Nb) transition-edge sensor (TES) bolometer, which was cooled by a pulse tube cooler. One of the pump beams was chopped at a frequency of 713 Hz to lock in the detection of THz waves, resulting in high sensitivity and long-term signal stability. The maximum S/N ratio for the spectrometer exceeded 1,000, and S/N ratios > 10 were achieved in the frequency range from 0.6 to 6.0 THz. As the wavelengths of the two pump beams were monitored by a two-channel wavelength meter and feedback-controlled, the absolute frequency accuracy and resolution were 3.0 and 8.0 MHz, respectively, in all bands. The sample was set in a liquid refrigerant-blown cryostat (Oxford Instruments, Abingdon, UK) to obtain temperature-dependent spectra in the range of 4–400 K (temperature stability: $< \pm 0.05$ K). Because absorption lines due to water vapor are sensitively observed by high-frequency accuracy spectroscopy, the entire optical path of the THz wave was purged with dry air. The spectrometer constructed here basically operated non-stop. The measurement sequence was controlled by in-house software. Typically, for one sample, five temperature-dependent spectra could be obtained after approximately 24 h.

A THz time domain setup (Aispec Instruments, Fukui, Japan) using a photoconductive antenna system to generate and detect THz radiation was applied to record the THz spectra in the 5–80 cm^{-1} frequency range. A liquid nitrogen cryostat (Oxford Instruments) was used to produce a low-temperature environment. A far-IR spectrometer (FT/IR-6X; JACSO, Tokyo, Japan) was used to measure the spectra in the 100–700 cm^{-1} frequency range.

10.2.2 Calculations

The geometry optimizations were performed by implementing the periodic boundary condition [43]. The frequencies were calculated by diagonalizing the Hessian matrix under the harmonic approximation at the gamma point. The IR intensities were calculated through the Berry-phase approach [44–46]. The B3LYP functional [47, 48] augmented by Grimme's dispersion correction D* [49, 50] was applied. The Gaussian-type 6-311G(d,p) basis set [51] was employed for H, C, N, and O atoms in scPLA and $MAPbBr_3$. A pseudopotential and Gaussian-type basis set Pb_ECP60MDF-6111(51d) was used for Pb [52], and the Gaussian-type pob_TZVP_rev2 basis set was used for Br [53] in $MAPbBr_3$. The Gaussian-type 6-311G(2df,2pd) basis set was used for all atoms in diflunisal [51, 54].

The Gaussian-type 6-31G(d,p) basis set [55] was used for all atoms in PGA. The calculations for scPLA and Form I of diflunisal were carried out using the CRYSTAL14 software package [56, 57], while the calculations for $MAPbBr_3$ and PGA were performed in CRYSTAL17 [58, 59]. The SCF convergent thresholds for total energy were set to 10^{-9} and 10^{-11} Hartree for the geometry and frequency calculation, respectively [57].

The GSAS-II software package was used to calculate the neutron/X-ray powder diffraction peaks [60]. The PDFgui software package was used to calculate the pair distribution functions (PDFs) of neutron scattering [61].

10.3 Determination of the Positions of H Atoms in SCPLA

Symmetry conservation has been applied for determining polymer conformations in crystals [62]. The equivalence postulate formulated by the early pioneers of polymer science (Bunn [63], Huggins [64], and Pauling [65]) claims that the constitutional repeating units, i.e., "the smallest constitutional unit, the repetition of which constitutes a regular macromolecule" [66], should be related by symmetry. Under this postulate, many polymers have been regarded to conserve helical symmetries. Despite being used as such a fundamental principle, the equivalence postulate should be subjected to verifications whenever new experimental criteria are available.

ScPLA provides a prototype system for examining the equivalence postulate. The crystal structure of scPLA has been resolved by the electron and X-ray diffraction methods [32, 33]. The crystal possesses *R3c* space group symmetry. In each primitive cell, a left-handed 3_1 PLLA helix and a right-handed 3_1 PDLA helix adopt a parallel packing conformation, as shown in Figure 10.1a. The *R3c* space group gives rise to three irreducible representations, A_1, A_2, and E [28]. A_1, which is general to all space groups, represents *IR* active modes with polarizations parallel to the chain axes. E is generated by the 3_1-screw symmetry, representing double-generated *IR* active modes with polarizations perpendicular to the chain axes. A_2 originates from the glide plane symmetry, representing *IR* inactive but Raman active modes. Using the THz spectroscopic method, we were able to gain direct access to the A_1 and E representation by polarizing the THz radiation parallel and perpendicular to the chain axes of the polymers, respectively. It was then possible to determine whether the corresponding symmetry elements were good or not.

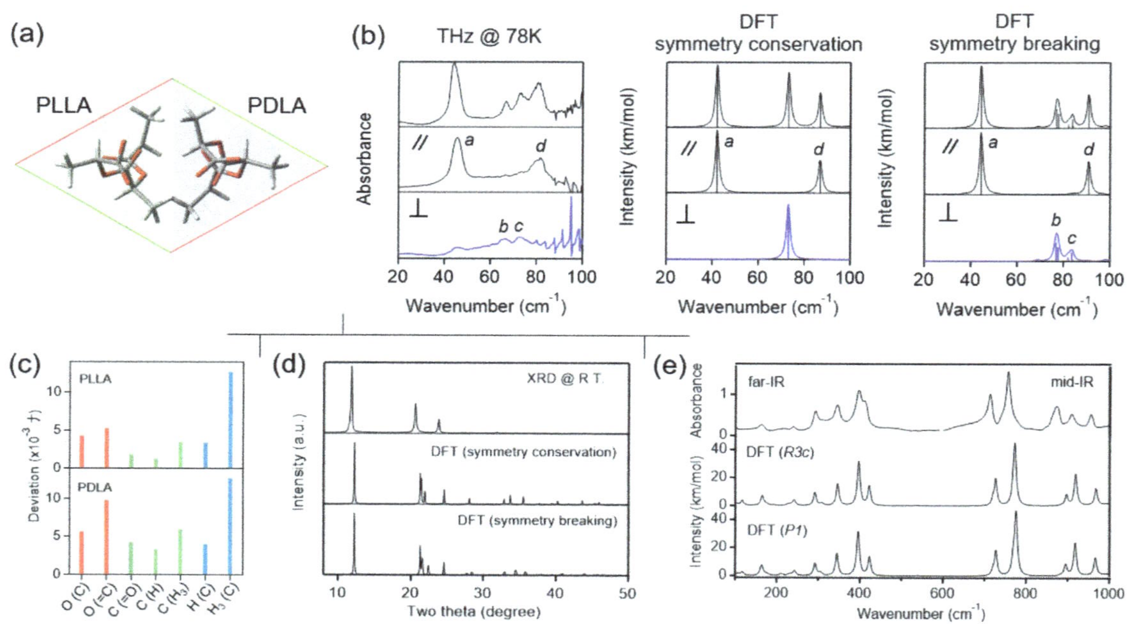

Figure 10.1 Crystal-structure and spectroscopic information of scPLA. (a) View of the unit cell along the *z*-axis. (b) Comparison between the experimental THz spectra (left) and spectra calculated with the *R3c* space-group symmetry conserved (middle) and broken (right). (c) The RMSDs of all of the chemically irreducible atoms from the 3_1-screw symmetry for PLLA and PDLL. (d) Comparison between the experimental XRD spectra (top) and spectra calculated with the *R3c* space-group symmetry conserved (middle) and broken (bottom). (e) Comparison between the experimental far-IR and mid-IR spectra and the calculated spectra with the *R3c* space-group symmetry conserved (middle) and broken (bottom).

As shown in the left panel of Figure 10.1b, scPLA displayed four THz bands in the 5–85 cm^{-1} frequency range. Bands *a* and *d* possessed polarizations parallel to the chain axis, while bands *b* and *c* had polarizations perpendicular to the chain axis. As a result, the first pair belonged to the A_1 representation; while the later pairs belonged to the *E* representation if 3_1 helical symmetry existed. We first calculated the THz modes by preserving the *R3c* space-group symmetry. As shown in the middle panel of Figure 10.1b, the two A_1 modes were reproduced correctly. However, the *E* representation gave rise to only one mode, despite the two-mode criterion observed in the experiment. This observation indicated that *E* was not a good irreducible representation, and the underpinning 3_1-screw symmetry was not a good element. We then reoptimized the geometry by degrading the *R3c* space-group symmetry to *P1*, i.e., breaking all of the symmetric restrictions. As shown in the right panel of Figure 10.1b, the *P1*-simulation qualitatively reproduced all four experimental bands. Compared with the *R3c*-simulation, the symmetry relegation barely affected the reproduction of normal modes *a* and *d* with a polarization parallel to the chain axes, but it substantially improved the reproduction of normal modes *b* and *c* with a polarization perpendicular to the chain axes.

We next quantified the root-mean-square deviations (RMSDs) of the atoms in the symmetry-broken configuration from their ideal sites in the *R3c* configuration, for both PLLA and PDLA. The RMSD evaluations of the 3_1 screw symmetry breaking were taken for all of the chemically irreducible atoms comprising the constitutional repeating units. Figure 10.1c shows that the hydrogen atoms of the CH_3 groups underwent the most substantial deviations in the symmetry-breaking process. Because it is invisible to hydrogen atoms, the XRD method cannot distinguish the symmetry-conserved (*R3c*) and -breaking (*P1*) structures, as shown in Figure 10.1d. We also examined the far-IR spectrum of scPLA in the 100–700 cm^{-1} frequency range. As shown in Figure 10.1e, both the *R3c* and *P1* configurations could effectively reproduce the far-IR spectrum. Compared with THz spectroscopy, far-IR spectroscopy probes more localized atomic vibrations, and is therefore, less sensitive to the structural changes associated with the symmetry on an extended scale.

10.4 Analysis of the F/H Occupation in Form I of Diflunisal

Diflunisal is a chiral molecule composed of a biphenyl backbone with 2,4-difluoro-substitutions on one phenyl ring and 4-hydroxyl and 3-carboxylic-acid substitutions on another phenyl ring. Previous X-ray analysis studies have reported that diflunisal has at least six polymorphs depending on the solvents used for crystallization [39, 40]. In the crystallization process from toluene leading to Form I of diflunisal, the fluorine-containing ring can exist in two configurations related to the two-fold flipping freedom about the single bond connecting the two phenyl rings [40]. The hydrogen and fluorine pair, occupying the two 2,6-ortho sites of the fluorine-containing ring, were disordered; they both had an occupancy factor of 0.5. The disordered ortho sites are highlighted in light blue in Figure 10.2a. A pair of enantiomers formed an *SR* dimer via the carboxylic acid hydrogen-bond connection and comprised the smallest building block. Each *SR* dimer had four disordered sites, specified as $2^S6^S2^R6^R$, where the superscripts denote the chirality of the subject enantiomer. As shown in Figure 10.2b, the pairwise occupations of 2^S6^S and 2^R6^R by fluorine and hydrogen resulted in four unit-cell configurations, *#1–4*, corresponding to the combinations of *HFHF*, *HFFH*, *FHHF*, and *FHFH*, respectively. Among the four unit-cell configurations, *#2* and *#3* had an inverse relationship, and their energy thus degenerated. In summary, the goal of structural analysis of disorder is to determine the spatial distributions of the four types of *SR*-dimers.

We first optimized the four unit-cell configurations under the periodic boundary condition. All four models satisfactorily reproduced the unit cell parameters, covalent bonds, dihedral angles of the biphenyl backbone, intramolecular and intermolecular H-bonds, weak CH···F bonds between ordered atoms, and layer-layer stacking distance [67]. This implied that the variation of the four unit-cell configurations did not induce substantial changes in the atomic packing. We then calculated the THz modes associated with the four unit-cell configurations. As shown in Figure 10.2c, the four unit-cell configurations displayed fingerprint peaks in the 70–110 cm^{-1} frequency range. Configurations #2 and #3 yielded the same spectrum because they had degenerated.

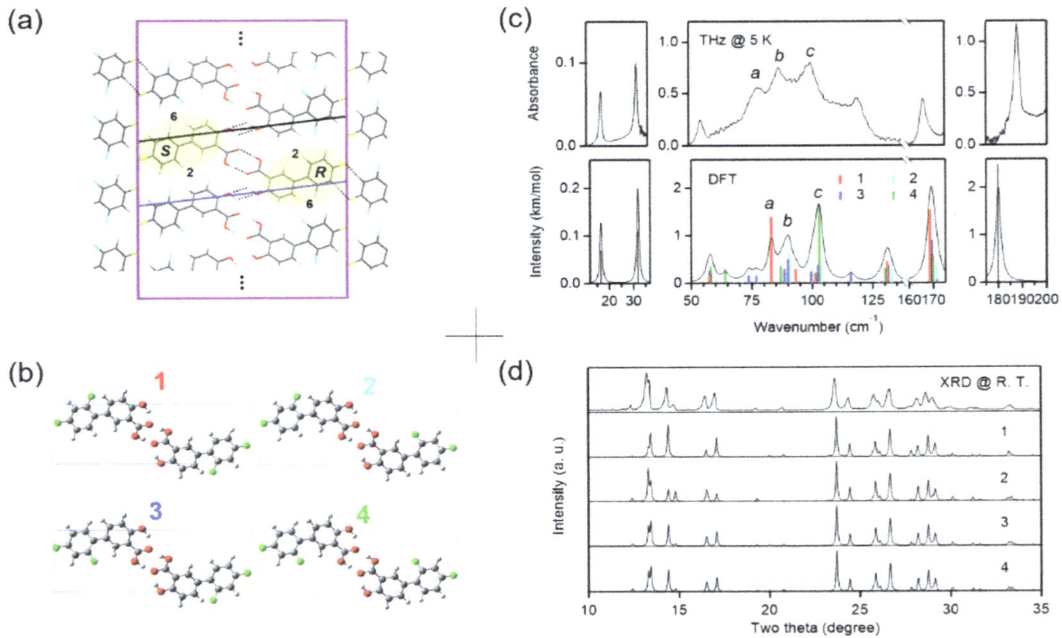

Figure 10.2 Crystal-structure and spectroscopic information of Form I of diflunisal. (a) Intermolecular bonding patterns along the *a*-axis. (b) The four unit-cell structures caused by the occupational disorder of F and H atoms. (c) Comparison between the experimental THz spectrum and calculations with the four types of unit-cell structures. (d) Comparison between the experimental XRD and four types of unit-cell structures.

We could unambiguously assign the three fingerprint peaks *a*, *b*, and *c* to the unit-cell configurations #1, #2 and #3, and #4, respectively. Based on the above observation, we concluded that the four unit-cell configurations coexisted in Form I of diflunisal. In contrast, the four unit-cell configurations led to similar XRD patterns (Figure 10.2d), implying that the X-ray method could not distinguish the subtle structural variation.

10.5 Analysis of the Orientation of MA in HOI Perovskite

Hybrid organic-inorganic (HOI) perovskite materials have the potential for fabricating inexpensive and high-efficiency solar cells [68]. Optimizing the crystal structures of perovskites is crucial for improving the light-electron conversion efficiency. In the case of $MAPbBr_3$, the lead-centered octahedral form the inorganic frame, and the MA cations sit in cuboctahedron cages. The MA cations have a dipole moment of 2.3 D and are bound to the inorganic frame via hydrogen bonds [69]. Theoretical investigations have clarified that the MA cations do not directly contribute to the electronic structure around the band edges because the molecular electronic level is lower than that of the inorganic frames [70]. The spatial arrangement of the MA cations plays an essential role in determining the fine structure of the inorganic frame that impacts the band structure and creates the dielectric property [71]. Because the C and N atoms differ from each other by only one electron, it is difficult to use XRD to distinguish them and resolve the orientation of the MA cations. Because each unit cell contains four MAs, each of which has two possible orientations, there are 16 combinations for their collective orientations. Half of the 16 unit-cell configurations are degenerate due to an inversion symmetry relationship. We, therefore, needed to consider only eight irreducible configurations, where each MA was represented by a dipole vector, as shown in Figure 3b. Configurations #1 and #7 did not have net dipole moments due to cancellations, while all the other configurations produced dipole moments with equal amplitude but variable directions [72].

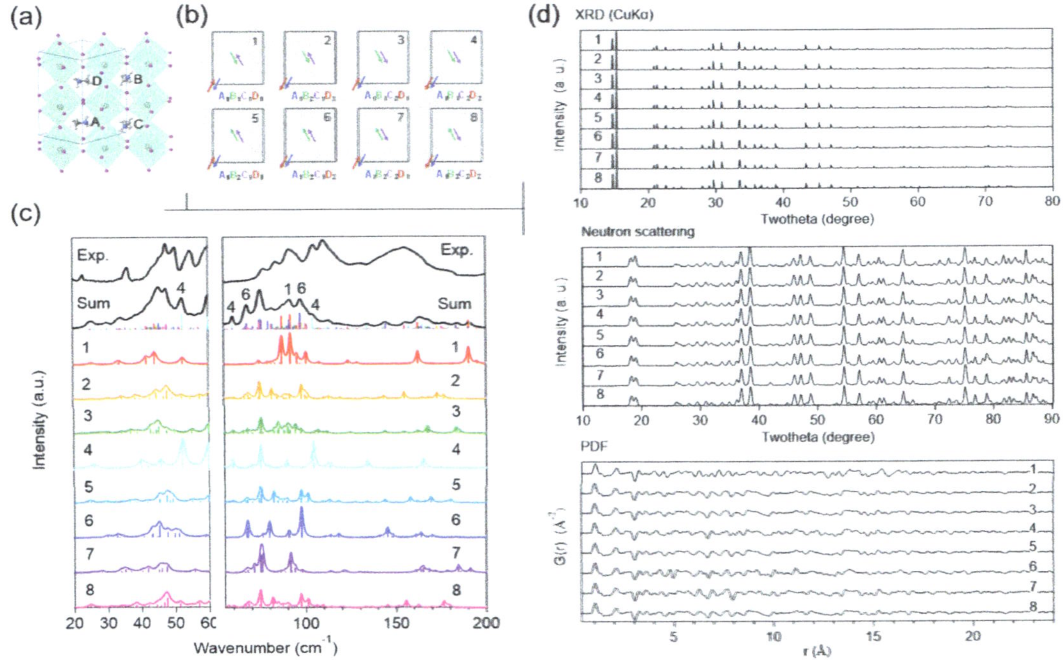

Figure 10.3 Crystal-structure and spectroscopic information of the low-temperature orthorhombic phase perovskite. (a) Interpretation of the four MA cations, A–D, in the unit cell and their cuboctahedron cage environment. (b) Orientations of the four MA cations in each of the eight unit-cell configurations. (c) Comparison between the experimental THz spectrum and spectra calculated with the eight unit-cell configurations. (d) Comparison between the experimental data and data calculated with the eight unit-cell configurations for XRD, neutron scattering, and PDFs.

We compared the experimental THz spectrum recorded at 10 K and the calculated spectra using the eight irreducible unit-cell configurations in Figure 10.3c. The experimental data is shown in the top panel, and the sum of the line shapes of the eight unit-cell configurations is displayed in the second panel from the top. In the presence of the eight unit-cell configurations, the number and frequency sequence of all characteristic THz peaks could be accurately reproduced. The band correspondence between the experimental and calculated data could be assessed. Moreover, configurations #1, #4, and #6 show fingerprint peaks, as labeled in Figure 10.3c. The coexistence of all eight forms of unit-cell configurations would essentially induce the short-range ordered distribution domains, which have recently been determined by piezoresponse force microscopy [73–78], atomic force microscopy [79], scanning electron microscopy [79, 80], electron backscattered diffraction [74], and atomic-resolution transmission electron microscopy observations [81, 82] in both polycrystalline and single-crystal HOI perovskites.

In comparison, the eight irreducible unit-cell configurations gave rise to similar X-ray diffraction peaks (Figure 10.3d), although there were some differences in terms of a few very weak peaks. A similar result was observed for the simulated neutron-scattering peaks. We also calculated the PDFs of neutron scattering in the 0.1–24 Å range for these unit-cell configurations. As shown in Figure 10.3d, although distinct patterns could be identified in specific ranges, they were very similar across the entire range.

Regarding the reproduction of the experimental THz bands, the frequencies of the bands in the 70–120 cm^{-1} frequency range were underestimated, as were the IR intensities of the two bands in the 100–120 cm^{-1} frequency range, and a broadband in the 140–180 cm^{-1} frequency range. There were three possible reasons for these discrepancies. First, we ignored the anharmonicity of the potential surfaces, which not only affected the frequencies and line shapes of the THz modes but also yielded the overtone and combination bands [83–85]. Second, we ignored the interactions between different structural domains at their interfaces. Third, we did not take defects into account. The HOI perovskite materials, synthesized via the chemical route, always contained a large number of point, line, planar, and bulk defects. The defects not only altered the frequencies and IR intensities of the THz modes but also induced localized vibrations that added additional features to the spectra [86, 87]. Nevertheless, we reproduced all of the observed vibrational bands below 120 cm^{-1}. To ensure their assignment, the eight irreducible unit-cell configurations were indispensable in terms of the collective orientation of MA cations.

10.6 Characterization of the Order and Disorder Zones in PGA Films

PGA is a biocompatible polyester with good mechanical and degradative properties. The structures of highly oriented PGA fibers have been characterized by XRD, small and wide-angle X-ray scattering, and differential scanning calorimetry studies [34–36]. We prepared highly oriented PGA fibers by melting the amorphous PGA and then drawing the fibers to extend their lengths sixfold at 50 °C. Finally, we annealed the fibers at 180 °C for 1.5 h. After annealing, the fibers showed sharp XRD peaks (Figure 10.4a), indicating the existence of highly crystalline domains; in contrast, the nonannealed samples displayed a diffuse band. According to a study by Oca and Ward, the structures of the annealed samples can be described by the Prevorsek model, which features alternating crystalline and amorphous domains along the fiber axis, as shown in Figure 10.4b [34]. The atomic packing in the crystalline zones has *Pcmn* space-group symmetry, and the PGA polymers adopted a zigzag configuration. In each unit cell, two polymer chains were aligned in parallel and extended along the *c*-axis (Figure 10.4c). The unit-cell dimensions were a = 5.22 Å, b = 6.19 Å, and c = 7.02 Å.

We measured the far-IR spectra of both the nonannealed and annealed samples at room temperature and present the results in the top and middle panels of Figure 10.4d, respectively. Unlike the XRD observation, the nonannealed sample showed an abundance of features in the far-IR spectrum. These features were generated by the atomic vibrations in the amorphous structures.

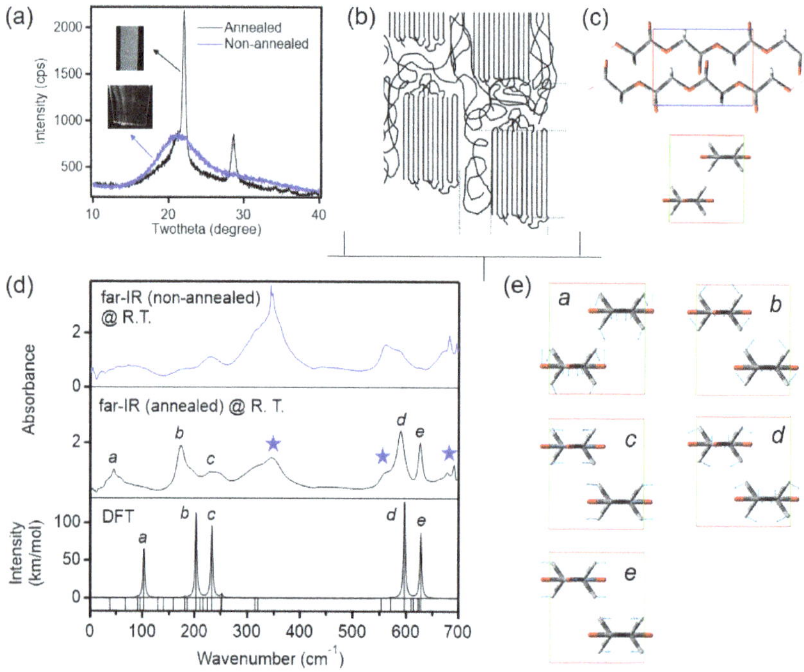

Figure 10.4 Structure and spectroscopic information of PGA. (a) XRD results for annealed and nonannealed PGA. (b) Schematic representation of the structure of the annealed PGA adopted from Ref. [34]. Copyright permission was granted by Elsevier. (c) The 3D packing of PGA in the crystalline zone. The unit cell axes *a–c* are shown in red, green, and blue, respectively. (d) Comparison between the far-IR spectra of annealed and nonannealed PGA and the calculations for the crystal structure shown in panel (b). (e) Atomic vibration schemes of the five THz modes labeled in panel (d).

Due to the lack of long-range symmetry, all of the vibrational modes were IR active and could therefore be probed in experiments. As a result, we observed the density of the vibrational state (DOVS) of the amorphous structures [88]. Because such amorphous domains were also present in the annealed samples, the same DOVS outline appeared in the far-IR spectrum of the annealed sample. In addition to the amorphous outline, the annealed sample displayed sharp peaks labeled *a–e* in the frequency sequence. We found that these sharp peaks could be reproduced using the crystal structure resolved by Oca and Ward, as shown in the bottom panel of Figure 10.4d. This phenomenon indicated that these sharp peaks originated from the crystalline domains. The atomic vibration schemes of the five modes are provided in Figure 10.4e. All of them feature the internal motions of the polymer chain, as predicted by Yamamoto et al. using low-frequency Raman spectroscopy [89].

Finally, it should be noted that very few studies have been conducted to obtain microscopic information for the polymer packing in the amorphous domain, largely due to the lack of structural information provided by XRD measurements. The abundance of features observed in the far-IR spectra of the nonannealed sample may reveal the microscopic structures of the amorphous domains. We intend to address this in future studies.

10.7 Conclusion

The crystal-structure determination is one of the central issues in drug production and biopolymer development. Many bio-related molecules contain a large proportion of hydrogen atoms and disordered atoms. However, analyzing hydrogen atoms and disorder is currently challenging due to the inherent limits of X-ray crystallography. Terahertz spectroscopy is an emerging technique that has the potential to solve the above two problems. Through the combination of THz spectroscopy and solid-state density-functional theory (DFT) calculations, we have presented several case studies of crystal-structure determination. We have obtained THz evidence of the symmetry-broken structure associated with hydrogen atoms in scPLA, the existence of four unit-cell configurations induced by F/H occupational disorder in Form I of diflunisal, and the eight irreducible unit-cell configurations generated by the orientational disorder of MA in $MAPbBr_3$. It is difficult for XRD to capture such subtle structural changes. THz spectroscopy provides a new opportunity to determine the fine structures of crystals. We also presented a preliminary study of the far-IR spectra of highly orientated PGA films. The amorphous domains showed an abundance of far-IR spectroscopy features, which can be used to retrieve microscopic structural information regarding the disorder.

Acknowledgments

We thank the Research Center for Computational Science, Okazaki Research Facilities, National Institutes of Natural Science in Japan for providing the computational resource. This study was supported by the Cooperative Research Project of Research Center for Biomedical Engineering.

References

1. Hangyo, M.; Tani, M.; Nagashima, T. Terahertz Time-Domain Spectroscopy of Solids: A Review. *J. Infrared Millim. Terahertz Waves* **2005**, *26*, 1661–1690.
2. Nishizawa, S.; Sakai, K.; Hangyo, T.; Nagashima, T.; Takeda, M. W.; Tominaga, K.; Oka, A.; Tanaka, K.; Morikawa, O. Terahertz Time-Domain Spectroscopy. In *Terahertz Optoelectronics*, Sakai, K. Ed.; Topics in Applied Physics, Vol. 97; 2005; pp. 203–269.
3. Sasaki, T.; Sakamoto, T.; Otsuka, M. Detection of Impurities in Organic Crystals by High-Accuracy Terahertz Absorption Spectroscopy. *Anal. Chem.* **2018**, *90*, 1677–1682.
4. Neu, J.; Nikonow, H.; Schmuttenmaer, C. A. Terahertz Spectroscopy and Density Functional Theory Calculations of Dl-Norleucine and Dl-Methionine. *The Journal of Physical Chemistry A* **2018**, *122*, 5978–5982.
5. Tan, N. Y.; Zeitler, J. A. Probing Phase Transitions in Simvastatin with Terahertz Time-Domain Spectroscopy. *Molecular Pharmaceutics* **2015**, *12*, 810–815.
6. https://www.rie.shizuoka.ac.jp/~thz/shizuoka_univ_sasaki_lab_database/group_absorbance_index.html.
7. Banks, P. A.; Burgess, L.; Ruggiero, M. T. The Necessity of Periodic Boundary Conditions for the Accurate Calculation of Crystalline Terahertz Spectra. *Physical Chemistry Chemical Physics* **2021**, *23*, 20038–20051, 10.1039/D1CP02496E.
8. Zhang, F.; Wang, H.-W.; Tominaga, K.; Hayashi, M.; Sasaki, T. High-Resolution Thz Spectroscopy and Solid-State Density Functional Theory Calculations of Polycyclic Aromatic Hydrocarbons. *Journal of Infrared, Millimeter, and Terahertz Waves* **2020**, *41*, 1378–1392.
9. Dampf, S. J.; Korter, T. M. Crystalline Molecular Standards for Low-Frequency Vibrational Spectroscopies. *Journal of Infrared, Millimeter, and Terahertz Waves* **2020**, *41*, 1284–1300.

10. BēRziņš, K. R.; Sutton, J. J.; Fraser-Miller, S. J.; Rades, T.; Korter, T. M.; Gordon, K. C. Solving the Computational Puzzle: Toward a Pragmatic Pathway for Modeling Low-Energy Vibrational Modes of Pharmaceutical Crystals. *Crystal Growth & Design* **2020**, *20*, 6947–6955.

11. Ruggiero, M. T.; Zhang, W.; Bond, A. D.; Mittleman, D. M.; Zeitler, J. A. Uncovering the Connection between Low-Frequency Dynamics and Phase Transformation Phenomena in Molecular Solids. *Phys. Rev. Lett.* **2018**, *120*, 196002.

12. Zhang, F.; Wang, H.-W.; Hayashi, M.; Pan, S. Origins of Thz Modes and Their Ir Intensities in $LiNbO_3$. *J. Phys. Chem. C* **2022**.

13. Zhang, F.; Tominaga, K.; Hayashi, M.; Tani, M. A Quantitative Interpretation for the Difference of Terahertz Spectra of Dl- and L-Alanine: Origins of Infrared Intensities in Terahertz Spectroscopy. *J. Phys. Chem. C* **2021**, *125*, 16175–16182.

14. Zhang, F.; Tominaga, K.; Hayashi, M.; Nishino, T. Effects of Non-Covalent Interactions on Molecular and Polymer Individuality in Crystals Studied by Thz Spectroscopy and Solid-State Density Functional Theory. In *Molecular Spectroscopy: A Quantum Chemistry Approach*, Wiley-VCH Verlag GmbH & Co. KGaA, 2019; pp. 459–495.

15. Zhang, F.; Wang, H.-W.; Tominaga, K.; Hayashi, M. Mixing of Intermolecular and Intramolecular Vibrations in Optical Phonon Modes: Terahertz Spectroscopy and Solid-State Density Functional Theory. *Wiley Interdiscip. Rev. Comput. Mol. Sci.* **2016**, *6*, 386–409.

16. Zhang, F.; Hayashi, M.; Wang, H.-W.; Tominaga, K.; Kambara, O.; Nishizawa, J.-i.; Sasaki, T. Terahertz Spectroscopy and Solid-State Density Functional Theory Calculation of Anthracene: Effect of Dispersion Force on the Vibrational Modes. *J. Chem. Phys.* **2014**, *140*, 174509.

17. Palatinus, L.; Brázda, P.; Boullay, P.; Perez, O.; Klementová, M.; Petit, S.; Eigner, V.; Zaarour, M.; Mintova, S. Hydrogen Positions in Single Nanocrystals Revealed by Electron Diffraction. *Science* **2017**, *355*, 166–169.

18. Keen, D. A.; Goodwin, A. L. The Crystallography of Correlated Disorder. *Nature* **2015**, *521*, 303–309.

19. Welberry, T. R.; Weber, T. One Hundred Years of Diffuse Scattering. *Crystallography Reviews* **2016**, *22*, 2–78.

20. Born, M.; Huang, K. *Dynamical Theory of Crystal Lattice*; Clarendon Press, Oxford: 1998.

21. Davydov, A. S. *Theory of Light Absorption in Molecular Crystals, Translated from Acad. Sci. of Ukrssr, Kiev, 1951 in (Russian)*; McGRAW-Hill Book COMPANY, INC: 1962.
22. Zhang, F.; Wang, H.-W.; Tominaga, K.; Hayashi, M. Intramolecular Vibrations in Low-Frequency Normal Modes of Amino Acids: L-Alanine in the Neat Solid State. *The Journal of Physical Chemistry A* **2015**, *119*, 3008–3022.
23. Zhang, F.; Wang, H.-W.; Tominaga, K.; Hayashi, M.; Lee, S.; Nishino, T. Elucidation of Chiral Symmetry Breaking in a Racemic Polymer System with Terahertz Vibrational Spectroscopy and Crystal Orbital Density Functional Theory. *The Journal of Physical Chemistry Letters* **2016**, *7*, 4671–4676.
24. Davydov, A. S. The Theory of Molecular Excitons. *Soviet Physics Uspekhi* **1964**, *7*, 145.
25. Bhagavantam, S.; Venkatarayudu, T. *Theory of Groups and Its Application to Physical Problems*; Academic Press: 1969.
26. Halford, R. S. Motions of Molecules in Condensed Systems: I. Selection Rules, Relative Intensities, and Orientation Effects for Raman and Infra-Red Spectra. *J. Chem. Phys.* **1946**, *14*, 8–15.
27. Hornig, D. F. The Vibrational Spectra of Molecules and Complex Ions in Crystals. I. General Theory. *J. Chem. Phys.* **1948**, *16*, 1063–1076.
28. Rousseau, D. L.; Bauman, R. P.; Porto, S. P. S. Normal Mode Determination in Crystals. *J. Raman Spectrosc.* **1981**, *10*, 253–290.
29. Ashbrook, S. E.; Dawson, D. M. Exploiting Periodic First-Principles Calculations in Nmr Spectroscopy of Disordered Solids. *Acc. Chem. Res.* **2013**, *46*, 1964–1974.
30. Moran, R. F.; Dawson, D. M.; Ashbrook, S. E. Exploiting Nmr Spectroscopy for the Study of Disorder in Solids. *Int. Rev. Phys. Chem.* **2017**, *36*, 39–115.
31. Sakellariou, D.; Brown, S. P.; Lesage, A.; Hediger, S.; Bardet, M.; Meriles, C. A.; Pines, A.; Emsley, L. High-Resolution Nmr Correlation Spectra of Disordered Solids. *Journal of the American Chemical Society* **2003**, *125*, 4376–4380.
32. Okihara, T.; Tsuji, M.; Kawaguchi, A.; Katayama, K.; Tsuji, H.; Hyon, S. H.; Ikada, Y. Crystal-Structure of Stereocomplex of Poly(L-Lactide) and Poly(D-Lactide). *Journal of Macromolecular Science-Physics* **1991**, *B30*, 119–140.
33. Cartier, L.; Okihara, T.; Ikada, Y.; Tsuji, H.; Puiggali, J.; Lotz, B. Epitaxial Crystallization and Crystalline Polymorphism of Polylactides. *Polymer* **2000**, *41*, 8909–8919.

34. Montes de Oca, H.; Ward, I. M. Structure and Mechanical Properties of PGA Crystals and Fibres. *Polymer* **2006**, *47*, 7070–7077.

35. Chatani, Y.; Suehiro, K.; Ôkita, Y.; Tadokoro, H.; Chujo, K. Structural Studies of Polyesters. I. Crystal Structure of Polyglycolide. *Die Makromolekulare Chemie* **1968**, *113*, 215–229.

36. Hirono, K.; Wasai, G.; Saegusa, T.; Furukawa, J. II. Structure of Polyglycolide. *The Journal of the Society of Chemical Industry, Japan* **1964**, *67*, 604–607.

37. Brittain, H. G. *Polymorphism in Pharmaceutical Solids*; CRC Press: 2009. Boca Raton.

38. Censi, R.; Di Martino, P. Polymorph Impact on the Bioavailability and Stability of Poorly Soluble Drugs. *Molecules* **2015**, *20*, 18759–18776.

39. Kim, Y. B.; Park, I.-Y. Disordered Crystal Structure of Diflunisal. *Journal of Pharmaceutical Investigation* **1996**, *26*, 55–59.

40. Cross, W. I.; Blagden, N.; Davey, R. J.; Pritchard, R. G.; Neumann, M. A.; Roberts, R. J.; Rowe, R. C. A Whole Output Strategy for Polymorph Screening: Combining Crystal Structure Prediction, Graph Set Analysis, and Targeted Crystallization Experiments in the Case of Diflunisal. *Crystal Growth & Design* **2003**, *3*, 151–158.

41. Sasaki, T.; Tanabe, T.; Nishizawa, J.-I. Development of Continuous Wave Terahertz Signal Generator based on Difference Frequency Generation in Gallium Phosphide Crystal. *Journal of the Japan Society of Infrared Science and Technolog* **2016**, 26, 74–81.

42. Sasaki, T.; Tanabe, T.; Nishizawa, J.-I. Frequency Stabilized Gap Continuous-Wave Terahertz Signal Generator for High-Resolution Spectroscopy. *Optics and Photonics Journal* **2014**, *4*, 8–13.

43. Swainson, I. P.; Hammond, R. P.; Soullière, C.; Knop, O.; Massa, W. Phase Transitions in the Perovskite Methylammonium Lead Bromide, $CH_3ND_3PbBr_3$. *J. Solid State Chem.* **2003**, *176*, 97–104.

44. Dall'Olio, S.; Dovesi, R.; Resta, R. Spontaneous Polarization as a Berry Phase of the Hartree-Fock Wave Function: The Case of $KnBO_3$. *Phys. Rev. B* **1997**, *56*, 10105–10114.

45. Resta, R. Macroscopic Polarization in Crystalline Dielectrics: The Geometric Phase Approach. *Rev. Mod. Phys.* **1994**, *66*, 899–915.

46. King-Smith, R. D.; Vanderbilt, D. Theory of Polarization of Crystalline Solids. *Phys. Rev. B* **1993**, *47*, 1651–1654.

47. Becke, A. D. Density-Functional Thermochemistry. III. The Role of Exact Exchange. *J. Chem. Phys.* **1993**, *98*, 5648–5652.

48. Lee, C.; Yang, W.; Parr, R. G. Development of the Colle-Salvetti Correlation-Energy Formula into a Functional of the Electron Density. *Phys. Rev. B* **1988**, *37*, 785–789.
49. Grimme, S. Accurate Description of Van Der Waals Complexes by Density Functional Theory Including Empirical Corrections. *J. Comput. Chem.* **2004**, *25*, 1463–1473.
50. Civalleri, B.; Zicovich-Wilson, C. M.; Valenzano, L.; Ugliengo, P. B3lyp Augmented with an Empirical Dispersion Term (B3LYP-D*) as Applied to Molecular Crystals. *Crystengcomm* **2008**, *10*, 405–410.
51. Krishnan, R.; Binkley, J. S.; Seeger, R.; Pople, J. A. Self-Consistent Molecular Orbital Methods. Xx. A Basis Set for Correlated Wave Functions. *J. Chem. Phys.* **1980**, *72*, 650–654.
52. Sophia, G.; Baranek, P.; Sarrazin, C.; Rérat, M.; Dovesi, R. First-Principles Study of the Mechanisms of the Pressure-Induced Dielectric Anomalies in Ferroelectric Perovskites. *Phase Transitions* **2013**, *86*, 1069–1084.
53. Vilela Oliveira, D.; Laun, J.; Peintinger, M. F.; Bredow, T. Bsse-Correction Scheme for Consistent Gaussian Basis Sets of Double- and Triple-Zeta Valence with Polarization Quality for Solid-State Calculations. *J. Comput. Chem.* **2019**, *40*, 2364–2376.
54. Frisch, M. J.; Pople, J. A.; Binkley, J. S. Self-Consistent Molecular Orbital Methods 25. Supplementary Functions for Gaussian Basis Sets. *J. Chem. Phys.* **1984**, *80*, 3265–3269.
55. Harihara PC; Pople, J. A. Influence of Polarization Functions on Molecular-Orbital Hydrogenation Energies. *Theor. Chim. Acta* **1973**, *28*, 213–222.
56. Dovesi, R.; Orlando, R.; Erba, A.; Zicovich-Wilson, C. M.; Civalleri, B.; Casassa, S.; Maschio, L.; Ferrabone, M.; De La Pierre, M.; D'Arco, P.; et al. Crystal14: A Program for the Ab Initio Investigation of Crystalline Solids. *Int. J. Quantum Chem.* **2014**, *114*, 1287–1317.
57. R. Dovesi; V. R. Saunders; C. Roetti; R. Orlando; C. M. Zicovich-Wilson; F. Pascale; B. Civalleri; K. Doll; N. M. Harrison; I. J. Bush. *Crystal14 User's Manual*; University of Torino: 2014. Torino.
58. Dovesi, R.; Saunders, V. R.; Roetti, C.; Orlando, R.; Zicovich-Wilson, C. M.; Pascale, F.; Civalleri, B.; Doll, K.; Harrison, N. M.; Bush, I. J.; et al. Crystal17 Munual. University of Torino, Torino: 2017.
59. Dovesi, R.; Erba, A.; Orlando, R.; Zicovich-Wilson, C. M.; Civalleri, B.; Maschio, L.; Rérat, M.; Casassa, S.; Baima, J.; Salustro, S.; et al. Quantum-Mechanical Condensed Matter Simulations with Crystal. **2018**, *8*, e1360.

60. Toby, B. H.; Von Dreele, R. B. Gsas-II: The Genesis of a Modern Open-Source All Purpose Crystallography Software Package. *J. Appl. Crystallogr.* **2013**, *46*, 544–549.

61. Farrow, C. L.; Juhas, P.; Liu, J. W.; Bryndin, D.; Božin, E. S.; Bloch, J.; Proffen, T.; Billinge, S. J. L. Pdffit2 and Pdfgui: Computer Programs for Studying Nanostructure in Crystals. *J. Phys.: Condens. Matter* **2007**, *19*, 335219.

62. De Rosa, C.; Auriemma, F. Packing of Macromolecules in Polymer Crystals. In *Crystals and Crystallinity in Polymers*, John Wiley & Sons, Inc., 2013; pp. 88–122.

63. Bunn, C. W. Molecular Structure and Rubber-Like Elasticity. II. The Stereochemistry of Chain Polymers. *Proceedings of the Royal Society of London A: Mathematical, Physical and Engineering Sciences* **1942**, *180*, 67–81.

64. Huggins, M. L. Comparison of the Structures of Stretched Linear Polymers. *J. Chem. Phys.* **1945**, *13*, 37–42.

65. Pauling, L.; Corey, R. B.; Branson, H. R. The Structure of Proteins: Two Hydrogen-Bonded Helical Configurations of the Polypeptide Chain. *Proc. Natl. Acad. Sci.* **1951**, *37*, 205–211.

66. Meille, S. V.; Allegra, G.; Geil, P. H.; He, J.; Hess, M.; Jin, J.-I.; Kratochvil, P.; Mormann, W.; Stepto, R. Definitions of Terms Relating to Crystalline Polymers (Iupac Recommendations 2011). *Pure Appl. Chem.* **2011**, *83*, 1831–1871.

67. Zhang, F.; Wang, H.-W.; Tominaga, K.; Hayashi, M.; Sasaki, T. Terahertz Fingerprints of Short-Range Correlations of Disordered Atoms in Diflunisal. *The Journal of Physical Chemistry A* **2019**, *123*, 4555–4564.

68. Kojima, A.; Teshima, K.; Shirai, Y.; Miyasaka, T. Organometal Halide Perovskites as Visible-Light Sensitizers for Photovoltaic Cells. *Journal of the American Chemical Society* **2009**, *131*, 6050–6051.

69. Whalley, L. D.; Frost, J. M.; Jung, Y.-K.; Walsh, A. Perspective: Theory and Simulation of Hybrid Halide Perovskites. *J. Chem. Phys.* **2017**, *146*, 220901.

70. Brivio, F.; Butler, K. T.; Walsh, A.; Van Schilfgaarde, M. Relativistic Quasiparticle Self-Consistent Electronic Structure of Hybrid Halide Perovskite Photovoltaic Absorbers. *Phys. Rev. B* **2014**, *89*.

71. Frost, J. M.; Butler, K. T.; Walsh, A. Molecular Ferroelectric Contributions to Anomalous Hysteresis in Hybrid Perovskite Solar Cells. *APL Materials* **2014**, *2*, 081506.

72. Zhang, F.; Karimata, I.; Wang, H.-W.; Tachikawa, T.; Tominaga, K.; Hayashi, M.; Sasaki, T. Terahertz Spectroscopic Measurements

and Solid-State Density Functional Calculations on $CH_3NH_3PbBr_3$ Perovskites: Short-Range Order of Methylammonium. *J. Phys. Chem. C* **2022**, *126*, 339–348.

73. Kutes, Y.; Ye, L.; Zhou, Y.; Pang, S.; Huey, B. D.; Padture, N. P. Direct Observation of Ferroelectric Domains in Solution-Processed $CH_3NH_3Pbi_3$ Perovskite Thin Films. *The Journal of Physical Chemistry Letters* **2014**, *5*, 3335–3339.

74. Leonhard, T.; Schulz, A. D.; Röhm, H.; Wagner, S.; Altermann, F. J.; Rheinheimer, W.; Hoffmann, M. J.; Colsmann, A. Probing the Microstructure of Methylammonium Lead Iodide Perovskite Solar Cells. *Energy Technology* **2019**, *7*, 1800989.

75. Rossi, D.; Pecchia, A.; Maur, M. A. D.; Leonhard, T.; Röhm, H.; Hoffmann, M. J.; Colsmann, A.; Carlo, A. D. On the Importance of Ferroelectric Domains for the Performance of Perovskite Solar Cells. *Nano Energy* **2018**, *48*, 20–26.

76. Vorpahl, S. M.; Giridharagopal, R.; Eperon, G. E.; Hermes, I. M.; Weber, S. A. L.; Ginger, D. S. Orientation of Ferroelectric Domains and Disappearance Upon Heating Methylammonium Lead Triiodide Perovskite from Tetragonal to Cubic Phase. *ACS Applied Energy Materials* **2018**, *1*, 1534–1539.

77. Hermes, I. M.; Bretschneider, S. A.; Bergmann, V. W.; Li, D.; Klasen, A.; Mars, J.; Tremel, W.; Laquai, F.; Butt, H.-J.; Mezger, M.; et al. Ferroelastic Fingerprints in Methylammonium Lead Iodide Perovskite. **2016**, 5724–5731.

78. Röhm, H.; Leonhard, T.; Hoffmann, M. J.; Colsmann, A. Ferroelectric Domains in Methylammonium Lead Iodide Perovskite Thin-Films. *Energy & Environmental Science* **2017**, *10*, 950–955.

79. Liu, Y.; Collins, L.; Proksch, R.; Kim, S.; Watson, B. R.; Doughty, B.; Calhoun, T. R.; Ahmadi, M.; Ievlev, A. V.; Jesse, S.; et al. Chemical Nature of Ferroelastic Twin Domains in $CH_3NH_3PbI_3$ Perovskite. *Nat. Mater.* **2018**, *17*, 1013–1019.

80. De Quilettes, D. W.; Vorpahl, S. M.; Stranks, S. D.; Nagaoka, H.; Eperon, G. E.; Ziffer, M. E.; Snaith, H. J.; Ginger, D. S. Impact of Microstructure on Local Carrier Lifetime in Perovskite Solar Cells. *Science* **2015**, *348*, 683–686.

81. Zhang, D.; Zhu, Y.; Liu, L.; Ying, X.; Hsiung, C.-E.; Sougrat, R.; Li, K.; Han, Y. Atomic-Resolution Transmission Electron Microscopy of Electron Beam–Sensitive Crystalline Materials. *Science* **2018**, *359*, 675–679.

82. Rothmann, M. U.; Li, W.; Zhu, Y.; Bach, U.; Spiccia, L.; Etheridge, J.; Cheng, Y.-B. Direct Observation of Intrinsic Twin Domains in Tetragonal $CH_3NH_3PbI_3$. *Nature Communications* **2017**, *8*, 14547.

83. Carbonnière, P.; Erba, A.; Richter, F.; Dovesi, R.; Rerat, M. Calculation of Anharmonic Ir and Raman Intensities for Periodic Systems from DFT Calculations: Implementation and Validation. *Journal of Chemical Theory and Computation* **2020**, *16*, 3343–3351.

84. Erba, A.; Maul, J.; Ferrabone, M.; Carbonnière, P.; Rérat, M.; Dovesi, R. Anharmonic Vibrational States of Solids from DFT Calculations. Part I: Description of the Potential Energy Surface. *Journal of Chemical Theory and Computation* **2019**, *15*, 3755–3765.

85. Erba, A.; Maul, J.; Ferrabone, M.; Dovesi, R.; Rérat, M.; Carbonnière, P. Anharmonic Vibrational States of Solids from DFT Calculations. Part II: Implementation of the VSCF and VCI Methods. *Journal of Chemical Theory and Computation* **2019**.

86. Montroll, E. W.; Potts, R. B. Effect of Defects on Lattice Vibrations. *Phys. Rev.* **1955**, *100*, 525–543.

87. Dettmann, K.; Ludwig, W. Localized Vibration States in Molecular Lattices. *Phys. Status Solidi B* **1965**, *10*, 689–707.

88. Zhang, F.; Wang, H.-W.; Tominaga, K.; Hayashi, M.; Hasunuma, T.; Kondo, A. Application of THz Vibrational Spectroscopy to Molecular Characterization and the Theoretical Fundamentals: An Illustration Using Saccharide Molecules. *Chemistry – An Asian Journal* **2017**, *12*, 324–331.

89. Yamamoto, S.; Miyada, M.; Sato, H.; Hoshina, H.; Ozaki, Y. Low-Frequency Vibrational Modes of Poly(Glycolic Acid) and Thermal Expansion of Crystal Lattice Assigned on the Basis of DFT-Spectral Simulation Aided with a Fragment Method. *The Journal of Physical Chemistry B* **2017**, *121*, 1128–1138.

Chapter 11

Organic Molecule-Containing Electrically Conductive Electron Beam Resist for Organic Biosensors with Nanostructures

Anri Nakajima

Research Institute for Nanodevices, Hiroshima University, 1-4-2 Kagamiyama, Higashihiroshima, Hiroshima 739-8527, Japan

anakajima@hiroshima-u.ac.jp

This chapter gives an overview of nanocomposite organic electron beam (EB) resist polymers from the viewpoint of advanced technology for biology and medicine. One of the serious remaining issues with organic devices is difficulty in simultaneous control of lateral size and position of their structures at nanometer scales. The problem can be solved if organic EB resists themselves are made electrically conductive and are used for the constituent materials of main nanoscale electronic devices. Therefore, here, we propose organic molecule-containing electrically conductive EB resists and discuss their applicability to biosensors with high functionality. First, the nanocomposite EB organic resist of ZEP520A containing [6,6]-phenyl-C_{61} butyric acid methyl ester (PCBM) is described. Capacitance-voltage (C-V) characteristics

Biomedical Engineering: Imaging Systems, Electric Devices, and Medical Materials
Edited by Akihiro Miyauchi and Hiroyuki Kagechika

ISBN 978-981-5129-16-8 (Hardcover), 978-1-003-46404-4 (eBook)
www.jennystanford.com

for the fabricated capacitors of the nanocomposite resist layer showed an excellent memory effect, which indicates the electrical conductivity of the proposed nanocomposite material. Structures of the material having line and dot patterns with sizes less than 200 nm were successfully fabricated by using an extremely simple process with only EB exposure and development. Semispherical PCBM aggregations whose base diameters and base center-to-center distance between adjacent aggregations are about 60 and 80 nm were observed in the nanocomposite resist. Next, descriptions are given for the nanocomposite EB organic resist of ZEP520A containing 8-hydroxyquinoline aluminum (Alq_3). After the simple process with EB exposure and development for the nanocomposite resist, square pattern structures somewhat less than 1.0 μm in lateral length were clearly formed. Greenlight emissions were observed from the electroluminescence (EL) devices with the nanocomposite resist. Biosensors with light-emitting nanowire channels of ZEP520A containing Alq_3 have the ability to estimate the precise number and position of biomolecules attached near the channel. These results open the door to the simple fabrication of densely integrated highly sensitive and functional biosensors with electrically conductive nanostructures for multiplexed and simultaneous diagnoses.

11.1 Introduction

Field-effect transistors (FETs) are used in biosensors for medical and life sciences since their usage realizes label-free and real-time detections and quantifications of biological species. The carrier density of the channel of FET biosensors is modulated by the change of charge on the gate insulator surface due to the adsorption of charged specific bio-species in buffer solution. After the first report of ion-sensitive FET (ISFET) [1], biosensors having a FET have widely been developed based on Si metal-oxide-semiconductor FETs (MOSFETs) [2–5]. Later on, FET biosensors having a channel with carbon or organic materials have also been developed [6, 7]. Organic devices generally have unique advantages of low weight, high mechanical flexibility, cost-effectiveness, and good chemical structural versatility in comparison with inorganic ones.

On the other hand, there is growing interest in applications of biosensors having nanostructures or nanomaterials. There are many kinds of nanometer-size biomaterials such as proteins or lipids. There are possibilities to get information precisely and in detail about such biomaterials if we use biosensors with nanostructures or nanomaterials because the size of the target biomaterials in detection is almost the same as that of the detector region for the biomaterial to attach. In fact, biosensors having a nanowire channel or a single electron transistor (SET) have been reported to have high detection sensitivity for nanometer-size biomaterials [8]. Biosensors having nanostructures have been fabricated based on Si in many cases because of the ability to use the mature LSI fabrication processes, which enables to miniaturize devices.

There are roughly two types of fabrication process of nanostructures for biosensors. One is the bottom-up process, which uses the self-assembled mechanism of atoms and molecules. The other is the top-down process utilizing the electron beam (EB) lithography technique, which enables the simultaneous control of the lateral size and position of fabricating structures at nanometer scales. Utilizing the bottom-up process, biosensors having a Si nanowire channel have been fabricated. For example, the nanowire structures were grown by using chemical vapor deposition with gold nanoclusters as catalysts [9–12], which is one of the bottom-up processes. As to the top-down process, on the other hand, many reports have also been published about the biosensors having Si nanowire channels [13–17]. Moreover, biosensors based on Si SET have been realized by the top-down process using EB lithography [18–21].

As to biosensors having nanostructures with carbon or organic materials, however, only bottom-up processes have been used for the fabrication. The most typical example is the biosensor with carbon nanotubes. Chen et al. demonstrated polyethylene oxide functionalized carbon-nanotube FET-based biosensors capable of selective detection of proteins in a solution [22]. Maehashi et al. also realized label-free protein biosensors based on aptamer-modified carbon nanotube FETs for detecting immunoglobulin E [23]. In contrast, few reports have been published on biosensors having carbon- or organic-material nanostructures fabricated by using EB lithography. The main reason is the difficulty in the application of EB lithography to the nanostructure fabrication of carbon or organic materials. Conventional EB lithography techniques have a lot of problems when they are used for carbon or organic materials. For example, it is difficult to remove only the mask organic resist by using oxygen plasma ashing or cleaning with a sulfuric acid – hydrogen peroxide mixture since there is only a small selective etching ratio between the resist and the organic object. There is also difficulty in obtaining a large selective ratio in dry etching between the resist and the organic object.

Based on the above background, we proposed the idea of utilizing the organic EB resist itself as a constituent material of electrically conductive nanometer-sized structures [24–26]. However, most of the EB resists are insulators having insufficient electrical conductivity for electron devices. Therefore, we mixed organic molecules such as [6,6]-phenyl-C_{61} butyric acid methyl ester (PCBM) or 8-hydroxyquinoline aluminum (Alq_3) as a filler in a matrix EB resist. These molecules have the lowest unoccupied molecular orbital (LUMO) level near the Fermi energy of the negative electrode of devices and/or the highest occupied molecular orbital (HOMO) level near the Fermi level of the positive electrode. We used a positive type EB resist of ZEP520A as a matrix material. In these nanocomposite organic polymers, carriers (electrons and/or holes) transfer through the LUMO levels and/or HOMO levels of the filler molecules, leading to electrical conduction. Moreover, if we mix light-emitting molecules into the EB resist, there is a possibility of realizing current-drivable light-emitting organic structures having nanometer sizes. Alq_3 is a typical light-emitting molecule used for electro-luminescence (EL) devices. Indeed, green EL attributed to the emission was observed from Alq_3 in the Alq_3-containing ZEP520A layer we fabricated.

Therefore, in this chapter, electrically conductive EB resists containing organic molecules we fabricated are introduced with their applicability to biosensors having high and/or new functionality. Following this section, first, the results and applicability of PCBM-containing ZEP520A are described. Next, those of Alq_3-containing ZEP520A are shown. Then, we summarize this chapter.

11.2 PCBM-Containing ZEP520A

As described in the introduction, one of the remaining issues in organic devices is the difficulty in simultaneous control of the lateral size and position of the structures in the nanometer region. In regions with lateral dimensions larger than 5 μm, in contrast, photosensitive electrically conductive organic polymer composites have been reported. They consist of photopolymerizable matrix material and electrically conducting fillers. One example is that high-aspect-ratio structures with a minimum lateral size of 5 μm have been fabricated using a photosensitive negative resist of SU8 as a matrix polymer and silver particles as fillers [27, 28]. Also, a pattern having a line width of 10 μm was obtained with an electrically conductive SU8 resist embedding carbon black particles [29]. Since these composite resist materials are electrically conductive themselves, it is not necessary to use an additional mask resist for determining their lateral sizes and positions in the micrometer size region.

In the nanometer region, in contrast, such electrically conductive composite resist materials had not been reported. There were reports of organic resist polymers in which fullerene derivatives are incorporated in a conventional EB resist of ZEP520 [30–32]. However, these resist polymers were only used as a mask resist with high resistance for dry etching and were not used as carrier conducting materials for electronic devices. Their characteristics related to carrier transport had not been investigated.

On the other hand, nanocomposites of gate-insulating organic polymers containing fullerene derivative molecules were reported as promising materials for organic memories [33–37]. It was found that electrons or holes are injected into and stored in the LUMO or HOMO levels of the fullerene derivatives and the carriers are transferred through the levels in the nanocomposite organic polymers.

Then, an idea has come to our mind that there is a possibility of creating EB-patternable electrically conductive nanocomposite organic polymers if organic EB resists themselves can be used for the matrix polymers of gate-insulating organic polymers containing electrically conductive fillers. Here, we chose a positive-type EB resist of ZEP520A as a matrix polymer and [6,6]-phenyl-C_{61} butyric acid methyl ester (PCBM) as an electrically conducting filler [24, 25].

11.2.1 Results

The proposed composite resist was found to be electrically conductive. To show this, we fabricated capacitors and measured capacitance-voltage (C-V) characteristics. Figure 11.1a shows a schematic diagram of the capacitor structure. A ZEP520A layer containing PCBM was formed on a 20-nm SiO_2 layer on an n-type Si substrate. PCBMs were dissolved in a ZEP520A solution with an anisole solvent, and the mixture was ultrasonicated for a sufficiently long time for obtaining a uniform solution. The mole ratio of PCBM relative to the monomer of ZEP520A was 1:10. Then the resist solution was spin-coated on the underlying SiO_2 layer and then baked at 165°C for 10 min. Since ZEP520A is a positive resist and the remaining part after development is the region where EBs were not exposed, no EB exposures were carried out for the sample of C-V measurements. After development, we deposited the Al gate and back electrodes. The thickness of the ZEP520A containing PCBM layer is 150 nm. Figure 11.1b shows the band diagram of ZEP520A containing PCBM molecules with an Al gate electrode in the equilibrium state under the assumption that the PCBM molecules are uniformly dispersed.

Figure 11.2 shows the C-V characteristics of the fabricated capacitor. A large flat band voltage shifts ΔV_F of more than 4 V and excellent retention characteristics were obtained after applying −10.0 V for 600 s to the ZEP520A containing PCBM. Here, the initial effective injected charge corresponds to -4.4×10^{-9} C. About 50% of the $|\Delta V_F|$ remained three days later, compared with the $|\Delta V_F|$ obtained immediately after programming.

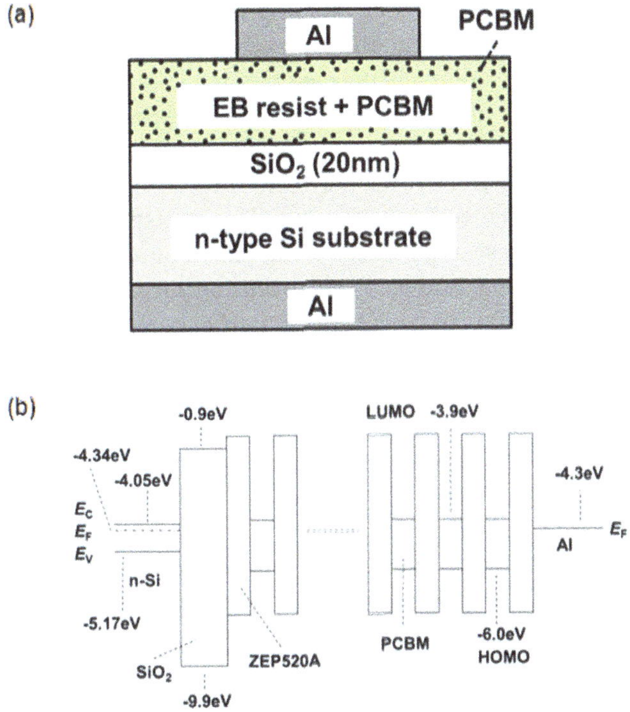

Figure 11.1 (a) Schematic diagram of a fabricated capacitor with Al/EB resist polymer containing PCBM/SiO_2/n-type Si substrate. (b) Band diagram of nanocomposite resist polymer containing PCBM in the equilibrium state.

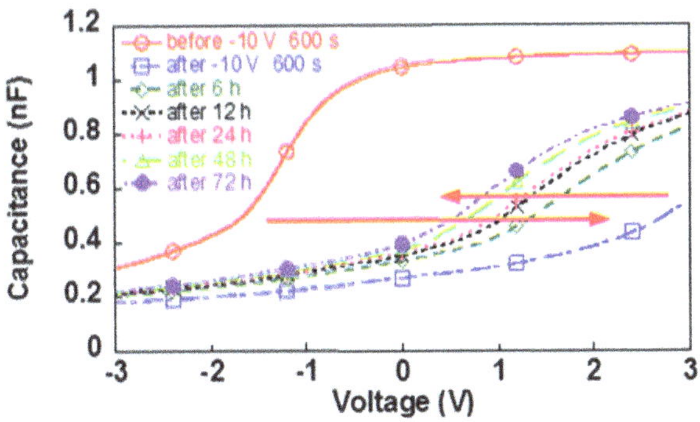

Figure 11.2 C-V retention characteristics for the capacitor of ZEP520A containing PCBM after writing at −10.0 V for 600 s. Arrows indicate the directions in which C-V curves shifted. Solid lines are for before applying the gate voltage and dashed and dash-dotted lines are for after applying the gate voltage. Reproduced from [24].

Since the LUMO level of PCBM is closer to the Fermi energy (E_F) of the gate Al than the HOMO level of PCBM is (Figure 11.1b), electrons are preferentially injected into the LUMO levels of PCBM, and transferred through the levels at negative programming voltages. This leads to electrical conductivity in the proposed nanocomposite organic resist polymer.

Regarding the resist patterning characteristics, it was found that line patterns of ZEP520A containing PCBM with widths of less than 200 nm can be made by using an extremely simple process with only EB exposure and development [24]. Square patterns of ZEP520A containing PCBM were also found to be made with side lengths of less than 200 nm by using the process [24]. Figure 11.3 shows a cross-sectional transmission electron microscopy (TEM) image of ZEP520A containing PCBM for the line and space pattern. The designed pitch and line width were 400 nm and 200 nm, respectively. A very clear pattern was formed. The width of the formed line was 140 nm and no resist remained in the space regions on the SiO_2 layer where the EB exposures occurred.

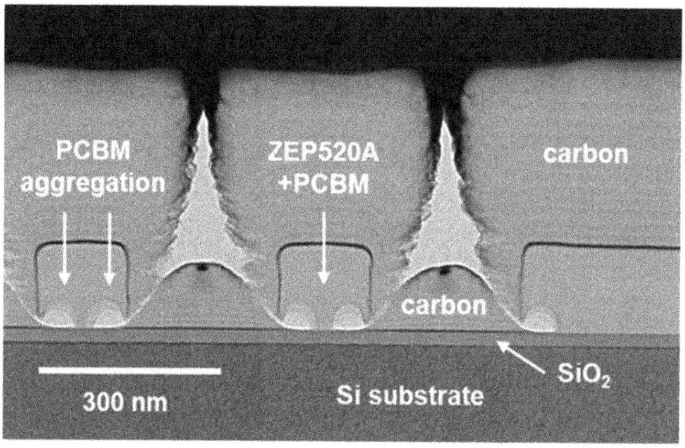

Figure 11.3 Cross-sectional TEM micrograph of ZEP520A containing PCBM after EB exposure and development for the design pattern of lines and spaces with a line width of 200 nm. After a thin platinum (Pt) layer a few nm thick was deposited, carbons were evaporated to protect the line and space structure from damage by the Ga ion beam during the TEM sample processing. The purpose of the thin Pt layers is to clearly distinguish the structure from the evaporated carbons.

Aggregations were clarified in ZEP520A containing PCBM. There are white regions, indicated by arrows, near the bottom edges of the resist pattern in Figure 11.3. These regions are considered to be empty and no resist nor PCBM exists due to the dissolution of PCBM in the developer (ZED-N50) or isopropyl alcohol (IPA) used for rinsing during the development. Since no such white empty regions were observed in the region far from the edge of the line pattern with large width (the pattern of the most right-hand side in Figure 11.3), the PCBM aggregations near the edge regions of the line pattern are considered to be preferentially dissolved due to the permeation of ZED-N50 or IPA. Since there are no white regions in the upper region of the resist pattern, PCBM molecules preferentially aggregated in the bottom region of the line pattern.

The base diameters of the semispherical PCBM aggregation are about 60 nm, and the base center-to-center distances between adjacent aggregations are about 80 nm. There is a possibility of remaining the dispersed PCBMs in the upper region in a molecular state or in much smaller aggregations than those of the bottom region. Taking the base diameter and center-to-center distance of these large bottom PCBM aggregations into consideration, the minimum side length of the EB pattern for a memory cell or the minimum width of a conducting line is necessary to be 200–250 nm. Optimization of the kind and concentration of incorporated fullerene derivatives as well as of the baking conditions of ZEP520A containing fullerene derivative will make it possible to reduce the size of the aggregation for a further reduction in lateral device size.

11.2.2 Application to Biosensor

The above results open the door to the simple fabrication of flexible nanodevices such as highly integrated flexible memories or single-electron or quantum information devices as well as sensitive nanowire biosensors for multiplexed and simultaneous diagnoses [24, 25].

Here, explanations are given especially for the application to the nanowire channel FET biosensor. Nanowire channel FET biosensors have high sensitivity especially when the concentration of target species in solution is small [8]. When a charged target biomolecule attaches to the surface of the nanowire channel made of PCBM-containing ZEP520A near a PCBM aggregation (Figure 11.4a), the LUMO level of the aggregation near the target changes as shown in Figure 11.4b and the conductivity of the channel varies. Therefore, the proposed nanowire FET biosensor is considered to be applied to disposable sensitive biosensors for multiplexed and simultaneous diagnoses.

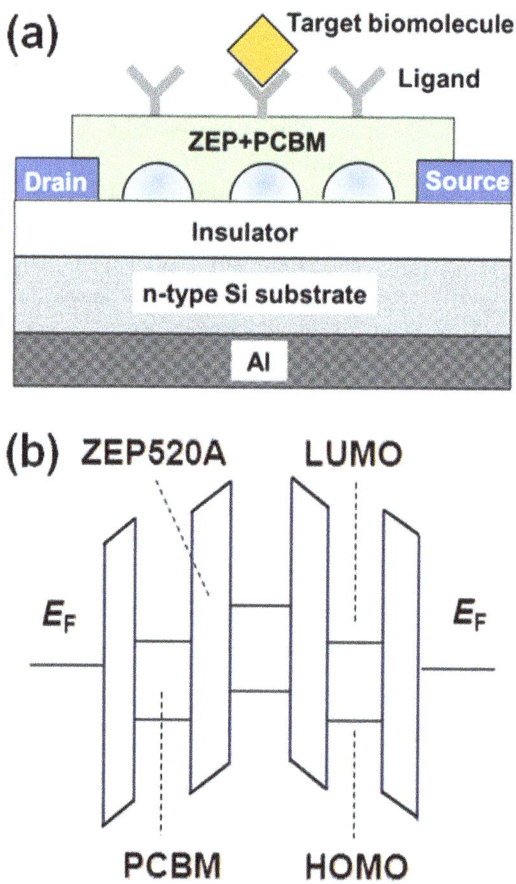

Figure 11.4 (a) Schematic diagram of the detection of a target biomolecule attaching to the surface of the nanowire FET channel made of PCBM-containing ZEP520A near a PCBM aggregation. (b) Band diagram of the nanowire channel when a negatively charged target biomolecule attaches to the ligand as shown in (a).

11.3 ALQ_3-Containing ZEP520A

Organic optical devices have also advantages in view of weight, mechanical flexibility, cost-effectiveness, and chemical structural versatility. Moreover, the miniaturization of optoelectronic organic components has attracted extensive attention. The organic light-emitting diodes (OLEDs) fabricated with their lateral sizes in nanometer region have potential applications to organic quantum-information devices, near-field optical microscopy, highly sensitive biosensor, as well as high-resolution OLEDs and nanoscale photo-patterning [26]. However, most of the light-emitting layers in OLEDs are over 10 μm in lateral size. The difficulty of simultaneous control of lateral sizes and positions of the structures in the nanometer region is one of the remaining issues also for organic optoelectronic devices. To solve the issue, we recently proposed an idea of replacing the fullerene derivatives in ZEP520A described in the previous section with current drivable light-emitting molecules generally used for OLEDs [26]. Here, Alq_3 was used as the filler molecule.

11.3.1 Results

First, we make a solution containing ZEP520A, Alq_3, and a solvent (such as chloroform or a mixture of chloroform and anisole). After the solution was ultrasonicated followed by filtration, the solution was spin-coated on a Si substrate and baked at 165 °C for 10 min.

In the nanocomposite resist layer thus fabricated, many thin planar crystals appear approximately with the shapes of rectangle, parallelogram, or trapezoid with side lengths less than 1 μm and a thickness much smaller than 0.1 μm [26].

EB exposure experiments were carried out on the composite-resist layer formed on a p-type Si substrate at an acceleration voltage of 100 kV. After the EB exposure, the samples were developed using the ZEP developer (ZED-N50). Figure 11.5 shows plan-view optical microscope images of the square patterns for the 5:1 mol ratio of ZEP520A to Alq_3. The design mask patterns were squares of side-length 1.0–5.0 μm. The area dose was 280 μC cm^{-2}. The pale-colored regions in the images are those where the nanocomposite resist was removed, and the dark-colored regions are those where the resist remained after development. Square patterns somewhat less than 1.0 μm in lateral length clearly formed.

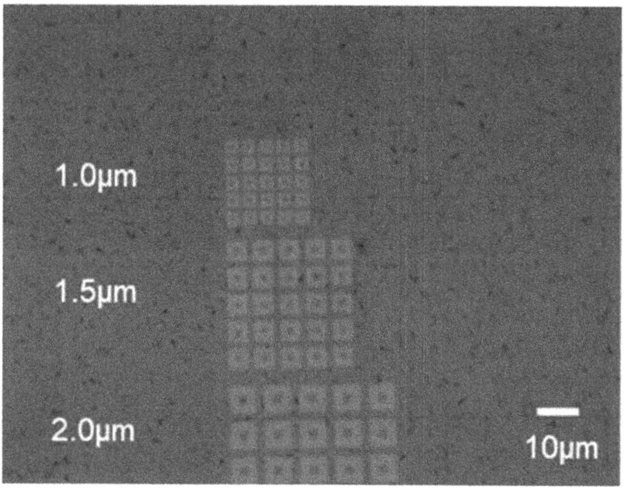

Figure 11.5 Optical microscopy images of the square-pattern structures for the mol ratio of ZEP520A copolymer to Alq_3 of 5:1 after EB exposure and development. Reproduced with permission from [26].

Next, we performed EL experiments by using these composite-resist layers as light-emitting layers. A multilayer structure was formed on indium-tin-oxide (ITO) electrodes on a glass substrate to observe EL from the light-emitting layer. Figure 11.6 shows the possible energy levels of the multilayer structure.

Optical micrographs of a square region (2×2 mm^2) where the positive and negative electrodes cross confirmed greenlight emissions from the EL devices with the 5:1 mol ratio (Figure 11.7).

A remaining problem for the realization of the light-emitting device having such a dot structure with nanometer lateral size is how to electrically insulate the upper contact layer from the bottom contact layer around the dot region. One possible way for the realization is the usage of an appropriate water-soluble insulating polymer for spin-coating after the formation of the light-emitting dot layer. A more detailed description is given in the supporting information of Ref. [26].

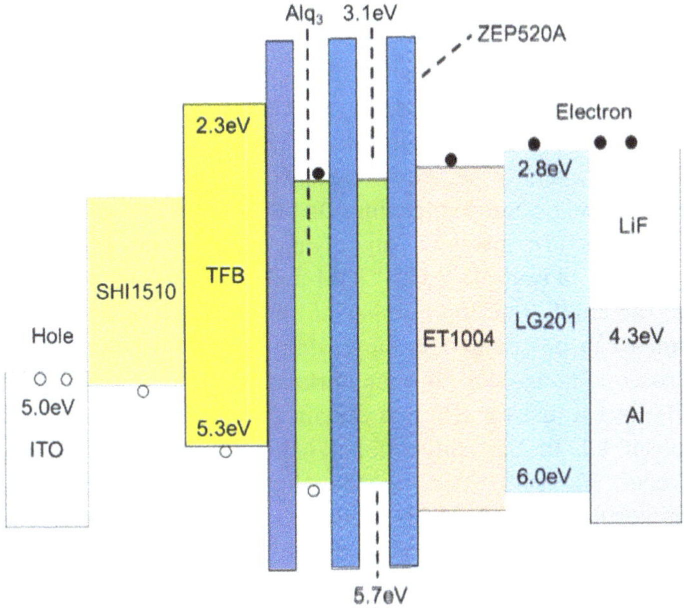

Figure 11.6 Schematic illustration of the energy levels of the multilayer structure of OLED.

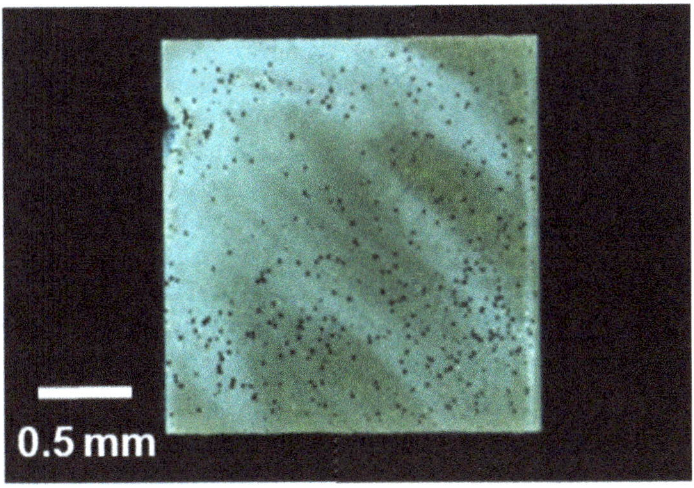

Figure 11.7 Optical micrograph of a square region (2 mm × 2 mm) for EL of the mole ratio of ZEP520A copolymer to Alq$_3$ of 5:1. Reproduced with permission from [26].

11.3.2 Application to Biosensor

The nanometer-size organic light-emitting diodes fabricated using the above nanocomposite resist have potential applications for organic quantum-information devices, near-field optical microscopy, highly sensitive biosensor, high-resolution OLEDs, and nanoscale photo-patterning. Detail descriptions of the above applications are given in supporting information of Ref. [26]. Especially, biosensors with light-emitting nanowire channels have the ability that the number of biomolecules attaching to the channel can be counted by observing the contrast of the optical microscope image due to biomaterials around the channel of the field-effect transistor where a certain threshold voltage (V_{th}) shift is observed. In the conventional nanowire channel biosensors, however, V_{th} shifts become the same no matter how many biomolecules are attached to the nanowire channel in series [8]. Besides the merit, biosensors with light-emitting nanowire channels have the advantage that the charge of the target biomolecule can be estimated precisely. Since the detection with a nanowire biosensor is based on the long-range electrostatic interaction, a small V_{th} shift occurs even when a target molecule is attached apart from the nanowire channel. If the V_{th} shift is observed using the conventional nanowire biosensor, the charge of the target molecule will be underestimated because the observed V_{th} shift is smaller than the one observed in the case when the target is attached right above the nanowire channel. Even in this case, however, the distance between the target biomolecule and the nanowire channel can be measured if the distance is not too long by using biosensors with a light-emitting nanowire channel by means of observing the position of the contrast due to biomaterials in the optical microscope image. This leads to the precise estimation of the charge of a target molecule.

11.4 Summary

In this chapter, an overview is given for nanocomposite organic EB resists and their applicability to high functional biosensors. Two types of nanocomposite organic EB resist are introduced. One is the nanocomposite resist, which consists of ZEP520A containing PCBM, and the other comprises ZEP520A containing Alq_3. These nanocomposite resists are indeed electrically conductive. Line or dot patterns could be fabricated with their width or side length in nanometer size by using an extremely simple process only with EB exposure and development. In the nanocomposite layers, nanoscale aggregations or crystals consisting of their filler materials exist. The above results open the door to the simple fabrication of flexible nanodevices such as highly integrated flexible memories or single-electron or quantum information devices as well as sensitive biosensors for multiplexed and simultaneous diagnoses. Especially, biosensors with light-emitting nanowire channels made of ZEP520A containing Alq_3 have the ability to estimate the precise number and position of biomolecules attaching near the channel.

References

1. Bergveld, P. (1970). Development of an ion-sensitive solid-state device for neurophysiological measurements, *IEEE Trans. Biomed. Eng.*, **17**, pp. 70–71.
2. Matsuo, T., Esashi, M. (1981). Methods of ISFET fabrication, *Sens. and Actuators*, **1**, pp. 77–96.
3. Gotoh, M., Tamiya, E., Karube, I., Kagawa, Y. (1986). A microsensor for adenosine-5′-triphosphate pH-sensitive field effect transistors, *Anal. Chim. Acta,* **187**, pp. 287–291.
4. Park, K.-Y., Kim, M.-S., Choi, S.-Y. (2005). Fabrication and characteristics of MOSFET protein chip for detection of ribosomal protein, *Biosens. Bioelectron.*, **20**, pp. 2111–2115.
5. Kim, D.-S., Jeong, Y.-T., Park, H.-J., Shin, J.-K., Choi, P., Lee, J.-H., Lim, G. (2004). An FET-type charge sensor for highly sensitive detection of DNA sequence, *Biosens. Bioelectron.*, **20**, pp. 69–74.
6. Mohanty, N., Berry, V. (2008). Graphene-based single-bacterium resolution biodevice and DNA transistor: Interfacing graphene derivatives with nanoscale and microscale biocomponents, *Nano Lett.*, **8**, pp. 4469–4476.
7. Khan, H.U., Roberts, M.E., Johnson, O., Förch, R., Knoll, W., Bao, Z. (2010). In situ, label-free DNA detection using organic transistor sensors, *Adv. Mater.*, **22**, pp. 4452–4456.

8. Nakajima, A. (2022). *Biomedical Engineering*, eds. Miyauchi, A. and Miyahara, Y., Chapter 2 "Biosensors based on FETs containing nanostructures," (Jenny Stanford Publishing Pte. Ltd., Singapore) pp. 17–32.
9. Cui, Y., Wei, Q., Park, H., Lieber, C.M. (2001). Nanowire nanosensors for highly sensitive and selective detection of biological and chemical species, *Science*, **293**, pp. 1289–1292.
10. Patolsky, F., Zheng, G., Hayden, O., Lakadamyali, M., Zhuang, X., Lieber, C.M. (2004). Electrical detection of single viruses, *Proc. Natl. Acad. Sci. USA*, **101**, pp. 14017–14022.
11. Wang, W.U., Chen, C., Lin, K.-H., Fang, Y., Lieber, C.M. (2005). Label-free detection of small-molecule-protein interactions by using nanowire nanosensors, *Proc. Natl. Acad. Sci. USA*, **102**, pp. 3208–3212.
12. Zheng, G., Patolsky, F., Cui, Y., Wang, W.U., Lieber, C.M. (2005). Multiplexed electrical detection of cancer markers with nanowire sensor arrays, *Nat. Biotechnol.*, **23**, pp. 1294–1301.
13. Stern, E., Klemic, J.F., Routenberg, D.A., Wyrembak, P.N., Turner-Evans, D.B., Hamilton, A.D., LaVan, D.A., Fahmy, T.M., Reed, M.A. (2007). Label-free immunodetection with CMOS-compatible semiconducting nanowires, *Nature*, **445**, pp. 519–522.
14. Li, Z., Chen, Y., Li, X., Kamins, T.I., Nauka, K., Williams, R.S. (2004). Sequence-specific label-free DNA sensors based on silicon nanowires, *Nano Lett.*, **4**, pp. 245–247.
15. Kim, A., Ah, C.S., Yu, H.Y., Yang, J.-H., Baek, I.-B., Ahn, C.-G., Park, C.W., Jun, M.S., Lee, S. (2007). Ultrasensitive, label-free, and real-time immunodetection using silicon field-effect transistors, *Appl. Phys. Lett.*, **91**, 103901. doi:10.1063/1.2779965.
16. Kudo, T., Kasama, T., Ikeda, T., Hata, Y., Tokonami, S., Yokoyama, S., Kikkawa, T., Sunami, H., Ishikawa, T., Suzuki, M., Okuyama, K., Tabei, T., Ohkura, K., Kayaba, Y., Tanushi, Y., Amemiya, Y., Cho, Y., Monzen, T., Murakami, Y., Kuroda, A., Nakajima, A. (2009). Fabrication of Si nanowire field-effect transistor for highly sensitive, label-free biosensing, *Jpn. J. Appl. Phys.*, **48**, 06FJ04. doi:10.1143/JJAP.48.06FJ04.
17. Knopfmacher, O., Tarasov, A., Fu, W., Wipf, M., Niesen, B., Calame, M., Schönenberger, C. (2010). Nernst limit in dual-gated Si-nanowire FET sensors, *Nano Lett.*, **10**, pp. 2268–2274.
18. Kudo, T., Nakajima, A. (2011). Highly sensitive ion detection using Si single-electron transistors, *Appl. Phys. Lett.*, **98**, 123705. doi:10.1063/1.3569148.

19. Kudo, T., Nakajima, A. (2012). Biomolecule detection based on Si single-electron transistors for highly sensitive integrated sensors on a single chip, *Appl. Phys. Lett.*, **100**, 023704. doi:10.1063/1.3676664.

20. Nakajima, A., Kudo, T., Furuse, S. (2013). Biomolecule detection based on Si single-electron transistors for practical use, *Appl. Phys. Lett.*, **103**, 043702. doi:10.1063/1.4816267.

21. Nakajima, A. (2016). Application of single-electron transistor to biomolecule and ion sensors, *Appl. Sci.*, **6**, 94. doi:10.3390/app6040094.

22. Chen, R.J., Bangsaruntip, S., Drouvalakis, K.A., Kam, N.W.S., Shim, M., Li, Y., Kim, W., Utz, P.J., Dai, H. (2003). Noncovalent functionalization of carbon nanotubes for highly specific electronic biosensors, *Proc. Natl. Acad. Sci. USA*, **100**, pp. 4984–4989.

23. Maehashi, K., Katsura, T., Kerman, K., Takamura, Y., Matsumoto, K., Tamiya, E. (2007). Label-free protein biosensor based on aptamer-modified carbon nanotube field-effect transistors, *Anal. Chem.*, **79**, pp. 782–787.

24. Nakajima, A., Tabei, T., Yasukawa, T. (2017). Fullerene-containing electrically conducting electron beam resist for ultrahigh integration of nanometer lateral-scale organic electronic devices, *Sci. Rep.*, **7**, 4306. doi:10.1038/s41598-017-04451-9.

25. Nakajima, A. (2018). Short review on fullerene-containing electrically conducting electron beam resist for organic biosensors with nanostructures, *Adv. Tech. Biol. Med.*, **6**, 1000257. doi:10.4172/2379-1764.1000257.

26. Nakajima, A., Sakurai, H., Abe, S. (2020). Electroluminescence from Alq_3-containing electron-beam resists for light-emitting organic nanometer-scale devices, *ACS Appl. Nano Mater.*, **3**, pp. 11688–11694.

27. Jiguet, S., Bertsch, A., Hofmann, H., Renaud, P. (2004). SU8-silver photosensitive nanocomposite, *Adv. Eng. Mater.*, **6**, pp. 719–724.

28. Jiguet, S., Bertsch, A., Hofmann, H., Renaud, P. (2005). Conductive SU8 photoresist for microfabrication, *Adv. Funct. Mater.*, **15**, pp. 1511–1516.

29. Hauptman, N., Žveglič, M., Maček, M., Gunde, M.K. (2009). Carbon based conductive photoresist, *J. Mater. Sci.*, **44**, pp. 4625–4632.

30. Ishii, T., Nozawa, H., Tamamura, T. (1997). Nanocomposite resist system, *Appl. Phys. Lett.*, **70**, pp. 1110–1112.

31. Ishii, T., Tamamura, T., Shigehara, K. (2000). Fullerene-derivative nanocomposite resist for nanometer pattern fabrication, *Jpn. J. Appl. Phys.*, **39**, pp. L1068–L1070.

32. Ishii, T., Murata, Y., Shigehara, K. (2001). Contrast enhancement of ZEP520 resist by fullerene-derivative incorporation, *Jpn. J. Appl. Phys.*, **40**, pp. L478–L480.
33. Nakajima, A., Uchino, M. (2012). Charge redistribution in a charge storage layer containing C_{60} molecules and organic polymers for long electron retention, *Appl. Phys. Lett.*, **101**, 213301. doi:10.1063/1.4767132.
34. Nakajima, A., Fujii, D., Uchino, M. (2013). Excellent retention characteristics of nanocomposite gate insulator consisting of fullerene-containing polystyrene, *Appl. Phys. Lett.*, **103**, 013302. doi:10.1063/1.4812840.
35. Nakajima, A., Fujii, D. (2015). Memory operation mechanism of fullerene-containing polymer memory, *Appl. Phys. Lett.*, **106**, 103302. doi:10.1063/1.4914881.
36. Nakajima, A., Shoji, A., Nagano, K., Kajihara, J. (2015). Dependence of memory characteristics of fullerene-containing polymer on the kind of gate metal, *Jpn. J. Appl. Phys.*, **54**, 100303. doi:10.7567/JJAP.54.100303.
37. Ham, J.H., Jung, J.H., Kim, H.J., Lee, D.U., Kim, T.W. (2008). Electrical properties and operating mechanisms of nonvolatile organic memory devices fabricated utilizing hybrid poly(*N*-vinylcarbazole) and C_{60} composites, *Jpn. J. Appl. Phys.*, **47**, pp. 4988–4991.

Chapter 12

mRNA Medicines and mRNA Vaccines

Hideyuki Nakanishi and Keiji Itaka

Department of Biofunction Research, Institute of Biomaterials and Bioengineering, Tokyo Medical and Dental University, Japan

itaka.bif@tmd.ac.jp

Messenger RNA (mRNA) is attracting much attention as a new drug modality. Artificially, synthesized mRNA is administered to the body as a therapeutic agent or vaccine. mRNA vaccine was first developed for COVID-19, demonstrating excellent efficacy in reducing the incidence and aggravation of infections. Since mRNA has advantages such as the capability of producing any protein by simply changing the nucleic acid sequences, and the negligible risk of insertional mutagenesis, it is also used for various applications including vaccines for other infectious diseases, cancer vaccines, and therapeutic agents. In this part, the methodology to prepare the mRNAs and their delivery systems is described.

12.1 Design and Construction of Template DNAs for In Vitro Transcription (IVT)

To prepare mRNAs by IVT, first, template DNAs should be designed and constructed. Template DNAs are usually linear

Biomedical Engineering: Imaging Systems, Electric Devices, and Medical Materials
Edited by Akihiro Miyauchi and Hiroyuki Kagechika

ISBN 978-981-5129-16-8 (Hardcover), 978-1-003-46404-4 (eBook)
www.jennystanford.com

DNAs, which are prepared by restriction digestion of plasmid DNAs (pDNAs) or PCR (Figure 12.1) [1]. When preparing template DNAs by restriction digestion of pDNAs, restriction enzymes that create 3′ protruding ends (e.g., PstI) should not be used, since template DNAs with 3′ protruding ends tend to increase by-products during IVT [2]. If the pDNAs must be digested by 3′ protruding end-producing restriction enzymes, the 3′ protruding end should be changed to the blunt end by T4 DNA polymerase. Type IIS restriction enzymes (e.g., SapI), whose cleavage sites exist outside of their recognition sequence, enable avoiding the addition of extra bases downstream of poly(A) tail and may help produce mRNAs with higher translation efficiency [3].

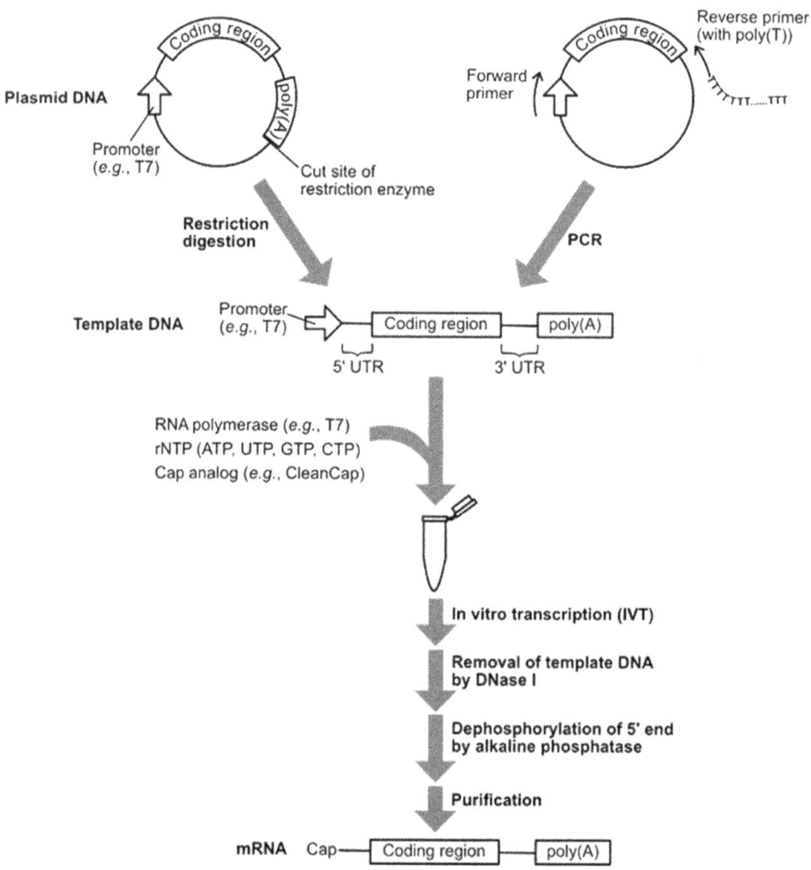

Figure 12.1 Procedure of mRNA preparation by IVT.

After the preparation of template DNAs by restriction digestion or PCR, the size of template DNAs should be confirmed by agarose gel electrophoresis. Template DNAs are usually purified by conventional PCR clean-up kits. However, when undigested pDNAs or PCR by-products are observed by agarose gel electrophoresis, only proper size template DNAs should be purified by gel extraction.

Template DNAs should contain four components: promoter, protein-coding region, 5' and 3' untranslated regions (UTRs), and poly(A) tail. Details of each component are described below.

12.1.1 Promoter

Promoters in template DNAs should be compatible with DNA-dependent RNA polymerase used in IVT. For example, if you use T7 RNA polymerase in IVT, template DNAs should contain the T7 promoter sequence. T7, T3, and SP6 promoters (Table 12.1) are mainly used in IVT, and the T7 promoter is the most popular. It should be noted that promoters for transcription in mammalian cells such as CAG promoter are generally not applicable for IVT. Inserting an AT-rich sequence (e.g., ATAAT) immediately downstream of the T7 promoter may increase the transcription efficiency [4].

Table 12.1 Sequences of promoters used in IVT

Promoter	Sequence (transcription start sites are underlined)
T7 (conventional)	TAATACGACTCACTATA<u>G</u>GG
T7 (for CleanCap AG reagent)	TAATACGACTCACTATA<u>A</u>GG
T3 promoter	AATTAACCCTCACTAAA<u>G</u>GG
SP6 promoter	ATTTAGGTGACACTATA<u>G</u>AA

12.1.2 Protein-Coding Region

Codon optimization is the most important point in designing protein-coding regions since non-optimal codons decrease not only the translation elongation rate but also mRNA stability [5].

Currently, many commercially available artificial gene synthesis services (e.g., GeneArt from ThermoFisher Scientific) provide codon optimization tools. In addition to avoiding non-optimal codons, the usage of codons with lower uridine and higher guanosine and cytidine contents is more desirable to decrease immunogenicity and increase translation efficiency [6, 7]. However, it should be noted that the high translation elongation rate sometimes causes misfolding of proteins [5]. Therefore, the codon usage that provides the highest translation elongation rate does not always result in the highest production of properly folded functional proteins. When multiple mRNA variants with different codon usages are compared, it is recommended to evaluate not only the production of encoded proteins but also their activities, since there is a possibility that misfolded proteins are produced.

12.1.3 UTR

As the names imply, UTRs are not translated to proteins, but they affect translation efficiency and mRNA stability.

A region between a 5′ end of an mRNA and a start codon of the protein-coding region is called 5′ UTR. The suitable length of 5′ UTR is 50 - 70 nt [8, 9], and stable RNA secondary structures in 5′ UTRs have negative effects on translation [10, 11]. The especially important sequence in 5′ UTRs is "GCCRCC" (R = A or G) immediately upstream of a start codon, which is a part of the Kozak consensus sequence (GCCRCCATGG) [12]. The lack of a Kozak consensus sequence can result in low translation efficiency. The presence of upstream open reading frames or upstream start codons in 5′ UTRs can cause the translation to start from unintended sites. To avoid an inefficient translation, 5′ UTRs should be devoid of such alternative translation start sites [13].

A region between a stop codon of the protein-coding region and a poly(A) tail is called 3′ UTR. To avoid low translation efficiency, the length of 3′ UTR should not be shorter than 27 nt [14], but too long 3′ UTR (e.g., 1500 nt) may decrease mRNA stability [15]. Different from 5′ UTR, stable secondary structures in 3′ UTRs have positive effects on translation [11].

While UTRs of α- or β-globin mRNA are widely used, there are several reports of UTRs that enable higher translation efficiencies and mRNA stability [3, 9, 16, 17]. However, it should be noted that the suitability of UTR can depend on cell types. The expression level of endogenous microRNAs and RNA binding proteins differ among cell types, and the binding of these endogenous biomolecules can positively or negatively affect translation efficiencies and mRNA stability. For example, 3′ UTR containing a binding site of HuR, an RNA binding protein, increases translation [9]. On the other hand, microRNA-binding sites in 5′ or 3′ UTRs decrease translation [16, 18]. Therefore, if a target cell type to be transfected is already determined, checking highly active microRNAs in the target cell type, and deleting binding sites of such microRNAs from UTRs may help to achieve higher translation.

12.1.4 Poly(A) Tail

To stabilize mRNAs, the 3′ ends of mRNAs are protected by poly(A) tails, which also have an important role in translation. In the preparation of mRNAs by IVT, there are two ways to add poly(A) tails at the 3′ ends of mRNAs. One is enzymatic polyadenylation after IVT, in which poly(A) polymerase is used. The other is adding a template sequence of poly(A) tail to an IVT template DNA and transcribing poly(A) tail by DNA-dependent RNA polymerase as well as other regions of the mRNA.

If poly(A) tails are added by enzymatic polyadenylation, IVT template DNAs do not have to contain template sequences for poly(A) tails. However, compared to the method using poly(A)-containing template DNAs, the enzymatic polyadenylation after IVT increases the step of mRNA preparation. In addition, poly(A) tails added by enzymatic polyadenylation tends to have variable length [3].

Therefore, the method using IVT template DNAs containing poly(A)-template sequences is currently more popular. This method allows adding poly(A) tails with consistent lengths. The length of the poly(A) tail is generally 100–120 adenosines, and the shorter poly(A) tail results in less efficient translation [3]. A previous study reported that a further longer poly(A) tail, which consists of 300 adenosines achieved further higher translation efficiency [19]. However, preparing an IVT template DNA containing such a long poly(A) tail is difficult. When an IVT template DNA is prepared by PCR, a poly(A) tail-template sequence is added by using a reverse primer containing a poly(T) sequence (Figure 12.1). Therefore, the length of the poly(A) tail in PCR-prepared IVT template DNA cannot exceed the available primer length. Usually, the maximum length of commercially available primer is less than 200 nucleotides. On the other hand, when an IVT template DNA is prepared by restriction digestion of a pDNA, the pDNA should contain a poly(A) tail-template sequence. However, such repeated sequence tends to induce recombination and resulting truncation of poly(A) tail-template sequence in *Escherichia coli*. The insertion of interval sequences into poly(A) tail-template sequence or the usage of a linear pDNA can decrease such truncation [19, 20].

12.2 In Vitro Transcription and Purification of mRNAs

The preparation of mRNAs usually consists of five steps: IVT, digestion of template DNAs by DNase I, enzymatic capping (and enzymatic polyadenylation, if necessary), dephosphorylation, and purification.

In IVT, mRNAs are transcribed from template DNAs by DNA-dependent RNA polymerase (e.g., T7 RNA polymerase) using rNTPs (ATP, UTP, GTP, and CTP) as substrates. mRNAs containing modified nucleotides can be transcribed by replacing an unmodified nucleotide in the IVT reaction mixture with a modified nucleotide (e.g., N1-methyl-pseudoUTP). The incorporation of modified nucleotides can enhance the translation and decrease the immunogenicity of mRNAs [21, 22]. Especially, UTP is often replaced with N1-methyl-pseudoUTP, a modified nucleotide that is also used in COVID-19 vaccines [23, 24]. However, it should be noted that the effects of modified nucleotides can be affected by cell types, sequences, and delivery methods of mRNAs [6, 7, 11, 25].

When T7 RNA polymerase is used in IVT, the usual reaction time is 4–6 hours, but it depends on the type of RNA polymerase and reaction buffer. The longer reaction time can increase the total amount of transcribed mRNAs, but it sometimes produces shorter mRNAs due to the decrease in RNA polymerase activity. The reaction temperature of the canonical T7 RNA polymerase is 37 °C, but it is reported that IVT in 51–55 °C by the thermostable RNA polymerase can reduce the double strand RNA (dsRNA) by-product, which is immunogenic [26]. After the completion of IVT, template DNAs should be digested by DNase I or its derivative.

Poly(A) tail can be enzymatically added to 3′ ends of mRNAs by poly(A) polymerase, but as described in Section 12.1, using IVT template DNAs containing poly(A) tail-template sequences is a more popular method.

A cap structure at the 5′ end of mRNA is important for efficient translation and mRNA stability. There are two types of mRNA-capping methods. One is the enzymatic capping after IVT, and the other is the usage of a cap analog (e.g., anti-reverse cap analog (ARCA)) that enables co-transcriptional capping during IVT. In enzymatic capping, the vaccinia virus capping enzyme is generally used. Different from mammalian canonical mRNAs, mRNAs capped by vaccinia virus capping enzyme have no methyl group at the 2′-O position of the first nucleotide adjacent to the cap. Such a 2′-O-methyl-lacking cap structure is called "cap 0", which can induce translational repression of mRNAs [27, 28]. Therefore, converting "cap 0" to "cap 1", whose 2′-O position of the first nucleotide is methylated is recommended. This conversion can be catalyzed by 2′-O-methyltransferase. The co-transcriptional capping is a more convenient method since mRNAs can be capped by simply adding a cap analog to the IVT reaction mixture. While ARCA has been widely used for co-transcriptional capping, it produces cap 0-mRNAs, and its capping efficiency is less than 80% [29]. Therefore, an improved cap analog that can produce cap 1-mRNAs with 94% or higher capping efficiency has recently become popular [30].

Generally, capping efficiency is not 100%, and uncapped mRNAs have triphosphate (ppp) at their 5′ ends. As such 5′ ppp-mRNAs are immunogenic, the removal of 5′ ppp by alkaline phosphatase is necessary [31]. DsRNA by-products, which are produced during IVT, are also immunogenic. Therefore, the removal of these dsRNA by-products by purification using HPLC or cellulose is recommended [32, 33].

12.3 Carriers for mRNA Delivery

Since mRNA is very unstable under the physiological condition, due to RNase that exists abundantly in tissues and blood, mRNA usually requires its delivery systems for delivering the mRNA stably and efficiently to the target cells. Since mRNA is negatively charged, the formulation of mRNA-loaded carriers is generally based on electrostatic interaction with cationic-charged materials. At present, cationic lipids or lipid nanoparticles (LNPs) are mostly used for mRNA delivery including COVID-19 vaccines.

LNPs consist of cores and outer lipid membranes, and the cores contain both mRNAs and lipids. LNPs typically consist of cholesterol, helper lipid (e.g., 1,2-dioleoyl-*sn*-glycero-3-phosphoethanolamine (DOPE)), polyethyleneglycol (PEG)-modified lipid, and ionizable lipid, while many groups developed their original LNPs with different lipid constituents [34–36]. Each constituent of LNPs has an important role. For example, PEG-modified lipids are added to prevent LNPs from aggregating and non-specifically interacting with serum proteins. Ionizable lipids, which become cationic in low pH conditions such as endosomes, are used to help mRNAs in endosomes to enter cytosols by disrupting endosomal membranes. In addition to lipid-based carriers such as LNPs, polymer or peptide-based carriers are also developed for mRNA delivery [36, 37].

Constituents of carriers affect the physicochemical properties (e.g., size and surface charge) of the mRNA-carrier complex, and organ mRNAs are delivered depending on these physicochemical properties. Therefore, for efficient mRNA delivery to the target organs or tissues, optimizing the constituents of the carrier is important. Modifying carriers by ligands that can bind proteins represented on the target cell surface is another effective approach for targeted mRNA delivery [35].

When the preparation of carriers is difficult due to the shortage of expertise or equipment, there are some lipid-based commercially available mRNA transfection reagents especially for in vitro transfection (e.g., Lipofectamine MessengerMAX (ThermoFisher Scientific) and TransIT-mRNA (Takara Bio)).

LNPs have another important role in stimulating immune responses. Indeed, mRNA vaccines do not contain adjuvants, but LNP itself works as an adjuvant. However, the current mRNA vaccines are prone to induce excessive immune responses, leading to side effects such as inflammatory pain and fever. Thus, it is strongly demanded to regulate the responses.

Other than LNPs, cationic polymer-based carriers are under development. Polyplex nanomicelle is based on the self-assembly of mRNA and a block copolymer comprising a polyethylene glycol (PEG)-poly(amino acid) block copolymer [38]. Since the nanomicelle has little or no effect on immune stimulation because of the surface covered by a dense PEG palisade, it would be better used for disease treatment. Indeed, therapeutic mRNA-loaded nanomicelles successfully produced the effects without inflammatory responses in the articular cartilage, intervertebral disc, spinal cord, and brain [39–44].

References

1. H. Nakanishi, T. Yoshii, S. Tsukiji, H. Saito, *STAR Protocols.* **3**, 101451 (2022).
2. E. T. Schenborn, R. C. Mierendorf, *Nucleic Acids Res.* **13**, 6223–6236 (1985).
3. S. Holtkamp et al., *Blood.* **108**, 4009–4017 (2006).
4. T. Conrad, I. Plumbom, M. Alcobendas, R. Vidal, S. Sauer, *Commun Biol.* **3**, 1–8 (2020).
5. G. Hanson, J. Coller, *Nat Rev Mol Cell Biol.* **19**, 20–30 (2018).
6. A. Thess et al., *Molecular Therapy.* **23**, 1456–1464 (2015).
7. S. Vaidyanathan et al., *Molecular Therapy - Nucleic Acids.* **12**, 530–542 (2018).
8. S. A. Chappell, G. M. Edelman, V. P. Mauro, *Proc Natl Acad Sci U S A.* **103**, 18077–18082 (2006).
9. C. Zeng et al., *Advanced Materials.* **32**, 2004452 (2020).

10. J. R. Babendure, J. L. Babendure, J.-H. Ding, R. Y. Tsien, *RNA*. **12**, 851–861 (2006).
11. D. M. Mauger et al., *PNAS*. **116**, 24075–24083 (2019).
12. M. Kozak, *Nucleic Acids Res*. **15**, 8125–8148 (1987).
13. A. G. Hinnebusch, I. P. Ivanov, N. Sonenberg, *Science*. **352**, 1413–1416 (2016).
14. R. L. Tanguay, D. R. Gallie, *Molecular and Cellular Biology*. **16**, 146–156 (1996).
15. B. Schwanhäusser et al., *Nature*. **473**, 337–342 (2011).
16. A. G. Orlandini von Niessen et al., *Molecular Therapy*. **27**, 824–836 (2019).
17. S. Linares-Fernández et al., *Mol Ther Nucleic Acids*. **26**, 945–956 (2021).
18. H. Nakanishi, H. Saito, *Methods Mol Biol*. **2312**, 73–86 (2021).
19. A. E. Grier et al., *Mol Ther Nucleic Acids*. **5**, e306 (2016).
20. Z. Trepotec, J. Geiger, C. Plank, M. K. Aneja, C. Rudolph, *RNA*. **25**, 507–518 (2019).
21. K. Karikó, M. Buckstein, H. Ni, D. Weissman, *Immunity*. **23**, 165–175 (2005).
22. K. Karikó et al., *Molecular Therapy*. **16**, 1833–1840 (2008).
23. O. Andries et al., *Journal of Controlled Release*. **217**, 337–344 (2015).
24. K. D. Nance, J. L. Meier, *ACS Cent. Sci*. **7**, 748–756 (2021).
25. S. Uchida, K. Kataoka, K. Itaka, *Pharmaceutics*. **7**, 137–151 (2015).
26. M. Z. Wu, H. Asahara, G. Tzertzinis, B. Roy, *RNA*. **26**, 345–360 (2020).
27. T. Kimura et al., *Journal of Virology*. **87**, 9997–10003 (2013).
28. M. Habjan et al., *PLOS Pathogens*. **9**, e1003663 (2013).
29. J. Stepinski, C. Waddell, R. Stolarski, E. Darzynkiewicz, R. E. Rhoads, *RNA*. **7**, 1486–1495 (2001).
30. J. M. Henderson et al., *Current Protocols*. **1**, e39 (2021).
31. J. Devoldere, H. Dewitte, S. C. De Smedt, K. Remaut, *Drug Discovery Today*. **21**, 11–25 (2016).
32. K. Karikó, H. Muramatsu, J. Ludwig, D. Weissman, *Nucleic Acids Research*. **39**, e142–e142 (2011).
33. M. Baiersdörfer et al., *Molecular Therapy - Nucleic Acids*. **15**, 26–35 (2019).
34. X. Han et al., *Nat Commun*. **12**, 7233 (2021).

35. H. Mukai, K. Ogawa, N. Kato, S. Kawakami, *Drug Metab Pharmacokinet.* **44**, 100450 (2022).
36. M. Li et al., *Eur J Med Chem.* **227**, 113910 (2022).
37. M. L. Ibba, G. Ciccone, C. L. Esposito, S. Catuogno, P. H. Giangrande, *Advanced Drug Delivery Reviews.* **177**, 113930 (2021).
38. K. Itaka, K. Kataoka, *Curr. Gene Ther.* **11,** 457–465 (2011).
39. H. Aini et al., *Sci. Rep.* **6,** 18743 (2016).
40. C.Y. Lin et al., *Mol Ther Nucleic Acids.* **16**, 162–171 (2019).
41. S.T. Crowley et al., *Mol Ther Nucleic Acids.* **17**, 465–476 (2019).
42. Y. Fukushima et al., *Biomaterials.* **270**, 120681 (2021).
43. J. Deng et al., *Pharmaceutics.* **14**, 1785 (2022).
44. Y. Hashimoto et al., *Prog Neurobiol.* **216**, 102288 (2022).

Chapter 13

Fabrication of Decellularized Tissue for Biomedical Application

Tsuyoshi Kimura, Mika Suzuki, Yoshihide Hashimoto, and Akio Kishida

Institute of Biomaterials and Bioengineering, Tokyo Medical and Dental University, 2-3-10 Kanda-surugadai, Chiyoda-ku, Tokyo 101-0062, Japan

kimurat.mbme@tmd.ac.jp

Decellularized tissue is an extracellular matrix (ECM) obtained from living tissue by removing cellular components and is used as a new biomaterial for biomedical applications. Decellularized tissue products of sheets and powder of various decellularized tissues, such as dermis, urinary bladder matrix, and small intestinal submucosa, have already been used as covering and prosthetic materials clinically. Decellularized tissues show different characteristics from synthetic materials and tissue extracts because the decellularized tissue includes bioactive substances, such as growth factors, extracellular vesicles, and lipid mediators. Recently, decellularized tissue is called decellularized ECM (dECM) and various applications of dECM have been proposed. The dECM hydrogels are prepared from various tissue sources

Biomedical Engineering: Imaging Systems, Electric Devices, and Medical Materials
Edited by Akihiro Miyauchi and Hiroyuki Kagechika

ISBN 978-981-5129-16-8 (Hardcover), 978-1-003-46404-4 (eBook)
www.jennystanford.com

and attempted as injectable hydrogel and 3D-printing bioink. Also, the functionalization of decellularized tissue with synthetic materials, biofunctional molecules, and drugs is attempted while taking advantage of the features of decellularized tissue. In the future, decellularized tissue is expected to be applied to various biomedical fields.

13.1 Introduction

Decellularized tissues, in which cellular components are removed from living tissues, are used as alternative materials and scaffolds for tissue regeneration. Decellularized tissues are composed of extracellular matrices (ECMs), such as collagen and glycosaminoglycan (GAG), which is a major feature of decellularized tissues that maintains the complex three-dimensional tissue structure of living tissues. Many studies have been conducted to take advantage of this feature to regenerate tissues by implanting ECMs as scaffolds. Decellularized tissue is used to induce tissue regeneration/neogenesis, orthotopically, and ectopically. The development of decellularized organs, in which not only tissues but also organs are decellularized, is also underway. Currently, decellularized tissue products of about 50 are available in the US and European markets, and there is a wide variety of products derived from humans, porcine, bovine, and other allogeneic and xenogeneic animals. Many of the products are processed into sheets and powders, and are used in a variety of applications as transplant materials, such as tissue filling and covering. It is believed that various bioactive substances contained in decellularized tissues act on them to induce tissue regeneration. Recently, further applications of decellularized tissue, such as decellularized tissue ECM hydrogel, which is made by solubilizing decellularized tissue and forming a gel, are being considered for use as injectable materials, 3D printer materials, and cultured cell scaffolds. In addition, attempts are being made to add functionality to decellularized tissues by compounding drugs, bioactive molecules, and heterogeneous materials. This chapter describes the preparation, characterization, and fabrication of decellularized tissue and various applications of decellularized tissues.

13.2 Decellularization Methods

Decellularization processes generally consist of the cell destruction process and the washing process of cell debris. Many decellularization methods have been proposed and classified as chemical and physical methods (Figure 13.1). The features of these methods are described as the chemical method of perfect decellularization with heavy ECM damage and the physical method of minimal decellularization with small ECM damage. Also, it is required to choose the appropriate decellularization method for the tissue and purpose for which it is to be used because tissue varies from cell-based tissue, high cell-density and ECM-based tissue, and high ECM-density, with various sizes, thicknesses, and volumes.

Decellularization method		Decellularization process: Cell destruction	Decellularization process: Removal of cell debris	Decellularization effectiveness and ECM damages
Chemical	Surfactant Hypertonic/hypotonic Alcohol	Chemical	Washing (Enzyme)	Perfect decellularization Heavy damages
Physical	Freeze-thawing Pressurization Supercritical	Physic al	Washing (Enzyme)	Minimally decellularization Small damages

Figure 13.1 Chemical and physical decellularization methods.

13.2.1 Chemical Decellularization Method

The chemical decellularization method is a major method due to its easy processing. Tissue is immersed into solutions, such as surfactant solution, hypertonic and hypotonic solutions, and alcohol, and then washed to remove cell debris and surfactant. The amount of residual DNA in decellularized tissue is measured and 200 μg/mg tissue is a standard for decellularization. The cells in the tissue are effectively removed, but tissue is damaged because the surfactant can dissolve not only cells but also ECM in tissue. So, the control of surfactant type, concentration, and treatment time is required to obtain decellularized tissue for individual purposes. Various surfactants, such as sodium dodecyl sulfate (SDS), sodium deoxycholate (SDC), and Triton X-100®, are used for the decellularization of tissue [1]. SDS is the most used detergent and can effectively decellularize tissue. Although efficient decellularization is achieved, the dECM is strongly damaged. In the case of the structure of decellularized tissue that influences cellular functions, such as cell shape, growth, and differentiation, on tissue regeneration, the decellularization protocol is considered carefully. Also, it is needed to enough wash the SDS-treated tissue due to the cytotoxicity of SDS. SDC and Triton X-100 are often used for decellularization and allow for relatively mild decellularization because of these low surfactant activities. The cytotoxicity of these is lower than that of SDS. The combination of surfactants can effectively decellularize tissue. For example, tissue treated with SDS is treated with Triton X-100 in order to remove the residual SDS.

13.2.2 Physical Decellularization Method

In the physical decellularization methods, such as freeze-thawing, high hydrostatic pressure (HHP), and supercritical, destruct cells and the cell debris are washed out [2]. Special equipment is generally required for cell destruction. Also, for the washing process, the nuclease is often used to enhance the removal of DNA and RNA in the cell debris. For the freeze-thawing method, the conditions, such as time, temperature, and cycle, are adjusted to each tissue. The effect of decellularization generally increases with the increasing freeze-thawing cycle. Also, for HHP decellularization methods, it is known that the cell has died for hydrostatic pressurization of 200 MPa and the denaturing of proteins is induced by hydrostatic pressurization of more than 300 MPa. The effect of decellularization differs from the used tissue, it is needed that the conditions, such as pressure, time, and temperature, are adjusted to each tissue. After the process of cell destruction, the cell debris is removed for the washing process. The washing time is related to the size, thickness, and volume of used tissue, and long-term washing is required to remove cell debris at the deep site of tissue. The structure of decellularized tissue is generally remained compared to that of surfactant decellularized tissue, in which ECM is dissolved and washed out.

13.3 Properties of Decellularized Tissue

The properties of decellularized tissue including mechanical and chemical properties vary depending on the used tissue and the decellularization method. The mechanical properties, such as elastic modulus, tensile strength, and failure strain, of tissue generally reduce by decellularization. The degree of reduction in mechanical properties depends on the type of used tissue and the decellularization method. The tissue with low cell density and high ECM density, such as the aorta and dermis, relatively retained the mechanical properties; on the other hand, the mechanical property of tissue with high cell density and low ECM density, such as the lung and liver, decreased remarkably. Also, the mechanical properties of decellularized tissue are strongly affected by the decellularization method in relation to chemical properties, such as the amount of ECM and the degree of denaturation. The mechanical properties of surfactant decellularized tissue are decreased compared to that of HHP decellularized tissue because the structural ECMs, such as collagen and elastin, are removed. We have previously compared the mechanical properties of HHP decellularized aorta and SDS decellularized aorta. The HHP decellularized aorta was mechanically and structurally similar to the native aorta; however, for the SDS decellularized aorta, its structure was disordered, resulting in low mechanical properties [3]. In addition, other properties, such as permeability, optical property, and swelling property, should be considered for individual purposes.

13.4 Applications of Decellularized Tissue

Decellularized tissue is used as a scaffold material either orthotopically or ectopically (Figure 13.2). Orthotopic applications include the same tissue as the implant site is decellularized and implanted orthotopically and tissue is reconstructed (orthotopic tissue regeneration). Ectopic applications include two types of tissue reconstruction: the first is when decellularized tissue that is different from the implant site is used and reconstructed into tissue that is appropriate for the implant site (ectopic tissue regeneration). This is considered that the decellularized tissue acts as a scaffold and cells around the implant site regulate the tissue reconstruction, which is suitable to the implant site. These orthotopic and ectopic tissue regenerations constitute the majority of research on decellularized tissue [2]. Many decellularized tissue products are applied to both orthotopic and ectopic sites and promote tissue reconstruction of the implant site regardless of the origin of the decellularized tissue used. On the other hand, for the second ectopic application, when the decellularized tissue is applied to an ectopic site, tissue derived from the decellularized tissue is newly constructed ectopically (ectopic tissue generation). The tissue structure of the decellularized tissue strongly influences the cells, and the cells respond to the decellularized tissue, resulting in the formation of different tissues ectopically. Our group has focused on the fact that decellularized tissue prepared by the HHP method is less damaged than other chemical methods and maintains an ECM structure that is almost the same as that of the original tissue. We hypothesized that the HHP decellularized tissue shows high tissue reconstruction ability and attempted ectopic tissue generation using the HHP decellularized tissue. We have investigated ectopic bone formation by HHP-decellularized cortical bone [4] and hematopoiesis by HHP-decellularized bone marrow [5] in rats subcutaneously (ectopic). When HHP-decellularized cortical bone fragments were implanted subcutaneously, recipient cells infiltrated into the gaps between the HHP-decellularized cortical bone fragments and formed a bone-like collagen matrix between the cell layers, which became opaque on X-ray micro-CT observation. These findings suggest bone formation in the gaps between decellularized cortical bone fragments, which may represent ectopic tissue regeneration. For the HHP decellularized bone marrow, gross visual examination after subcutaneous (ectopic) implantation in mice revealed that the decellularized bone marrow, which became white-yellow by decellularization, turned red again, suggesting that hematopoietic cells grew within the HHP decellularized bone marrow and produced red blood cells. Histological findings showed a network-like structure of reticular tissue and spaces of fat droplets in the adipose tissue, and cells infiltrated the reticular tissue, resembling living bone marrow. These results suggest that the bone marrow microenvironment was ectopically constructed newly. This mechanism of induction of ectopic tissue generation as described above is still unknown in detail but assumed as follows. The maintenance of the undifferentiated state and differentiation of stem cells is regulated by the microenvironment (niche) consisting of supporting cells and their supporting ECMs. The HHP decellularized bone marrow maintains the structural factors of the spatial niche, such as the three-dimensional structure and surface characteristics unique to living organisms, and the recipient stem and supporting cells acted according to the microenvironment of the niche during cellular infiltration and adhesion. However, it is considered that such ectopic tissue generation is achieved under several limited conditions, such as the origin of the decellularized tissue and the site of implantation, as well as minimal damage to the ECM of the decellularized tissue. Further research is expected to identify the structural factors of the niche, and the clarification of these factors is expected to lead to the development of material-based tissue regeneration/generation, which is different from the cell-based tissue regeneration that has been achieved so far.

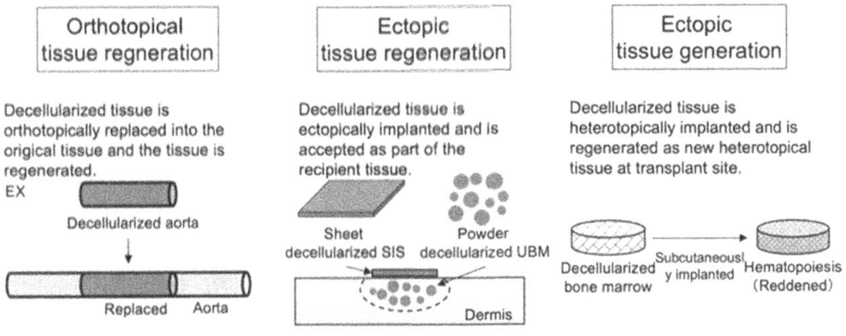

Figure 13.2 Orthotopic and ectopic application of decellularized tissues.

13.5 Decellularized Organs

Organ regeneration is studied using decellularized organs, such as the heart [6–8], liver [9–11], lungs [12, 13], and kidneys [14]. This is based on the fact that the complex morphology and structure of living organisms can be maintained even after decellularization. Generally, organs, which are connected by large blood vessels to capillaries, are decellularized by the perfusion of surfactant through the vascular network. Decellularized organs are used directly into the body or after recellularization with cells ex vivo. In the former case, the organ is connected to a large blood vessel in the body, and nutrients and new cells are supplied to the entire organ via blood circulation. In the latter, on the other hand, the cells are introduced via large blood vessels and placed throughout the entire organ through a preserved vascular network, and a perfusion culture technique is used. Regarding organ reconstruction using decellularized organs, H. Ott et al. first reported the successful reconstruction of the heart with some functions such as electrophysiological properties by seeding and culturing rat cardiomyocytes in decellularized rat hearts [6]. L. Yang et al. reported that human iPS cell-derived pluripotent cardiac vascular progenitor cells were seeded and cultured in decellularized mouse hearts, and the recellularized heart showed spontaneous contraction, electrophysiological properties, and normal responses to drugs. The recellularized decellularized heart has not yet achieved normal cardiac function, due to insufficient force required for blood circulation and insufficient electrical conductivity [7]. Since recellularization with iPS cell-derived cells overcome cell source issues and other problems, further research is expected in the future. Also, many recellularized decellularized organs with functionality have been reported [15]. In addition to iPS cells, cell sources suitable for organs are being explored for recellularization, including somatic stem cells, mesenchymal stem cells, and other stem cells, endothelial cells for vessel construction, and endothelial progenitor cells [16]. Development of decellularized organs in large animals is also attempted, and decellularization conditions and methods suitable for large-sized organs are being investigated to obtain decellularized organs maintaining their morphology, structure, and vascular network. Future progress is expected.

13.6 Application of Decellularized Tissue Powder

Decellularized tissue of powder is called dECM powder. Several decellularized tissue products are dECM powders. The dECM powder is adaptable to lacking sites with irregular shapes, and it is also expected to induce tissue regeneration because of including various bioactive substances. ECM powders of various tissues and organs, such as the bladder [17], small intestine [18], liver [19], brain [20], and cartilage [21], have been investigated. The mechanism of tissue regeneration using dECM powder has been studied by S. Badylak et al. In an immunological study of decellularized tissue, it was reported that the immune response differs depending on the source of decellularized tissue and the decellularization method, and that the polarization of macrophages into inflammatory and anti-inflammatory macrophages is one of the key factors in tissue regeneration [22]. In other words, it is considered that dECM powder implanted in the living body modulates inflammation and regeneration through appropriate infiltration of stem and progenitor cells. In addition to the direct implantation of dECM powder into a living body as described above, the application of dECM powder as a bioink for 3D printing is investigated [23]. In this case, dECM powder is often solubilized and gelatinized, which is described below.

13.7 Functionalization of Decellularized Tissue

Decellularized tissue products of powder and sheet are widely used for orthotopic and ectopic tissue regeneration with no limitation on the site of use. The next applications of decellularized tissue have been proposed and researched; dECM gels focusing on bioactive substances possessed by decellularized tissues and dECM composites with bioactive substances, drugs, and different materials to achieve higher functionality of decellularized tissues.

13.7.1 dECM Gels

dECM gels are prepared by solubilizing dECM powder with enzymatic treatment and readjusting pH, salt concentration, and temperature to physiological conditions (Figure 13.3). Unlike gels of single-component extracellular matrices (such as collagen) extracted and purified from animal tissues, dECM gels have compositions and bioactive substances similar to those of the original tissue and are expected to be a substitute material that mimics the in vivo environment. dECM gels have been prepared from decellularized tissues prepared by various decellularization methods using various tissues and organs as sources, such as dermis [24], fat [25], cartilage [26], brain [27], heart [28, 29], bladder [30], and small intestine [31, 32]. The main decellularization methods are surfactant methods such as SDS, SDC, and TritonX-100®, and the main solubilization method is enzymatic solubilization with pepsin. dECM gel is formed by incubating dECM solution under physiological conditions (37 °C, pH 7.4). The physical properties of the dECM gel, such as gelation rate and mechanical properties, depend on the used tissue/organ and decellularization method. This is because the tissue structure and composition of the obtained dECM are greatly influenced by the decellularization method. Using gels of the decellularized UBM and SIS by HHP and SDS decellularization methods, the elastic modulus and gelation time were measured by compression test and turbidity measurement (Table 13.1). Compared to porcine Type I collagen, the gelation time of dECM was shorter, and the elastic modulus was lower, indicating that dECM properties are dependent on decellularization treatment. Therefore, it is important to select the appropriate tissue according to the purpose based on the gel property data. The relationship between dECM gel properties and cell behavior has been studied from the viewpoint of mechanobiology. The behavior of dECM gels is different from that of synthetic gels or single-component gels such as collagen. We investigated the behavior of vascular endothelial cells on UBM-dECM and SIS-dECM gels by the HHP decellularization method. It was observed the formation of capillary-like networks of endothelial cells on UBM-dECM and SIS-dECM gels. This may be due to the influence of bioactive substances contained in the dECM gel. Also, the network formation differed between the low elastic modulus UBM-dECM gel and the high elastic modulus SIS-dECM gel, suggesting the influence of elastic modulus and source tissue (Figure 13.4). A wide range of applications for dECM gels has been investigated, including injectable materials [33] and 3D printing materials [23, 34]. The 3D printing of dECM gels is still in the basic exploration stage for the appropriate tissue for the cells, decellularization method, dECM solution concentration, physical properties, etc. The dECM gel fabricated by the 3D printer has a variety of applications, including being used as a cell scaffold for stem cells for implantation, organoid fabrication, and drug screening. The application of 3D-printed dECM gels is expected to expand rapidly in a variety of fields.

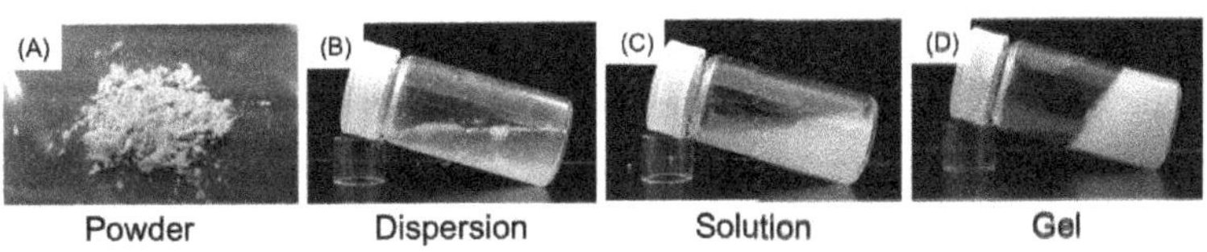

Figure 13.3 Photographs of powder, dispersion, solution, and gel of dECM.

Table 13.1 Characteristics of dECM gels of UBM and SIS

Tissue	Decellularization method	Elastic modulus (Pa)	Gelation time (min)
UBM (8 mg/ml)	HHP	682±50	26
	Detergent	879±91	71
SIS (8 mg/ml)	HHP	1438±122	26
	Detergent	774±135	61
Collagen (3 mg/ml)		1389±36	45

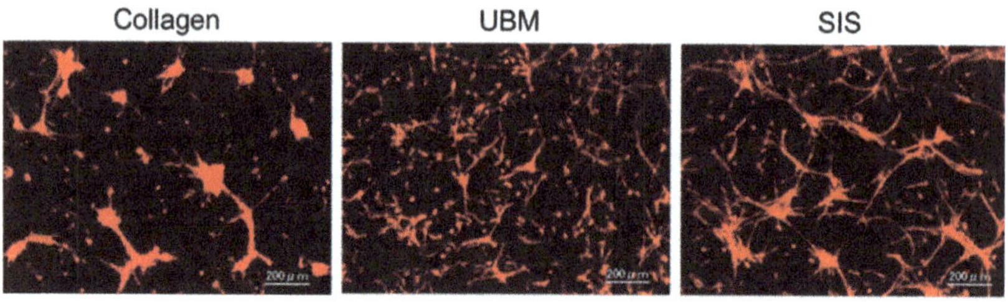

Figure 13.4 Culture of endothelial cells on dECM gels of UBM and SIS (3 days culture).

13.7.2 Composites

Regarding further functionalization with keeping advantage of the properties of decellularized tissue, decellularized tissue is combined with bioactive substances, drugs, artificial materials, etc. to functionalize decellularized tissue. As an example of adding functions that have been reduced by decellularization treatment, the immobilization of heparin on the endothelial side of decellularized blood vessels [35–37] and the immobilization of peptides that specifically act on vascular endothelial cells [38] to add anti-coagulant properties in order to prevent occlusion and blood clotting in decellularized blood vessels. Recently, immobilization of drug-encapsulated nanoparticles onto decellularized tissue was reported to add antithrombotic properties by sustained release of the drug [39].

Regarding the compositing of decellularized tissues with artificial materials to achieve high functionality, our group aims to apply decellularized tissues as novel devices by using artificial materials to cover the loss of functions by the decellularization process. Two studies are introduced below. One is the development of devices that artificial materials composite with decellularized tissues having biocompatibility. The percutaneous device is used for peritoneal dialysis catheter and artificial respirator catheter. As percutaneous devices, polymer materials (silicone rubber, Dacron, etc.) are used and show the down growth phenomenon, in which the epidermis falls off, because of low biocompatibility, resulting in infection. In order to improve the biocompatibility of polymeric materials, hydroxyapatite coating and titanium mesh coating on percutaneous devices are developed. Our group has proposed a device that integrates decellularized tissue with biocompatibility and polymeric materials partially and at the molecular level, resulting in integrating them with living tissue. We used polymethyl methacrylate (PMMA) as a polymeric material model. The decellularized dermis was gradient infiltrated and polymerized with methyl methacrylate (MMA) monomer to create a gradient-type PMMA/decellularized dermis composite (Figure 13.5(A)). Stress-strain (S-S) curves (compression test) of the gradient-type PMMA/decellularized dermis composite showed an increase in modulus at higher PMMA concentrations and a decrease in modulus at lower PMMA concentrations, and the shape of the curves also showed a straight line at higher PMMA concentrations and a J curve at lower PMMA concentrations (Figure 13.5(B)). These results suggest that the properties of the engineered material were added to the decellularized dermis, keeping with the mechanical properties of the dermis. It also indicated that PMMA was composited to the decellularized dermis in a gradient manner. The gradient-type PMMA/decellularized dermis/composite was prepared by pouring MMA monomer into the center of decellularized dermis formed on a doughnut (Figure 13.5(C)), which was gradient composited from the center. After subcutaneous implantation in rats, no integration with the surrounding tissue was observed in the PMMA portion, and down growth was observed, while integration with the surrounding tissue and cell infiltration were observed in the decellularized dermis portion (Figure 13.5(D)). These results suggest that the PMMA/decellularized dermis composites have the potential for application as a device to connect biological tissues and artificial materials [40–42].

The second is the development of small-diameter artificial blood vessels that are composites of decellularized tissue and synthetic material. So far, our group has investigated the tissue structure, mechanical properties, and permeability of the intima-media of decellularized aorta prepared by the SDS and HHP methods. The structure of the remaining ECM differed depending on the decellularization treatment method, with the HHP method maintaining relatively more structure than the SDS method. This difference in ECM structure affected the mechanical properties, with the SDS method showing reduced mechanical properties in circumferential and longitudinal tensile tests, while the HHP method showed mechanical properties similar to that of the untreated tissue [3]. The permeability of HHP decellularized intima-media was similar to that of untreated vessels [43]. In addition, the implantation of HHP decellularized aorta demonstrated long-term patency and endothelial cell lumen coverage, indicating high biocompatibility. The small-diameter decellularized blood vessels showed high patency and early endothelialization. In order to apply HHP decellularized blood vessels to ectopic sites, compliance with the target blood vessel is one of the issues to be considered, and composites of HHP decellularized blood vessels with synthetic materials are expected to be used to achieve mechanical compliance. An example of mechanical compliance is presented here [44]. This is a hybrid vascular technique in which the biocompatibility of the decellularized vessel is maintained and compliance is adapted by coating and compositing with synthetic fibers, with the aim of creating a small-diameter decellularized vessel from a large-diameter aorta. The intima-media of the decellularized aorta was used to create a small-diameter decellularized vessel by forming it into a tubular shape with an inner diameter of 2–4 mm. Segmented polyurethane (SPU) was wrapped around the small-diameter decellularized vessel by electrospinning (Figure 13.6). It is considered that reinforcement is possible while maintaining the high biocompatibility of the decellularized vessels on the lumen side. The SEM images show that the fibers uniformly coated the small-diameter decellularized blood vessels. The stiffness parameter (β) value, a measure of mechanical compliance of the vessel, was 9.4 ± 0.3 for the porcine aorta and 35.9 ± 7.5 for the porcine carotid artery, while the β value of the hybrid vessel was 24.4 ± 1.9, similar to that of native small diameter blood vessels. These results indicate that decellularized tissue can be used as parts and composited with artificial materials to provide high functionality.

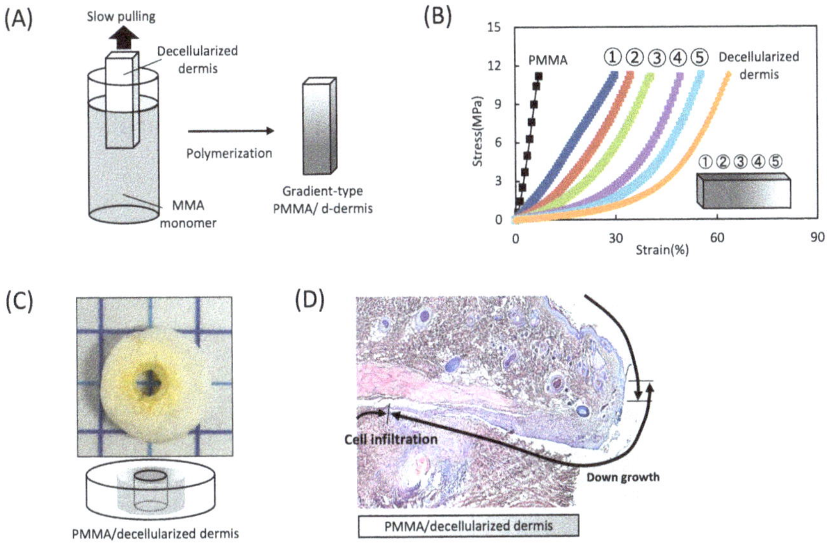

Figure 13.5 (A) Preparation of gradient-type PMMA/decellularized dermis. (B) Compression test of gradient-type PMMA/decellularized dermis. (C) Gradient-type PMMA/decellularized derimis. (D) HE staining of the implanted gradient-type PMMA/decellularied dermis subcutaneously.

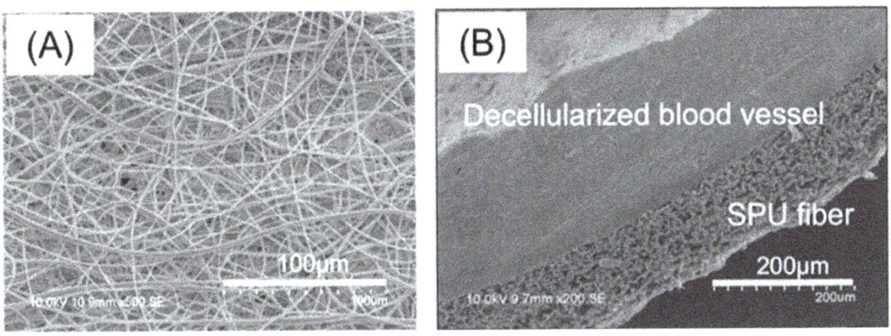

Figure 13.6 SEM photographs of (A) outer and (B) cross-sections of small-diameter decellularized blood vessels wrapped in the electrospun SPU fibers.

13.8 Conclusion

Thirty years have passed since the first paper on decellularized tissue was reported. Many decellularization methods have been proposed, and decellularized tissue from various tissues has been developed. The decellularized tissue has been used as a scaffold for regeneration medicine. Recently, various applications of decellularized tissue are attempted as new biomaterials. In the future, decellularized tissues are expected to be applied to biomedical fields.

References

1. Yao, Q. Zhang, Y.W. et al., Recent development and biomedical applications of decellularized extracellular matrix biomaterials, *Mater. Sci. Eng. C.*, 104, 109942 (2019).
2. Nakamura, N. Kimura, T. and Kishida, A. Overview of the development, applications, and future perspectives of decellularized tissues and organs, *ACS Biomater Sci Eng.*, 3(7), 1236–1244 (2017).
3. Wu, P. Kimura, T. et al., Decellularized porcine aortic intima-media as a potential cardiovascular biomaterial, *Intract. Cardiovasc. Thorac. Surg.*, 21(2), 189–194 (2015).
4. Nakamura, N. Sugano, K. et al., A basic study of osteogenesis between decellularized cortical bone pieces for bone graft construction, *Advanced Biomedical Engineering*, 2, 95–100 (2013).
5. Nakamura, N. Kimura, T. et al., Induction of in vivo ectopic hematopoiesis by a three-dimensional structured extracellular matrix derived from decellularized cancellous bone, *ACS Biomater Sci Eng.*, 5(11), 5669–5680 (2019).
6. Ott, H. C. Matthiesen, T. S. et al., Perfusion-decellularized matrix: using nature's platform to engineer a bioartificial heart, *Nat. Med.*, 14(2), 213–221 (2008).
7. Lu, T. Lin, Y. B. et al., Repopulation of decellularized mouse heart with human induced pluripotent stem cell-derived cardiovascular progenitor cells, *Nat Commun.*, 4, 2307 (2013).
8. Yasui, H. Lee, J. K. et al., Excitation propagation in three-dimensional engineered hearts using decellularized extracellular matrix, *Biomaterials*, 35(27), 7839–7850 (2014).
9. Uygun, B. E. Soto-Gutierrez, A. et al., Organ reengineering through development of a transplantable recellularized liver graft using decellularized liver matrix, *Nat Med.*, 16(7), 814–820 (2010).
10. Yagi, H. Fukumitsu, K. et al., Human-scale whole-organ bioengineering for liver transplantation: a regenerative medicine approach, *Cell Transplant.*, 22(2), 231–242 (2013).

11. Kadota, Y. Yagi, H. et al., Mesenchymal stem cells support hepatocyte function in engineered liver grafts, *Organogenesis*, 10(2), 268–277 (2014).
12. Ott, H. C. Clippinger, B. et al., Regeneration and orthotopic transplantation of a bioartificial lung, *Nat Med.*, 16(8), 927–933 (2010).
13. Petersen, T. H. Calle, E. A. et al., Tissue-engineered lungs for in vivo implantation, *Science*, 329(5991), 538–541 (2010).
14. Yu, Y. Cui, H. et al., Hypoxia-inducible Factor-1α directs renal regeneration induced by decellularized scaffolds, *Biomaterials*, 165, 48–55 (2018).
15. Yu, Y. Alkhawaji, A. et al., Decellularized scaffolds in regenerative medicine, *Oncotarget*, 7(36), 58671–58683 (2016).
16. Scarritt, M. Pashos, N. et al., A review of cellularization strategies for tissue engineering of whole organs, *Frontiers in Bioengineering and Biotechnology*, 3, article 43 (2015).
17. Badylak, S. Freytes, D. et al., Extracellular matrix as a biological scaffold material: structure and function, *Acta Biomaterialia*, 5 1–13 (2009).
18. Giobbe, G. G. Crowley, C. Extracellular matrix hydrogel derived from decellularized tissues enables endodermal organoid culture, *Nat. Commun.*, 10, 5658 (2019).
19. Tabuchi, M. Negishi, J. et al., Effect of decellularized tissue powders on a rat model of acute myocardial infarction, *Materials Science and Engineering C*, 56, 494–500 (2015).
20. DeQuach, J. A. Yuan, S. H. et al., Decellularized porcine brain matrix for cell culture and tissue engineering scaffolds, *Tissue Eng. A*, 17, 2583–2591 (2011).
21. Zahiri, S. Masaeli, E. et al., Chondrogenic response in presence of cartilage extracellular matrix nanoparticles, *Journal of Biomedical Materials Research Part A*, 106A, 2463–2471 (2018).
22. Huleihel, L. Dziki, J. et al., Macrophage phenotype in response to ECM bioscaffolds, *Seminars in Immunology*, 29, 2–13 (2017).
23. Jung, J. Bhujyan, D. et al., Solid organ fabrication: comparison of decellularization to 3D bioprinting, *Biomater. Res.*, 20(1), 27 (2016).
24. Wolf, M. Daly, K. et al., A hydrogel derived from decellularized dermal extracellular matrix, *Biomaterials*, 33(29), 7028–7038 (2012).

25. Young, D. Bajaj, V. et al., Decellularized adipose matrix hydrogels stimulate in vivo neovascularization and adipose formation, *J. Biomed. Mater. Res. A,* 102, 1641–1651 (2014).
26. Wu, J. Ding, Q. et al., An injectable extracellular matrix derived hydrogel for meniscus repair and regeneration, *Acta Biomaterialia,* 16, 49–59 (2015).
27. Medberry, C.J. Crapo, P. M. et al., Hydrogels derived from central nervous system extracellular matrix, *Biomaterials,* 34(4), 1033–1040 (2013).
28. Pati, F. Jang, J. et al., Printing three-dimensional tissue analogues with decellularized extracellular matrix bioink, *Nat Commun.,* 5, 3935 (2014).
29. Seif-Naraghi, S. B. Horn, D. et al., Injectable extracellular matrix derived hydrogel provides a platform for enhanced retention and delivery of a heparin-binding growth factor, *Acta Biomaterialia,* 8(10), 3695–3703 (2012).
30. Freytes, D. Martin, J. et al., Preparation and rheological characterization of a gel form of the porcine urinary bladder matrix, *Biomaterials,* 29(11), 1630–1637 (2008).
31. Fercana, G. Yerneni, S. et al., Perivascular extracellular matrix hydrogels mimic native matrix microarchitecture and promote angiogenesis via basic fibroblast growth factor, *Biomaterials,* 123, 142–154 (2017).
32. Wang, W. Zhang, X. et al., Preparation and characterization of pro-angiogenic gel derived from small intestinal submucosa, *Acta Biomater.,* 29, 135–148 (2016).
33. Spang, M. Christman, K. Extracellular matrix hydrogel therapies: in vivo applications and development, *Acta Biomaterialia,* 68, 1–14 (2018).
34. Garreta, E. Oria, R. et al., Tissue engineering by decellularization and 3D bioprinting, *Materials Today,* 20(4), 166–178 (2017).
35. Liao, D. Wang, X. et al., Covalent linkage of heparin provides a stable anti-coagulation surface of decellularized porcine arteries, *J Cell Mol. Med.,* 13(8B), 2736–2743 (2009).
36. Zhou, J. Ye, X. et al., Development of decellularized aortic valvular conduit coated by heparin–SDF-1α multilayer, *Ann. Thorac. Surg.,* 99(2), 612–618 (2015).

37. Bao, J. Wu, Q. et al., Hemocompatibility improvement of perfusion-decellularized clinical-scale liver scaffold through heparin immobilization, *Sci. Rep.*, 5, 10756 (2015).
38. A. Mahara, S. Somekawa et al., Tissue-engineered acellular small diameter long-bypass grafts with neointima-inducing activity, *Biomaterials*, 58, 54–62 (2015).
39. Zhou, M. Ding, J. et al., Surface biofunctionalization of the decellularized porcine aortic valve with VEGF-loaded nanoparticles for accelerating endothelialization, *Mater. Sci. Eng. C.*, 97, 632–643 (2019).
40. Matsushima, R. Nam, K. et al., Decellularized dermis-polymer complex provides a platform for soft-to-hard tissue interfaces, *Mater. Sci. Eng. C.*, 35, 354–362 (2014).
41. Nam, K. Matsushima, R. et al., In vivo characterization of a decellularized dermis-polymer complex for use in percutaneous devices, *Artif. Organs.*, 38(12), 1060–1065 (2014).
42. Nam, K. Shimatsu, Y. et al., In-situ polymerization of PMMA inside decellularized dermis using UV photopolymerization, *European Polymer Journal*, 60, 163–171 (2014).
43. Wu, P. Kimura, T et al., Relation between the tissue structure and protein permeability of decellularized porcine aorta, *Mater. Sci. Eng. C*, 43, 465–471 (2014).
44. Wu, P. Kimura, T. et al., A hybrid small-diameter blood vessel fabricated from decellularized aortic intima-media and reinforced with electrospun fibers, *Journal of Biomedical Materials Research Part A*, 107(5), 1064–1070 (2019).

Chapter 14

Bioengineering Challenges in Regenerative Medicine: Biofunctional Materials Design

Koichi Kato

Department of Biomaterials,
Graduate School of Biomedical and Health Sciences, Hiroshima University,
1-2-3 Kasumi, Minami-ku, Hiroshima 734-8553, Japan
Nanomedicine Research Division,
Research Institute for Nanodevices, Hiroshima University,
1-4-2 Kagamiyama, Higashi-Hiroshima 739-8527, Japan

kokato@hiroshima-u.ac.jp

Biofunctional materials have attracted increasing attention, owing to their ability to biologically interact with living cellular systems. These materials have various potential applications in medicine, particularly in tissue engineering and stem-cell-based regenerative therapy. This chapter focuses on the fabrication of biofunctional materials using artificial polypeptides that are rationally designed using recombinant DNA technology.

Biomedical Engineering: Imaging Systems, Electric Devices, and Medical Materials
Edited by Akihiro Miyauchi and Hiroyuki Kagechika

ISBN 978-981-5129-16-8 (Hardcover), 978-1-003-46404-4 (eBook)
www.jennystanford.com

14.1 Introduction

Various biomedical materials and devices have been fabricated using metals, ceramics, and organic polymers [1]. They are often required to be biologically inert and possess non-fouling surfaces. Alternatively, biomaterials used in direct contact with living tissues, such as titanium-based dental implants, often need to establish direct contact with tissues without the intervention of soft fibrous tissues. In contrast, more biologically active materials, such as hydroxyapatite coatings, are expected to promote mutual integration at the material–tissue interfaces. In these examples, conventional biomedical materials interact with living tissues at various levels, yet the mode of interaction is essentially passive because materials are not directly involved in biomolecular networks of living systems through biospecific interactions.

In recent years, there have been a rising number of studies on cell-based treatments for restoring damaged tissues [2]. The general scheme of regenerative therapy is shown in Figure 14.1. Various stem cell sources, such as mesenchymal stem cells (MSCs) [3] and induced pluripotent stem cells (iPSCs) [4], have been used to regenerate various tissues. Notably, scaffolding materials are often combined with tissue-forming cells, especially when a large volume of new tissues is required. Such scaffolding materials are not only used to maintain spaces for cells to form new tissues but also provide biological stimuli via protein–protein interactions for positively regulating cell behaviors. Conventional biomedical materials, however, cannot exert such biofunctional effects.

To biologically regulate cellular functions, scaffolding materials should be able to specifically interact with cells and optimize their activities through physiological pathways. The most practical pathways include integrin-mediated cell adhesion and growth factor receptor-mediated intracellular signaling, both of which lead to alterations in various cellular processes. To exert such abilities, scaffolding materials should carry polypeptides with functions similar to those of natural extracellular matrices (ECMs) and growth factors.

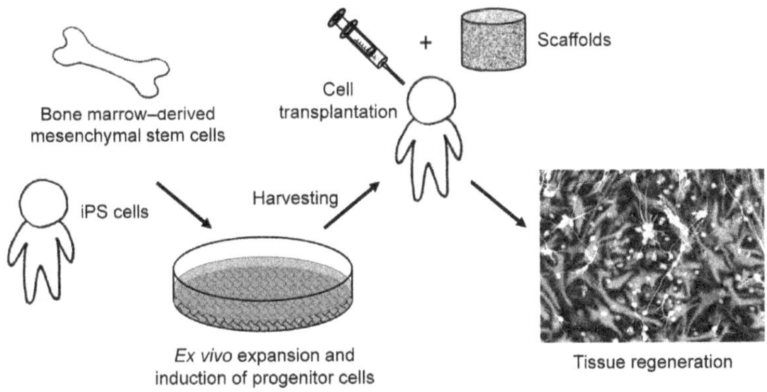

Figure 14.1 General scheme of stem cell-based regenerative therapy.

Recombinant DNA technology is effective in preparing polypeptide building blocks for assembling scaffolding materials with the desired biological, chemical, and physical properties. Based on the expected properties, polypeptide chains are designed and recombinantly synthesized in living organisms. This method allows the synthesis of artificial proteins with non-natural sequences as well as natural proteins. Thus, the polypeptide building blocks can be used to assemble materials with biofunctional properties, such as the ability to interact with integrins or growth factor receptors and to form structural components.

This article introduces previous studies in which recombinant DNA technology is effectively used to assemble bioactive materials, especially for stem cell-based cell replacement therapy.

14.2 Bioengineering Challenges in Regenerative Medicine

Over the last decade, regenerative medicine has attracted increasing interest. This is primarily owing to remarkable advances in stem cell biology, with various scientific breakthroughs, such as the establishment of human iPSCs [4] and the invention of gene-editing technology [5]. Owing to diverse scientific and technological advances in the field of regenerative medicine, more than 2,000 clinical trials are currently registered worldwide [6], with many encouraging results.

However, there are still limitations that need to be addressed before the widespread clinical application of stem-cell-based regenerative medicine, as summarized in Table 14.1. The mass production and quality control of clinically acceptable cells are important bioengineering challenges. Various bioreactor systems have been examined to enable closed, well-controlled, and automated cultivation of stem cells [7]. In addition, quality control of cellular products has been discussed in terms of safety and reproducibility [8].

Table 14.1 Bioengineering challenges in stem-cell-based regenerative medicine

Steps of regenerative therapy	Bioengineering challenges
1. Preparation of stem cells	Processes for the production of stem cells in a large quantity
2. Induction of progenitor cells	Technologies for safe and efficient induction
3. Cell purification	Processes for the non-invasive and efficient purification of cells
4. Quality control of cells	Methods and devices to analyze the quality of cells
5. Cell transplantation	Biomaterials for improving engraftment and functional integration of transplanted cells
6. Monitoring the therapeutic effect	Technologies for non-invasive cell tracking and functional monitoring

In contrast, developing methods for non-invasive tracking of transplanted cells and monitoring tissue regeneration is also a case in which a bioengineering approach plays a central role. For the non-invasive tracking of cells, many studies have been conducted on organic and inorganic nanoparticles that assist in in vivo imaging of transplanted cells using various techniques, such as magnetic resonance imaging, X-ray computed tomography, and optical imaging [9].

Another limitation is the difficulty in precisely directing cell survival and engraftment after transplantation, although the fate of transplanted cells significantly impacts the therapeutic outcomes. The low level of cell survival and poor engraftment following transplantation is of utmost concern with current treatments [10]. Combining cells with biofunctional materials is a rational strategy for increasing the survival rate of transplanted cells. The following sections introduce several attempts to develop biofunctional materials that can improve the survival of transplanted cells.

14.3 Engineered Polypeptides as Building Blocks for Biofunctional Materials

Before the details of biofunctional materials design are discussed, recombinant DNA technology is briefly introduced as a versatile pathway for synthesizing protein-based organic materials. Figure 14.2 shows an outline of recombinant polypeptide synthesis [11].

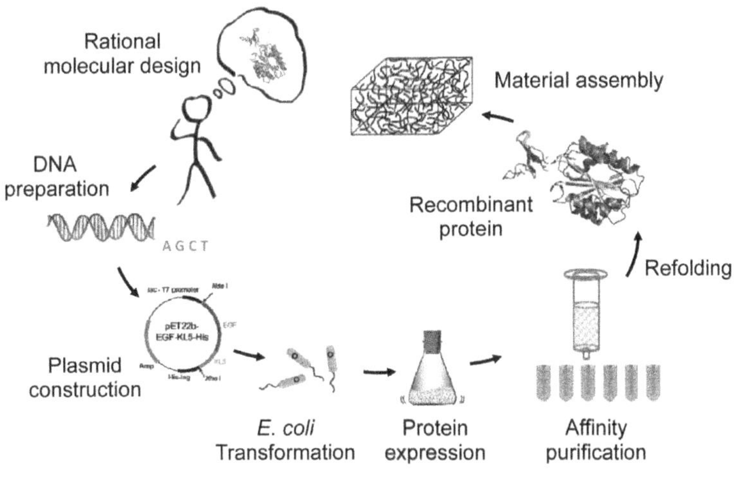

Figure 14.2 Outline of recombinant polypeptide synthesis.

In any organism, proteins are synthesized through the biosynthetic pathway. Genomic DNA encoding an amino acid sequence is first transcribed to messenger RNA (mRNA) by RNA polymerase. Then, the genetic code on the mRNA encoded as a nucleotide codon sequence is translated into a polypeptide by transfer RNA and the ribosome. Importantly, this flow is available even for artificial sequences designed on the table.

It is worthwhile to adopt the idea of modular polypeptides for the rational design of biofunctional materials. In nature, proteins or protein domains can be classified based on their function. Different classes of modular polypeptides can be considered as building blocks of biofunctional materials, such as adaptors, skeletal components, trophic factors, morphogenic factors, and enzymes. Depending on the design principles, more than two modules can be combined into a single polypeptide molecule. Fortunately, the structural information of these modular components is available in protein databases and can be utilized to design a DNA sequence corresponding to the polypeptide building block of interest.

For the recombinant synthesis of polypeptides, we first need to construct a plasmid DNA that contains a DNA sequence encoding the exogenous polypeptide of interest and promoter, replicator, and antibiotic resistance gene. Cells such as bacteria and mammalian cells are transformed with plasmid DNA and then cultivated to express exogenous polypeptides through a pathway similar to the biosynthesis of endogenous proteins. The polypeptide is purified using an appropriate method, such as affinity chromatography, and is used as a building block for biofunctional materials.

14.4 Biofunctional Materials Design Principles

There could be three major reasons for the poor survival of transplanted cells—induction of anoikis, attack by inflammatory cells, and poor microenvironment.

Most cells are adhesion-dependent; therefore, apoptosis is induced when cells lose their attachment to the ECM. This phenomenon is referred to as anoikis. Generally, cells are cultivated ex vivo in an adherent state and harvested for transplantation.

During these processes, cells temporarily lose their cell adhesion molecule-mediated physiological adhesion. This triggers the initiation of an apoptotic cascade.

Second, inflammatory reactions are activated at the transplantation site, where the tissues are often under pathological conditions. The mechanical stress caused by the transplantation procedure, such as the injection of cells with a needle, may also result in an inflammatory response. Consequently, inflammatory cells such as macrophages and activated microglia infiltrate the transplanted site to attack exogenous cells by phagocytosis and cytokine release.

Third, the microenvironment around the transplanted cells is not always appropriate for cells to proliferate, differentiate, and function as expected. This is because there are no necessary signaling molecules such as trophic factors, growth factors, and morphogens.

Considering the above reasons, attempts have been made to create biofunctional carriers that prevent cell death due to anoikis, inflammatory attack, and inappropriate microenvironments, thus leading to improved survival of transplanted cells. To molecularly design biofunctional carriers, genetically engineered polypeptides have been utilized. The following examples are mostly concerned with cell replacement therapy using neural stem cells (NSCs) for disorders of the central nervous system as an excellent example to demonstrate the feasibility of this strategy.

As shown in Figure 14.3, collagen hydrogels were first considered as a physical barrier against activated inflammatory microglia invading the transplanted site. Collagen is biodegradable and undergoes spontaneous gelation through the triple-helical association of collagen monomers under physiological conditions, even in the presence of cells. This property can be used to embed NSCs into hydrogels. Since collagen is more or less inert to NSCs, further attempts were made to incorporate polypeptides capable of interacting with integrins to avoid anoikis and growth factor receptors to optimize cellular microenvironments. Details of these modifications are described in the following sections.

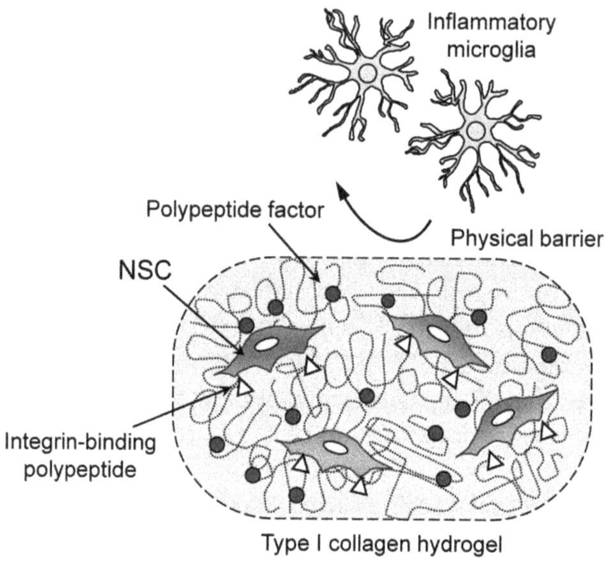

Figure 14.3 Design principles for biofunctional materials that serve to improve the survival of NSCs.

14.5 Incorporation of Integrin-Binding Polypeptides

Integrins are cell surface transmembrane proteins involved in cell adhesion to the ECM, and ECM–integrin binding activates intracellular signal transduction to prevent apoptosis [12]. Therefore, the incorporation of integrin-binding polypeptides into collagen hydrogels appears to be effective in improving cell survival. To tether an integrin-binding polypeptide to collagen networks in the presence of living cells, the hydrogel must be modified under mild conditions while avoiding chemical reactions in organic solvents.

To meet this requirement, attempts have been made to prepare a conjugate of integrin-binding polypeptides with a collagen-binding domain (CBD) derived from the von Willebrand factor (vWF), which recognizes the specific sequence of the collagen fibril assembly [13]. In a previous study [14], an integrin-binding peptide derived from the G3 domain of the laminin α3 chain (LNG3) was fused with the CBD from vWF to obtain the LNG3-CBD chimera (Figure 14.4a). It was demonstrated that the chimeric polypeptide LNG3-CBD effectively bound to collagen while promoting integrin-mediated adhesion of NSCs (Figure 14.4b).

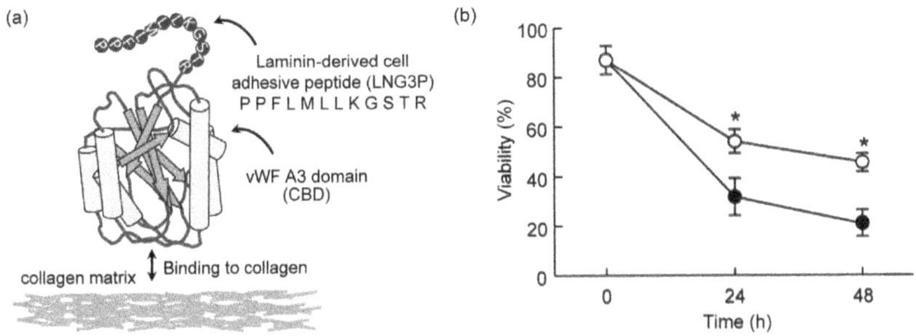

Figure 14.4 Incorporation of the integrin-binding peptide into collagen hydrogel. (a) Structure of LNG3–CBD. (b) Viability of NSCs in collagen hydrogels with and without LNG3–CBD incorporated. Adapted with permission from *Bioconjugate Chem.*, 2009; 20:976–983. ©2009 American Chemical Society [14].

A larger polypeptide domain could also be incorporated into collagen networks [15]. As shown in Figure 14.5a, the entire LNG3 domain was connected to the collagen-binding peptide derived from decorin (SYIRIADTNIT), with a helical linker inserted between them (CLG3). In addition, a separate polypeptide was prepared by connecting the C-terminal region of the laminin γ1 chain (LP), a helical peptide, and the collagen-binding peptide from decorin (CLP). According to a previous study [16], the C-terminal 9-residue peptide from the laminin γ1 chain modulates the integrin binding of globular domains of the laminin α chain in its vicinity. Therefore, the two polypeptides, CLG3 and CLP, were designed to spontaneously associate with each other through coiled-coil formation by helical linkers.

It was shown by circular dichroism spectroscopy that mixing CLG3 with CLP increased the α-helix content, indicating the spontaneous formation of a CLG3–CLP heterodimer. The CLG3–CLP complex was adsorbed onto the collagen-coated polystyrene surface at a density of 0.33 μg/cm^2. When NSCs obtained from fetal rats were cultured for 24 h on the CLG3–CLP-presenting collagen surface, the cell density reached a level similar to that on the laminin-coated surface (positive control). It was shown that integrins α6 and β1 were involved in NSC adhesion to the CLG3–CLP presenting surface. As shown in Figure 14.5b, the number of living NSCs in the collagen hydrogel incorporating CLG3–CLP increased 7-fold during 7 days. In contrast, in the pure collagen hydrogel, the living cell density remained constant for 7 days. These results suggest that incorporating the integrin-binding polypeptide complex into a collagen hydrogel increases the number of living NSCs.

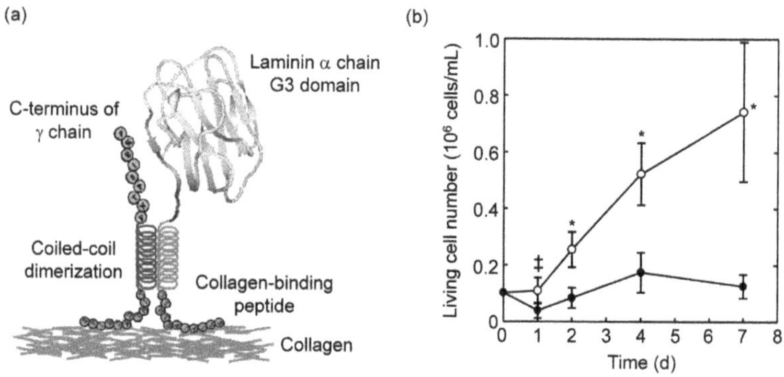

Figure 14.5 Incorporation of integrin-binding polypeptide domain into collagen hydrogel. (a) Structure of the CLG3–CLP heterodimer bound to collagen. (b) The number of living NSCs in CLG3–CLP-incorporated and control collagen hydrogel. Adapted with permission from *Bioconjugate Chem.*, 2012; 23:212–221. ©2012 American Chemical Society [15].

The modified collagen hydrogel was further examined in vivo to assess the feasibility of maintaining the number of transplanted NSCs in the recipient's brain [17]. This study used histidine-tag-fused LP (HLP) instead of collagen-binding LP (CLP). Enhanced green fluorescent protein (EGFP)-transformed NSCs were embedded in CLG3–HLP-incorporated collagen hydrogel and directly infused into the rat striatum. Figure 14.6a shows the results of the histological analysis performed 3, 7, and 15 days after transplantation. Tissue sections were immunostained with antibodies against EGFP (green) and Iba1 (microglial marker; red). EGFP-expressing cells transplanted with collagen and CLG3–HLP are prominently observed. On the 15th day, the cells had an extended shape. In contrast, when cells were embedded in a collagen hydrogel without CLG3 and HLP, EGFP-expressing cells were unremarkable 3 days after transplantation. On day 15th, it is difficult to visualize EGFP-expressing cells. Quantitative data for the number of EGFP-expressing cells (Figure 14.6b) are consistent with previously described observations. These results led us to conclude that the collagen hydrogel incorporating the engineered cell-adhesive polypeptides significantly improved the survival of NSCs transplanted into the brain by blocking the infiltration of inflammatory microglia and providing adhesive substrates for transplanted cells.

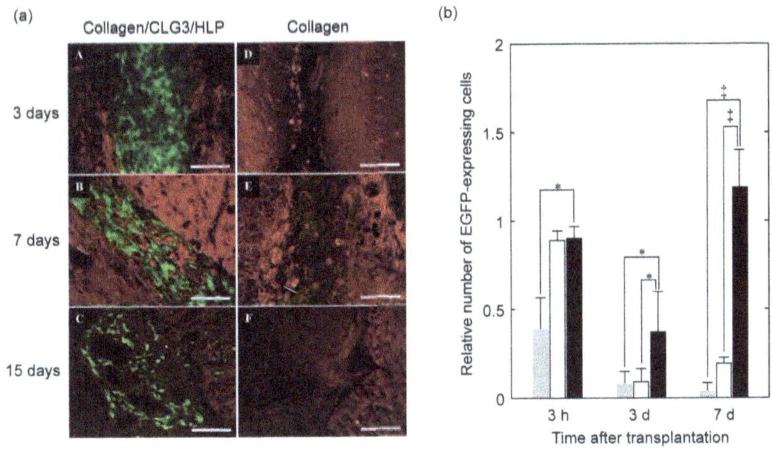

Figure 14.6 In vivo evaluation for the survival of NSCs suspended in collagen hydrogel with and without CLG3–HLP. (a) Immunofluorescence staining of the tissue sections using antibodies against EGFP (green) and Iba1 (red). Histological analysis was performed 3, 7, and 15 days after transplantation into the rat brain. Scale bar: 50 μm. (b) Relative number of EGFP-expressing cells. NSCs were suspended in collagen hydrogels (closed bar) with or (open bar) without CLG3–HLP or in the medium (hatched bar). Reproduced with permission from *Bioconjugate Chem.*, 2013; 24:1798–1804. ©2013 American Chemical Society [17].

Keratin can also be used to fabricate biofunctional materials that incorporate integrin-binding polypeptides. Keratins contain a long α-helical domain that is involved in the association of two keratin molecules via coiled-coil formation. The keratin dimers thus formed were further assembled into nanofilaments by lateral association. These processes have been used to prepare hydrogels [18]. As shown in Figure 14.7a, a laminin G3 domain was fused to the N-terminus of keratin-14 (LG3K14) [19]. The chimeric polypeptide, LG3K14, was mixed with wild-type keratins to obtain a hydrogel. NSCs cultured on the hydrogel proliferated considerably and extended dendrites in 3D (Figure 14.7b). This is in marked contrast to NSCs on the pure keratin hydrogel with no LG3K14. From these results, it was assumed that LNG3 fused with a keratin-derived helical polypeptide is also effective in improving the survival of NSCs in keratin networks. However, strong denaturants are required to dissolve keratin, making it difficult to disperse cells in the hydrogel before transplantation.

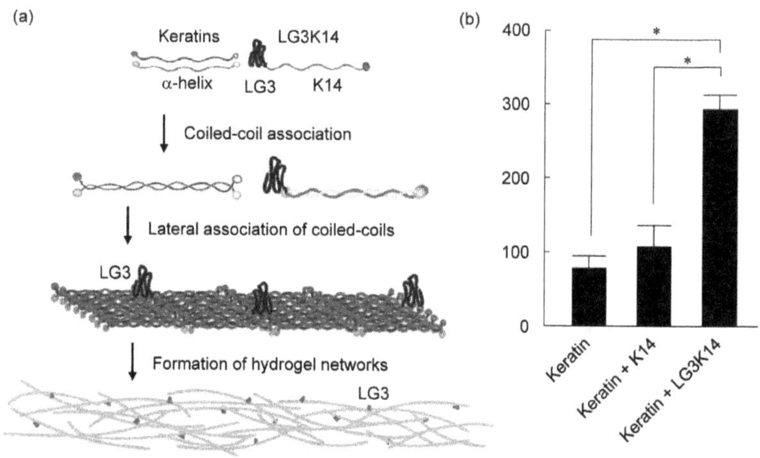

Figure 14.7 Keratin hydrogels modified with the integrin-binding polypeptide. (a) Schematic diagram showing the self-assembly of keratins in the presence of LG3K14. (b) Adhesion of NSCs to keratin hydrogel modified with LG3K14. Adapted with permission from *Biomacromolecules*, 2008; 9:1411–1416. ©2008 American Chemical Society [19].

14.6 Incorporation of Protein Factors

As described earlier, the site where cells are transplanted does not always provide optimal microenvironments for the cells to survive, proliferate, migrate, differentiate, and function. In this regard, incorporating protein factors such as growth factors, neurotrophins, and chemokines into cell carriers is effective for optimizing cellular microenvironments.

In a previous study [20], epidermal growth factor (EGF), known as a mitogen for NSCs [21], was fused with a vWF-derived CBD (EGF-CBD) (Figure 14.8a) and incorporated into a collagen hydrogel in the presence of NSCs isolated from fetal rats. The cells were cultured in the hydrogels for 7 days, and the number of cells was determined using the colorimetric method. The results showed that the proliferation of NSCs was significantly promoted in collagen hydrogels with incorporated EGF-CBD compared to control hydrogels (Figure 14.8b), demonstrating that EGF incorporation into cell carriers is effective in promoting the proliferation of NSCs.

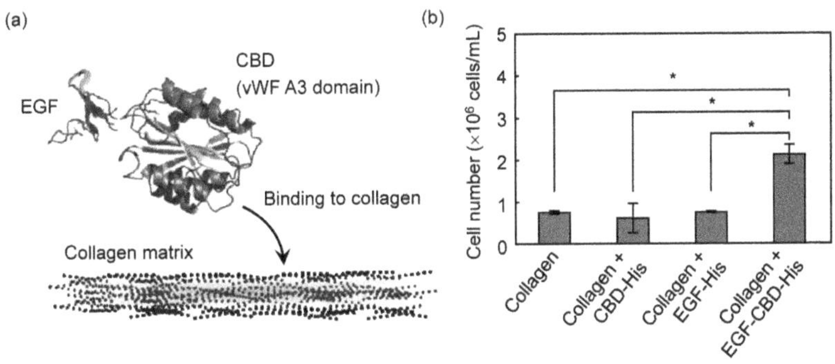

Figure 14.8 Incorporation of EGF chimera into collagen hydrogel. (a) Structure of the EGF–CBD binding to collagen. (b) Number of NSCs present in EGF–CBD-incorporated and control collagen hydrogels. In vitro culture period: 7 days. Adapted with permission from *Biomaterials*, 2011; 32: 4737–4743. ©2011 Elsevier Science [20].

Neurotrophins are another class of proteins that have a significant impact on the behavior of neural cells. Therefore, recombinant DNA technology was used to prepare brain-derived neurotrophic factor (BDNF) fused with a hexahistidine sequence capable of chelating metal ions, such as Ni(II) and Zn(II) [22]. The engineered BDNF was incorporated by chelation into a hyaluronic acid hydrogel modified with Zn(II) (Figure 14.9a). A 70-mer polypeptide possessing a hexahistidine sequence at both ends (CLP) was prepared and used to introduce cross-links in hyaluronic acid to form hydrogels under physiological conditions.

NSCs were cultured within the hydrogel, and cell viability was evaluated 1, 2, and 3 days after the onset of cell culture. The results showed that a significantly larger number of cells survived in the BDNF-incorporated hydrogel than in the control hydrogel (Figure 14.9b).

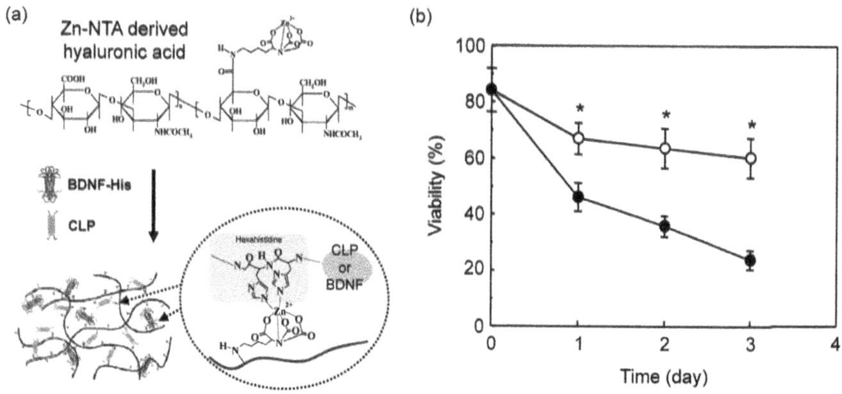

Figure 14.9 Incorporation of BDNF chimera into a hyaluronic acid hydrogel. (a) Schematic representation for the formation of BDNF-incorporated hyaluronic acid hydrogel. (b) Viability of NSCs cultured in the BDNF-incorporated (open symbol) and control (closed symbol) hydrogels. Adapted with permission from *Biomaterials*, 2009; 30:4581–4589. ©2009 Elsevier Science [22].

Kobayashi et al. demonstrated that a similar approach was effective for ectopically generating artificial lymph nodes with structural and functional similarities to their natural counterparts [23, 24]. In this study, multiple chemokines, including CXCL12, CXCL13, CCL19, and CCL21, were fused with a collagen-binding peptide from decorin and loaded in a spatially controlled manner within a collagen sponge for sustained release.

14.7 Summary

As discussed in this chapter, various building blocks for assembling biofunctional materials can be rationally prepared using recombinant DNA technology. Thus, biofunctional materials have a wide variety of potential applications, particularly in regenerative medicine. Since there is infinite freedom in designing polypeptide structures, increasing attention will be paid to this pathway for the fabrication of diverse biofunctional materials.

Acknowledgments

This work was supported by a Grant-in-Aid for Scientific Research, JSPS (No. 19KK0278).

References

1. Ratner, B. D., Hoffman, A. S., Schoen, F. J. and Lemons, J. E. (2004). *Biomaterial Science: An Introduction to Materials in Medicine*, 2nd Ed., eds. Ratner, B. D., Hoffman, A. S., Schoen, F. J. and Lemons, J. E., "Biomaterials science: A multidisciplinary endeavor" (Elsevier Academic Press, San Diego) pp. 1–9.
2. Ntege, E. H., Sunami, H. and Shimizu, Y. (2020). Advances in regenerative therapy: A review of the literature and future directions, *Regen. Ther.*, **14**, pp. 136–153.
3. Maqsood, M., Kang, M., Wu, X., Chen, J., Teng, L. and Qiu, L. (2020). Adult mesenchymal stem cells and their exosomes: Sources, characteristics, and application in regenerative medicine, *Life Sci.*, **256**, p. 118002.
4. Takahashi, K., Tanabe, K., Ohnuki, M., Narita, M., Ichisaka, T., Tomoda, K. and Yamanaka, S (2007). Induction of pluripotent stem cells from adult human fibroblasts by defined factors, *Cell*, **131**, pp. 861–872.
5. Khalil, A. M. (2020). The genome editing revolution: review, *J. Genet. Eng. Biotechnol.*, **18**, p. 68.
6. De Luca, M., Aiuti, A., Cossu, G., Parmar, M., Pellegrini, G. and Robey, P. G. (2019). Advances in stem cell research and therapeutic development, *Nat. Cell Biol.*, **21**, pp. 801–811.
7. Zhang, Y., Wang, X., Pong, M., Chen, L. and Ye, Z. (2017). Application of bioreactor in stem cell culture, *J. Biomed. Sci. Eng.*, **10**, pp. 485–499.
8. Samsonraj, R. M., Raghunath, M., Nurcombe, V., Hui, J. H., van Wijnen, A. J. and Cool, S. M. (2017). Concise review: Multifaceted characterization of human mesenchymal stem cells for use in regenerative medicine, *Stem Cells Transl. Med.*, **6**, pp. 2173–2185.

9. Peserico, A., Di Berardino, C., Russo, V., Capacchietti, G., Di Giacinto, O., Canciello, A., Camerano Spelta Rapini, C. and Barboni, B. (2022). Nanotechnology-assisted cell tracking, *Nanomaterials*, **12**, p. 1414.

10. Moeinabadi-Bidgoli, K., Babajani, A., Yazdanpanah, G., Farhadihosseinabadi, B., Jamshidi, E., Bahrami, S. and Niknejad, H. (2021). Translational insights into stem cell preconditioning: From molecular mechanisms to preclinical applications, *Biomed. Pharmacother.*, **142**, p. 112026.

11. Nakano, A. and Kato, K. (2022). Recombinant protein synthesis for nanomaterial assembly: Technical overview, *Bull. Soc. Nano Sci. Technol.*, **20**, pp. 31–37.

12. Desgrosellier, J. and Cheresh, D. (2010). Integrins in cancer: Biological implications and therapeutic opportunities, *Nat. Rev. Cancer*, **10**, pp. 9–22.

13. Kato, K., Sato, H. and Iwata, H. (2007). Ultrastructural study on the specific binding of genetically engineered epidermal growth factor to type I collagen fibrils, *Bioconjugate Chem.*, **18**, pp. 2137–2143.

14. Hiraoka, M., Kato, K., Nakaji-Hirabayashi, T. and Iwata, H. (2009). Enhanced survival of neural cells embedded in hydrogels composed of collagen and laminin-derived cell adhesive peptide, *Bioconjugate Chem.*, **20**, pp. 976–983.

15. Nakaji-Hirabayashi, T. Kato, K. and Iwata, H. (2012). Improvement of neural stem cell survival in collagen hydrogels by incorporating laminin-derived cell adhesive polypeptides, *Bioconjugate Chem.*, **23**, pp. 212–221.

16. Ido, H., Nakamura, A., Kobayashi, R., Ito, S., Li, S., Futaki, S. and Sekiguchi, K. (2007). The requirement of the glutamic acid residue at the third position from the carboxyl termini of the laminin gamma chains in integrin binding by laminins, *J. Biol. Chem.*, **282**, pp. 11144–11154.

17. Nakaji-Hirabayashi, T., Kato, K. and Iwata, H. (2013). In vivo study on the survival of neural stem cells transplanted into the rat brain with a collagen hydrogel that incorporates laminin-derived polypeptides, *Bioconjugate Chem.*, **24**, pp. 1798–1804.

18. Sierpinski, P., Garrett, J., Ma, J., Apel, P., Klorig, D., Smith, T., Koman, L., Atala, A. and Van Dyke, M. (2008). The use of keratin biomaterials derived from human hair for the promotion of rapid regeneration of peripheral nerves, *Biomaterials*, **29**, pp. 118–128.

19. Nakaji-Hirabayashi, T., Kato, K. and Iwata, H. (2008). Self-assembling chimeric protein for the construction of biodegradable hydrogels capable of interaction with integrins expressed on neural stem/progenitor cells, *Biomacromolecules*, **9**, pp. 1411–1416.

20. Egawa, E. Y., Kato, K., Hiraoka, M., Nakaji-Hirabayashi, T. and Iwata, H. (2011). Enhanced proliferation of neural stem cells in a collagen hydrogel incorporating engineered epidermal growth factor, *Biomaterials*, **32**, pp. 4737–4743.

21. Yamauchi, Y, Hirata, I., K. Tanimoto, K. and Kato, K. (2020). Epidermal growth factor-immobilized surfaces for the selective expansion of neural progenitor cells derived from induced pluripotent stem cells, *Biotechnol. Bioeng.*, **117**, pp. 2741–2748.

22. Nakaji-Hirabayashi, T., Kato, K. and Iwata, H. (2009). Hyaluronic acid hydrogel loaded with genetically-engineered brain-derived neurotrophic factor as a neural cell carrier, *Biomaterials*, **30**, pp. 4581–4589.

23. Kobayashi, Y., Kato, K. and Watanabe, T. (2011). Synthesis of functional artificial lymphoid tissues, *Discovery Med.*, **12**, pp. 351–362.

24. Kobayashi, Y., Kato, K., Nakamura, M. and Watanabe, T. (2016) *Synthetic Immunology*, eds. Watanabe, T. and Takahama, Y., "Synthesis of functional tertiary lymphoid organs," (Springer Nature, Berlin) pp. 151–169.

Chapter 15

Development of Etak, an Ethoxysilane-Based Immobilized Antibacterial and Antiviral Agent

Hiroki Nikawa[a] and Takemasa Sakaguchi[b]

[a]*Oral Biology & Engineering,*
Graduate School of Biomedical and Health Sciences, Hiroshima University,
1-2-3 Kasumi, Minami-ku, Hiroshima 734-8553, Japan
[b]*Graduate School of Biomedical and Health Sciences, Hiroshima University,*
1-2-3 Kasumi, Minami-ku, Hiroshima 734-8553 Japan

hirocky@hiroshima-u.ac.jp

Dr. Nikawa's original specialty is prosthodontics, and he has been studying microbial biofilms in the oral cavity. It is estimated that 700–800 kinds of microbes are present in the oral cavity, and approximately 10^{11} microbes are present in 1 g of plaque. Therefore, infectious diseases in the oral cavity such as dental caries, periodontal diseases, and oral candidiasis are caused by various microbes [1]. Furthermore, it has been pointed out that plaque microbes deposited in the oral cavity can serve as a reservoir, and cause aspiration pneumonia due to their aspiration, bacteremia due to transfer into the bloodstream during tooth extraction, and even thrombosis and other conditions. We have

Biomedical Engineering: Imaging Systems, Electric Devices, and Medical Materials
Edited by Akihiro Miyauchi and Hiroyuki Kagechika

ISBN 978-981-5129-16-8 (Hardcover), 978-1-003-46404-4 (eBook)
www.jennystanford.com

been studying the mechanism of microbial biofilm formation in the oral cavity, and have revealed that microbial biofilm formation is deeply related to the oral microbiome, the properties of substrate surfaces such as teeth and restorations, and biological components such as body fluids, like saliva or serum.

On the other hand, in the course of daily clinical practice, disabled patients were troubled by the fact that their teeth were getting worse and worse despite having them repaired, because they could not brush them adequately. In such a situation, conversely, we started to research the prevention of the growth of pathogenic microbes in the oral cavity by utilizing the microbiome, the properties of adherents such as teeth and restorations, and biological components [2], and one of the methods, we devised was to immobilize antimicrobial agents on intraoral restorations and dentures. In a series of such studies, the synthesis of Octadecyl dimethyl (3-triethoxysilylpropyl) ammonium chloride (hereafter, "Etak"), an ethoxy group, was commissioned to Manac Incorporated, a local company in Hiroshima, and a product was prepared.

15.1 Immobilized Antimicrobial Agent Etak and Its Antibacterial Effects

Etak is an antimicrobial agent classified as a quaternary ammonium salt, such as benzalkonium chloride, which is also used as a disinfectant in the medical field [3]. On the other hand, it is an ethoxysilane compound, which can be safely immobilized on various surfaces without generating toxic substances upon hydrolysis, such as methoxy groups (Figure 15.1). In other words, the disinfectant is immobilized on a surface at the same time as the surface is disinfected, and antibacterial and antiviral treatments are possible.

15.1.1 Immobilization on Towels and Antimicrobial Properties

Table 15.1 shows the relationship between Etak solution concentration and the antimicrobial properties and washing resistance of towels after Etak treatment. This test was conducted in accordance with the JIS L 1902:2002 test of antibacterial activity and efficacy on textile products. Gram-positive bacteria *Staphylococcus aureus*, methicillin-resistant *Staphylococcus aureus* (MRSA), and Gram-negative bacteria *Escherichia coli* were used as test strains. Approximately 10,000 of each kind of bacteria were inoculated on the surfaces of test towels and incubated for 18 hours. With the untreated towels, shown at the bottom of Table 15.1, each kind of test bacteria grew to 10^6–10^7 cells, but in the towels treated with 3% and 0.3% Etak for 2–3 minutes at room temperature, no bacteria were detected, suggesting a high probability that the inoculated bacteria were killed. Moreover, although bacteria grew on towels treated with 0.03% Etak, the bacteriostatic activity value was 2.2 or higher in the Log_{10} value, meeting the JIS standard for antibacterial treatment.

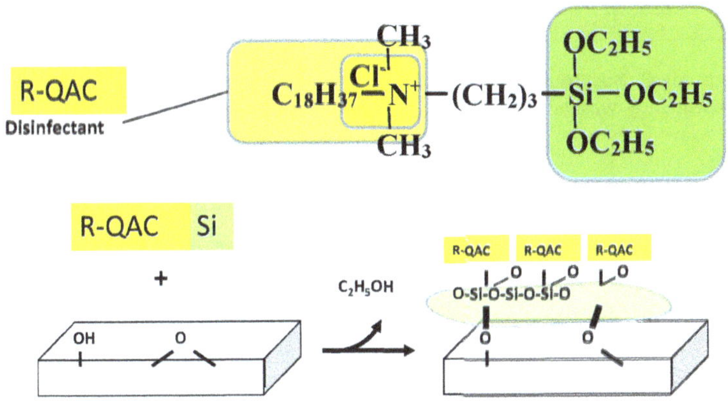

Figure 15.1 Structure of Etak and mode of binding to surfaces.

The number of washing resistance tests in JIS is also shown in the "Wash" column of the table, and in all cases, the antibacterial effect did not decrease even after 40 washing cycles, regardless of the Etak treatment concentration. In addition, for fibers such as cotton and cotton blends, the data show that the red mark for antibacterial treatment is 50 times or more for commercial washing resistance.

Based on these results, we set the concentration slightly higher than the low concentration during this testing and considered that it might be desirable to use it at a concentration of 0.06 to 3% for textile treatment and 0.06 to 0.09% for general use.

Table 15.1 Effects of concentration of Etak solution on antimicrobial properties and wash resistance of Etak-treated towels

Etak Conc.	Wash	*S. aureus*		MRSA		*E. coli*	
%	Number of repeat	Viable count (CFU)	Bacteriostatic activity	Viable count (CFU)	Bacteriostatic activity	Viable count (CFU)	Bacteriostatic activity
0.03%	0	65000	2.2	290000	2.55	44000	2.34
	10	25000	2.61	50000	4.32	8500	3.05
	40	27000	2.6	50000	4.32	5000	3.32
0.30%	0	—	7>	—	7>	—	7>
	10	—	7>	—	7>	—	7>
	40	—	7>	—	7>	—	7>
3.00%	0	—	7>	—	7>	—	7>
	10	—	7>	—	7>	—	7>
	40	—	7>	—	7>	—	7>
untreated control	0	13000000		27000000		1300000	
	10	61000000		77000000		86000000	
	40	41000000		63000000		59000000	

Each towel was treated with Etak solutions at room temperature for 3 min, subsequently washed with tapped water, dried in a desiccator, and sterilized by autoclave.

15.1.2 Antibacterial Spectrum of Etak

The antibacterial spectrum of Etak has been investigated in liquid formulations of 0.06–0.09% or textile treatment products, which are already in practical use, and a spectrum similar to that of quaternary ammonium salts has been obtained with Gram-positive bacteria, Gram-negative bacteria, and some kinds of fungi and molds. Specifically, for Gram-positive bacteria, it is effective against *Staphylococcus aureus* (both MRSA and MSSA), *Staph. epidermidis*, *Streptococcus mutans*, *Strep. sobrinus*, and *Bacillus cereus* (not effective against spores). For Gram-negative bacteria, it is effective against *Escherichia coli* (including O-157), *Salmonella enterica*, and *Corynebacterium xerosis* (body odor bacteria). Its bactericidal activity against these bacteria has been confirmed. Because it does not have a cell wall, it is also effective against mycoplasma, which has recently become a problem in the medical field because it is resistant to antibiotics. However, it is mostly ineffective against *Pseudomonas aeruginosa*, which causes problems such as nosocomial infections.

For fungi, it is effective against and kills *Malassezia* and *Candida*. For filamentous fungi, it is effective against *Aspergillus niger* and *Cladosporium* black mold. It shows bacteriostatic activity against the well-known athlete's foot fungus *Trichophyton rubrum*, and *Trichophyton tonsurans*, a new type of athlete's foot fungus.

15.1.3 Antiviral Spectrum of Quaternary Ammonium Salts and Anti-Influenza Effects of Etak

Quaternary ammonium salts are known for their antiviral spectrum and are generally capable of contact inactivation of viruses with envelopes. Since the disinfectant portion of Etak is a quaternary ammonium salt, it is thought to be effective against viruses with similar envelopes: influenza viruses (human [A/H3N2, A/H1N1], avian and swine), parainfluenza viruses, hepatitis viruses (types B and C), human immunodeficiency virus-1, SARS (corona) viruses, RS viruses, measles virus, herpes viruses, mumps virus, and rabies virus (Table 15.2).

Table 15.2 Antiviral spectra of quarterly ammonium salts

influenza viruses
parainfluenza viruses
hepatitis viruses (types B and C)
human immunodeficiency virus-1
SARS (corona) viruses
RS viruses
measles virus
herpes viruses
mumps virus
rabies virus

The antiviral spectrum of Etak has also been investigated, including liquid formulations and textile treatment products that are already in practical use. First, to determine the concentrations at which Etak is effective against influenza viruses, we present the results of an investigation of the antiviral activity of Etak against the H5N3 avian influenza virus using a solution of Etak diluted in distilled water (Milli-Q water). The results showed that all avian influenza viruses could be inactivated with a concentration of 20 ppm (Figure 15.2).

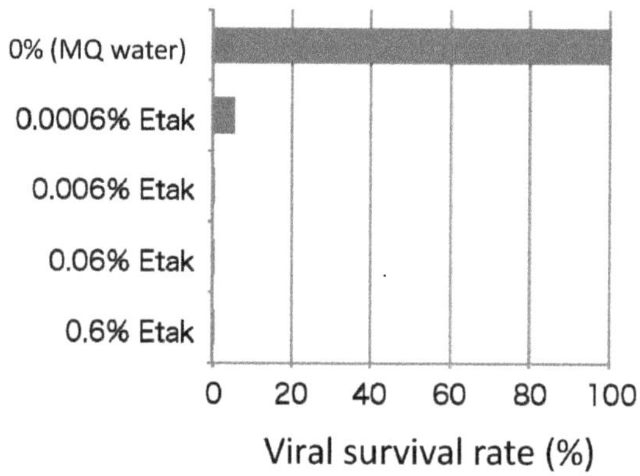

Figure 15.2 Antiviral effect of Etak solution against avian influenza virus. Etak was applied to avian influenza virus A/swan/Shimane/499/83 (H5N3) for 3 minutes, and the remaining virus titer was measured.

Next, we will investigate the inactivation of viruses on surfaces immobilized with Etak. Figure 15.3 shows the inactivation activity (residual) of using 0.12% Etak or 0.012% (70% ethanol solution) on towels against the pandemic 2009 influenza virus (A/H1N1) after treatment at room temperature for 3 minutes, then rinsing, drying, and autoclaving. In both cases of immobilization, more than 99% inactivation was observed in both samples. In addition, although the data is not presented here, even for SARS-CoV-2, which has caused the COVID-19 pandemic since 2020, the inactivation activity with the Etak solution itself and with fabrics and non-woven fabrics on which Etak was immobilized was confirmed to be greater than that of influenza viruses.

Etak is also effective against some non-enveloped viruses, such as human norovirus and adenovirus. Human norovirus is known as a non-enveloped RNA virus that causes acute nonbacterial gastroenteritis, and a major outbreak occurred in Japan at the end of 2012. Feline calicivirus is usually used as a surrogate to examine antiviral effects against human norovirus, and Etak shows high inactivation activity against feline calicivirus (Figure 15.4a).

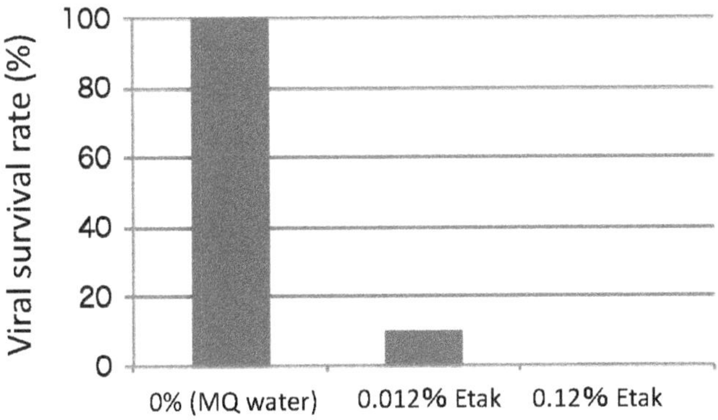

Figure 15.3 Effect of Etak against influenza virus (Pandemic 2009 (H1N1)). Inactivation effect (residual rate) against influenza virus on towel surface treated with Etak for 3 minutes at room temperature.

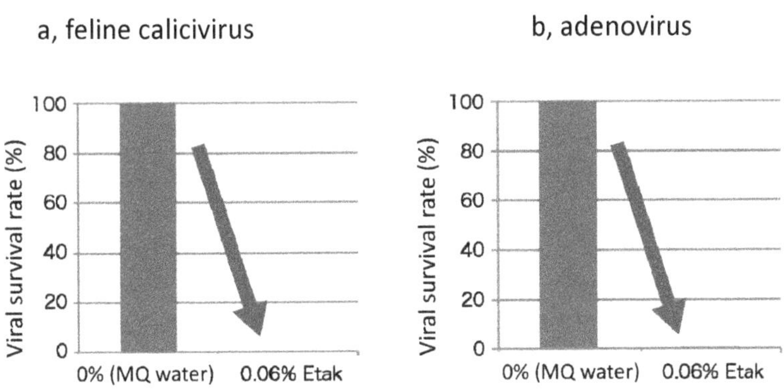

Figure 15.4 Effects of Etak against non-enveloped viruses (feline calicivirus, adenovirus).

It also shows high inactivation activity against adenoviruses, which, together with rhinoviruses and other viruses, cause "cold syndrome" and have attracted attention in the ophthalmologic field as a cause of epidemic keratoconjunctivitis and acute follicular conjunctivitis (Figure 15.4b).

Etak was allowed to act on feline calicivirus (a) and adenovirus (b) for 24 hours, and the remaining infectivity titer was measured.

15.2 Safety of Etak

15.2.1 Mutagenicity Test (Ames Test)

To investigate the mutagenic potential of Etak solution (60% Etak ethanol solution), the results of reversion mutation testing conducted using *Escherichia coli* WP2 *uvrA* and four strains of *Salmonella typhimurium* TA according to Ministry of Labour Notification No. 77 (September 1, 1988) were reported. The results of the study on specimens at doses ranging from 0.610 to 1,250 μg/plate showed no increase in the revertant colony count, and Etak was reported to be negative for mutagenic potential.

15.2.2 Acute Oral Toxicity Testing Using Mice

Etak 60% stock solution (ethanol solution) was diluted with an injectable solution to prepare test solutions of 400, 300, 200, and 100 mg/ml, and the results of a single oral administration of this solution to mice at a volume of 2,000 mg/kg and a single administration of the injectable solution water to a control group with observation for 14 days were reported. As a result, no abnormalities were observed after administration at 2,000 mg/kg, indicating that the LD50 value after a single oral dose in the specimen mice is greater than 2,000 mg/kg. In addition, although the study was conducted only with female mice, decreased spontaneous locomotion was observed in all cases with 8,000, 6,000, and 4,000 mg/kg doses and with two cases of 2,000 mg/kg doses from 5 minutes after administration, which recovered by 4 hours after administration, and subsequently no abnormalities were observed. The LD50 value for a single oral administration in the specimen female mice was reported to be 8,000 mg/kg or higher.

15.2.3 Primary Skin Irritation Test Using Rabbits

The results of the primary skin irritation test conducted using a 0.6% solution of Etak as a specimen in rabbits according to the OECD Guidelines for the Testing of Chemicals 404 (2002) were reported. Specimens were openly applied to the intact and injured skin of three rabbits for 24 hours. As a result, no irritant reaction was observed at 1, 24, 48, and 72 hours after removal. The primary irritation index (PII) obtained according to the Federal Register (1972) is 0, and the specimens were evaluated to be in the "non-irritant" category in the primary skin irritation test using rabbits.

15.2.4 Continuous Skin Irritation Test Using Rabbits

We have evaluated a continuous skin irritation test using four solutions of Etak in two concentrations of 0.15 and 1.5% with distilled water and 50% ethanol as solvents, and distilled water and 50% ethanol as controls, for 14 days of continuous open application to rabbit skin. As a result, it was reported that distilled water, 50% ethanol, 0.15% Etak distilled water solution, 0.15% Etak 50% ethanol solution, and 1.5% Etak distilled water solution were in the "negligible" category, while the 1.5% Etak 50% ethanol solution was in the "slightly" category.

15.2.5 Eye Irritation Test Using Rabbits

Eye irritation tests were conducted using Etak solution as a specimen in rabbits according to the OECD Guidelines for the Testing of Chemicals 405 (2002). Three rabbits received drops of 0.1 ml of the test solution (Etak concentration 0.09%) in one eye and 0.1 ml of water for injection in the other eye as solvent control, followed by a 30-second eye wash 30 seconds after the drops. As a result, in the test and control eyes, redness of the eyelid and conjunctiva were observed in all cases 1 hour after the eyedrops but disappeared in 24 hours. The maximum mean total score during the observation period, calculated according to the Draize method, was 2.0 in both the test and control eyes (1 hour after eyedrops). Based on these results, in the eye irritation test using rabbits, the test solution was evaluated to be in the category "non-irritant" when the eye was washed after the test solution was administered to the eye.

15.2.6 Human Patch Test

Forty healthy human subjects (11 males and 29 females; 25–67 years old) were tested, in which a 0.1 ml drop of Etak 50% ethanol solution adjusted to 1.5% was administered to a 2.0 by 2.0 cm square of the upper back and left until the skin surface dried. In addition, a 0.1 ml drop of saline solution was administered as a control substance in parallel with the test substance, and left until the skin surface dried. Skin symptoms at the contact site were visually determined 24 and 48 hours after contact, and observational evaluation was performed. The evaluation was based on the size and presence of irritant symptoms (erythema, edema, blistering) according to the Japanese criteria. As a result, no skin changes were observed in all 40 subjects at both 24 and 48 hours of contact.

From the results of these safety studies, Etak has been registered as an ingredient name in the International Nomenclature of Cosmetic Ingredients published by the Cosmetic Toiletry and Fragrance Association.

15.3 Applications of Etak as Cosmetics

15.3.1 Oral Cosmetics

In today's so-called aging and super-aging society, the number of patients complaining of xerostomia (dry mouth) is increasing along with the number of elderly patients in the dental field. Xerostomia is caused by a decrease in salivary secretory capacity due to a decline in physiological function, drug-related side effects due to an increase in the number of drugs taken, psychological factors such as stress, systemic diseases such as abnormal metabolism of body fluids and electrolytes, and structural changes in the salivary glands due to irradiation or Sjögren's syndrome. The causes are often overlapping. It is known that such xerostomia not only exacerbates dental caries and periodontal disease, but also interferes with eating and speaking due to decreased saliva production, which has lubricating, self-cleaning, and antibacterial actions, thus significantly impairing quality of life.

We are developing an oral moisturizing agent that can impart antibacterial properties to the surface of the tooth component hydroxyapatite as a moisturizer in the oral cosmetic category as shown in Fig. 15.5.

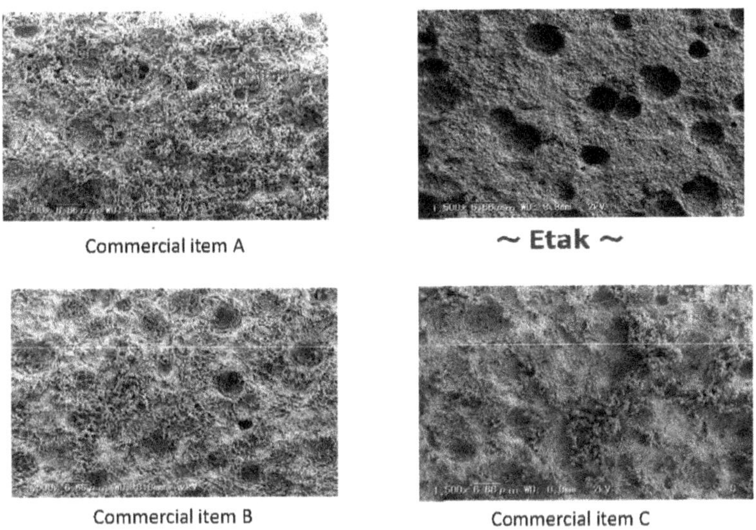

Figure 15.5 Aggregatibacter actinomycetemcomitans, which is a cause of periodontal disease, was used as a test bacterium, 5 minutes after applying an oral moisturizing agent, the bacterial solution was inoculated on the surface of hydroxyapatite that had been ultrasonically cleaned, and after static culture at 37 °C, it formed on the surface of each sample. The resulting biofilm was observed by SEM. No bacterial growth was observed on the Etak-treated surface.

15.3.2 Immobilization on the Skin

As shown in Figures 15.6 and 15.7, Etak can be immobilized on the skin. The antimicrobial agent is generally immobilized for one day and is not removed by washing with water and soap during the process. This kind of application of Etak could further reduce the risk of contact infection.

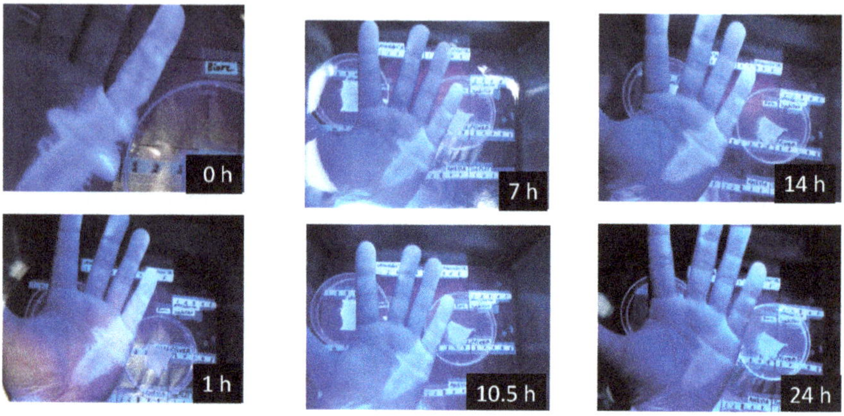

Figure 15.6 Immobilization of Etak on the skin.

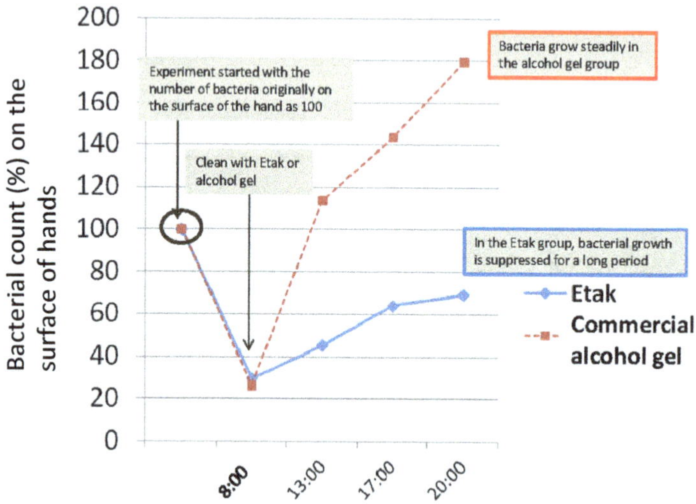

Figure 15.7 Antibacterial effect of Etak on the skin surface.

Although the image was taken immediately after hand washing with water, it was not removed for 14 hours. Twenty-four hours after bathing, the color became lighter due to desquamation, and it was confirmed that the amount of immobilization had decreased.

After hand disinfection with alcohol gel or Etak in the morning, microbiological changes were recorded. 40 participants cooperated in the study. At the first wash, both reduced the number of bacteria to the same level, but with alcohol gel, the number of bacteria increased rapidly after that, indicating that the effect was temporary. On the other hand, Etak suppresses subsequent contamination of fingers.

15.4 Conclusion

As described above, because Etak is highly safe and can be used in familiar situations, we believe that its use in the environment, in the oral cavity, and on the hands can significantly reduce the risk of infections of the digestive organs and respiratory system such as norovirus, mycoplasma, and influenza viruses.

References

1. Hamada T, Nikawa H, Yuda S. *Denture Cleaning: The Forefront of Plaque-Free Dentures.* Dental Diamond, Tokyo, 137, 2002. [In Japanese]
2. Nikawa H, Ishida K, Hamada T, Satoda T, Murayama T, Takemoto T, Tamamoto M, Tajima H, Shimoe S, Fujimoto H, Makihira S. Immobilization of octadecyl ammonium chloride on the surface of titan and its effects on microbial biofilm formation in vitro. *Dental Mater J*, 24, 570–582, 2005.
3. Nishimura T (ed.). *Basic Knowledge of Antimicrobials That Anyone Can Understand.* Techno System, Tokyo, 362, 1999. [In Japanese]
4. Sakudo A. General knowledge of virus inactivation and sterilization/ disinfection techniques. *J Antibact Antifung Agents,* 38, 81–88, 2010. [In Japanese]
5. Nikawa H, Yushita K, Hiramatsu M, Sakaguchi T. A compound that reduces the risk of influenza spreading. *Chemical Engineering,* 55 (8), 41–47, 2010. [In Japanese]

Chapter 16

A Real-Time Computer-Aided Diagnosis System with Quantitative Staging on Customizable Embedded Digital Signal Processor

Tetsushi Koide,[a] Masayuki Odagawa,[b,a] Toru Tamaki,[c] Shigeto Yoshida,[d] Shiro Oka,[e] and Shinji Tanaka[f]

[a]*Research Institute for Nanodevices, Hiroshima University, Higashi-Hiroshima, Hiroshima, Japan*
[b]*Cadence Design Systems, Japan*
[c]*Department of Computer Science, Nagoya Institute of Technology, Japan*
[d]*Department of Gastroenterology, JR Hiroshima Hospital, Japan*
[e]*Departments of Gastroenterology and Metabolism, Hiroshima University Hospital, Japan*
[f]*Department of Endoscopy, Hiroshima University Hospital, Japan*

koide@hiroshima-u.ac.jp

In this chapter, a hardware design of a quantitative staging classification in the computer-aided diagnosis (CAD) system for colorectal endoscopic images with narrow-band imaging (NBI) magnification is proposed. The proposed CAD system for real-time endoscopic video is implemented on a customizable embedded digital signal processor (DSP) to achieve high accuracy, high

Biomedical Engineering: Imaging Systems, Electric Devices, and Medical Materials
Edited by Akihiro Miyauchi and Hiroyuki Kagechika

ISBN 978-981-5129-16-8 (Hardcover), 978-1-003-46404-4 (eBook)
www.jennystanford.com

speed, and low power consumption. The proposed CAD system is also provided a quantitative and objective staging index to the doctor more accurately in magnified NBI endoscopic observation.

16.1 Introduction: Colorectal Cancer Classification

In recent years, the incidence and mortality of colorectal cancer is increasing in Japan and overseas. However, if colorectal cancer is detected and treated at an early stage, it can be recovered almost completely. The observation of endoscopic images with NBI magnification and the pathology are major methods of detection for colorectal cancer at the early stage. In the diagnosis by the NBI magnification endoscope, an expert clinical doctor diagnoses a tumor and the degree of cancer progression from the vessel pattern structure of the inner wall of the colon, etc. The clinical doctor for diagnosis requires high expertise and experience, and the number of expert clinical doctors is limited. Therefore, a CAD system is required for improving the accuracy of diagnosis by objective judgment using computer image analysis [1]. We aim to construct a CAD system with colorectal NBI magnification endoscopic image based on JNET (Japan NBI Expert Team) classification [2] (Figure 16.1).

Quantitative Staging Classification

	Non Cancer	Cancer (Type not 1)		
	Type 1	Type 2A	Type 2B	Type 3
Vessel pattern	•invisible	•Regular caliber •Regular distribution (meshed/spiral)	•Variable caliber •Irregular distribution	•Loose vessel areas •Interruption of thick vessels
Surface pattern	•Regular dark or white spots •Similar to surrounding normal mucosa	•Regular (tubular/branched/ papillary)	•Irregular or obscure	•Amorphous areas
Endoscopic image	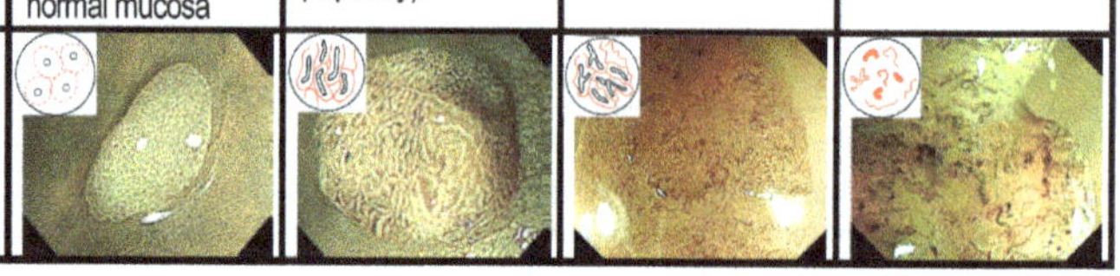			

Figure 16.1 The JNET classification for NBI magnification findings.

Research on CAD systems has been conducted, and reports have been made on the detection and classification of polyps for the purpose of preventing oversight by screening as shown in Figures 16.2 and 16.3 [3–9]. Figure 16.3 shows the difference in polyp detection, classification, and quantitative staging. Polyp detection provides the position of the polyp by bounding the box and label (Figure 16.3 (a)) [9]. Polyp classification classifies polyp type, adenoma, or hyperplastic with a quantitative index (Figure 16.3 (b)) [9]. On the other hand, we aim to realize a CAD system with a quantitative staging classification that provides a quantitative and objective index to recognize the degree of progression of colorectal cancer (Figure 16.3 (c)).

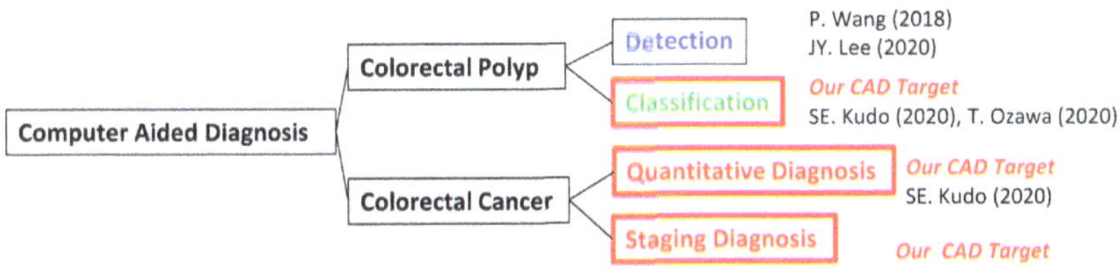

Figure 16.2 Purpose of CAD system.

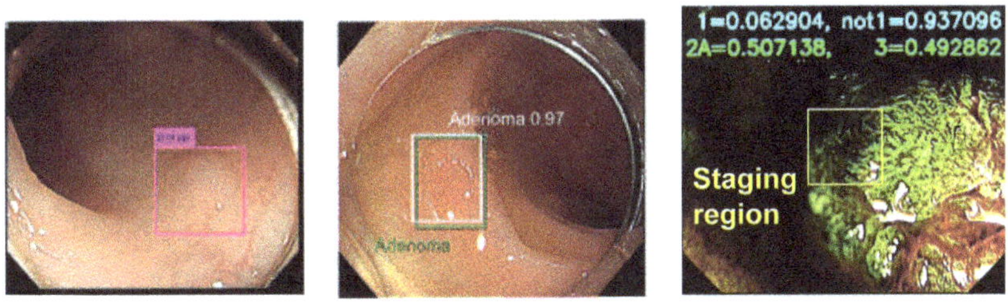

(a) Polyp Detection (JY. Lee 2020)

(b) Classification with Confidence Level of AI (T. Ozawa 2020)

(c) Quantitative Classification Measure (Our CAD Target)

Figure 16.3 Difference of detection, classification, and quantitative staging.

Machine learning has been applied to build CAD systems, with shallow learning and deep learning approaches, as shown in Figure 16.4 and Table 16.1. Figure 16.5 shows the comparison of performance, power, and diagnosis quality of previous studies [3–9]. While polyp detection and classification in CAD system are the main subjects, we aim to establish a diagnostic support method that provides a quantitative and objective index of cancer stage to doctors based on the standard JNET [2], not only classify cancer or not-cancer for real-time endoscopic video (30 fps). Our objects are realizing (a) the CAD system for real-time video (30 fps) on customizable embedded DSP, (b) real-time CAD with quantitative staging with over 90% accuracy, and (c) real-time navigation to improve quantitative staging quality.

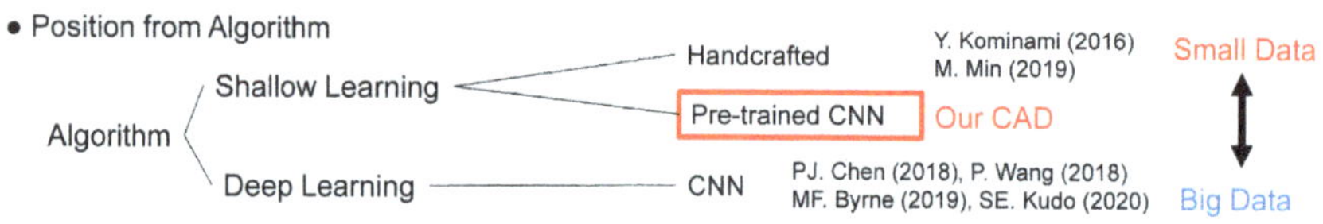

Figure 16.4 Positioning of CAD system (algorithm).

Table 16.1 Previous study using machine learning

	Machine Learning	Diagnosis Type	Endoscope	Training Data	Processing Time (fps)	Accuracy (%)	Sensitivity (%)	Platform
Y. Kominami (2016)	D-SIFT-SVM	Staging	Magnified NBI	2247 images	20	94.9	95.9	CPU
PJ. Chen (2018)	CNN	Classification	Magnified NBI	2157 images	2	90.1	96.3	-
P. Wang (2018)	CNN	Detection	White Light	5545 images	25	-	94.4	Server
MF. Byrne (2019)	CNN	Classification	NBI	223 videos	20	94.0	98.0	GPU
M. Min (2019)	GMM	Classification	BLI	208 images	-	78.4	83.3	-
SE. Kudo (2020) (Olympus)	CNN	Classification	Endocyto-NBI	25945 images	2.5	96.0	96.9	CPU
Our Target	Pre-trained CNN + SVM	Quantitative Staging + Navigation	Magnified NBI	10209 images	30	> 90 Video	> 90	Customizable DSP

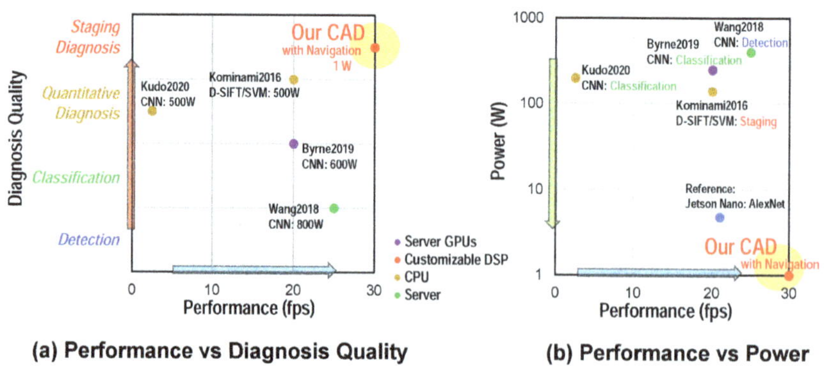

Figure 16.5 Comparison of (a) performance vs diagnosis quality and (b) performance vs power.

16.2 Computer-Aided Diagnosis System with Convolutional Neural Network

The convolutional neural network (CNN) was proposed by LeCun et al. [10] and is realized by local feature extraction by convolutional operation and repeating of resolution reduction of feature map using local area value by pooling. CNN is known to show high recognition performance in the field of general object recognition. We recognize the output of each layer of CNN as a multi-dimensional vector expressing the feature quantity of the input endoscopic image and use it as input data to classifier by SVM [21]. Figure 16.6 shows an overview of a CAD system with the bag of features (BoF) using handcraft feature amount, which is based on dense scale-invariant feature transform (D-SIFT) [1], and a CAD system with CNN feature extraction and support vector machine (SVM) classification [21], which is used in this study, respectively. In the proposed CNN-SVM method, the pre-trained AlexNet [11] is used. Specifically, the network model, which is pre-trained by the ImageNet dataset of 1,000 categories [12] provided by ImageNet, a large-scale visual recognition challenge (ILSVRC 2012) of the general object recognition contest, is used. In this data set, there is no endoscopic image data. Figure 16.7 shows the architecture of AlexNet. This has eight layers, five of them are convolution layers (***conv1*** to ***conv5***) with normalization (***norm1*** and ***norm2***) and pooling (***pool1***, ***pool2***, and ***pool5***), and two of them are fully connected layers (***fc6*** and ***fc7***) followed by a softmax layer (***fc8***).

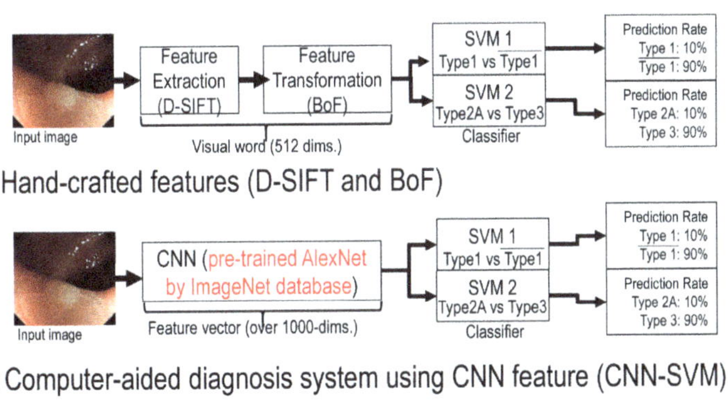

Figure 16.6 Overview of BoF-based and CNN-SVM CAD systems.

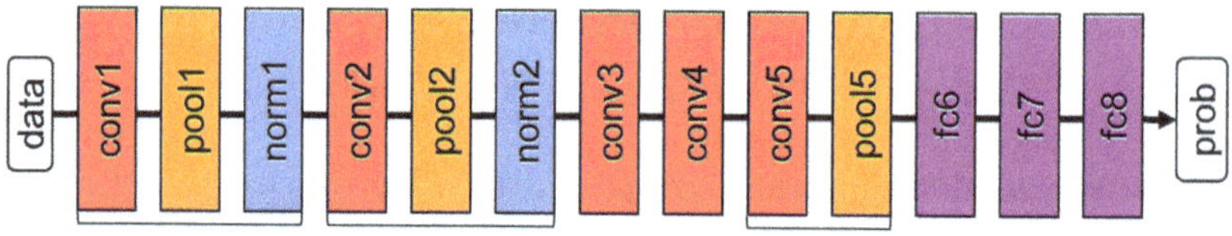

Figure 16.7 Architecture of AlexNet.

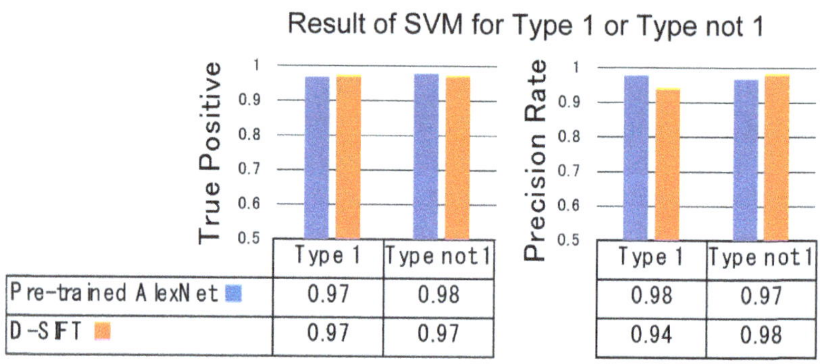

	True Positive: Type 1	True Positive: Type not 1	Precision Rate: Type 1	Precision Rate: Type not 1
Pre-trained AlexNet	0.97	0.98	0.98	0.97
D-SIFT	0.97	0.97	0.94	0.98

Figure 16.8 Comparison of pre-trained AlexNet (CNN-SVM) and D-SIFT (Type 1 and Type not 1).

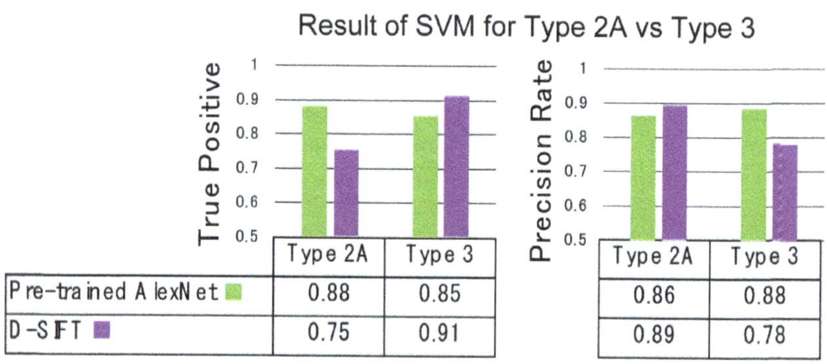

	True Positive: Type 2A	True Positive: Type 3	Precision Rate: Type 2A	Precision Rate: Type 3
Pre-trained AlexNet	0.88	0.85	0.86	0.88
D-SIFT	0.75	0.91	0.89	0.78

Figure 16.9 Comparison of pre-trained AlexNet (CNN-SVM) and D-SIFT (Type 2A and Type 3).

Figures 16.8 and 16.9 show the accuracy of the SVM trained by D-SIFT and the SVM trained by the output (1,000 dimensions) from ***prob*** of the pre-trained AlexNet. Figure 16.8 shows the result of Type 1 vs Type not 1 (Type 2A and Type 3) classification. The output from ***prob*** of the pre-trained AlexNet is comparable to the conventional D-SIFT-based approach. In

Figure 16.9, both the *True Positive* and *Precision Rate* of the SVM trained by the output from ***prob*** of the pre-trained AlexNet exceeded 85%, and these measures are improved from D-SIFT. Therefore, we decide on the CNN-SVM-based method to be used for quantitative staging classification [21].

16.3 Proposed CAD System Implementation to Embedded Customizable DSP Core

16.3.1 Multiply and Accumulate Calculation in CNN

CNNs are composed of different layers such as convolutional layers (***conv***), normalization layers (***norm***), pooling layers (***pool***), and fully connected layers (***fc***). A convolution calculation is shown in Eq. (16.1).

$$Y_{i,k,x,y} = \sum_{c=1}^{C}\sum_{v=1}^{r}\sum_{u=1}^{r} D_{i,c,x+u,y+v}\, G_{k,c,u,v} \# \qquad (16.1)$$

Table 16.2 The comparison of MAC calculations in CNN models

CNN models	AlexNet A. Krizhevsky (2012)	VGG-16 K. Simonyan (2015)	GoogLeNet C. Szegedy (2015)	ResNet 50 K. He (2016)
Input size	227 x 227	224 x 224	224 x 224	224 x 224
No. of conv layers	5	13	57	53
Depth of conv layers	5	13	21	49
Filter size	3,5,11	3	1,3,5,7	1,3,7
No. of channels	3-256	3-512	3-832	3-2048
No. of filters	96-384	64-512	16-384	64-2048
Strides	1,4	1	1,2	1,2
No. of weights in conv layers	2.3M	14.7M	6.0M	23.5M
No. of MACs in conv layers	666M	15.3G	1.43G	3.86G
No. of fc layers	3	3	1	1
No. of MACs in fc layers	58.6M	124M	1M	2M
Total weights	61M	138M	7M	25.5M
Total MACs	724M	15.5G (x21)	1.43G (x2)	3.9G (x5)

A convolution calculation is the multiplication and accumulation (MAC) of corresponding elements of an input feature map and a kernel to generate a single output pixel. The total number of parameters in AlexNet is 105,705,600 (290,400 × 364). Also, the number of multiplies and accumulates is 100 million. Table 16.2 shows the comparison of MAC calculations in CNN models. A convolutional layer computation consumes more than 90% of the total computation of CNNs [13]. AlexNet has the least number of total MAC operations, however, it is still over 700 million.

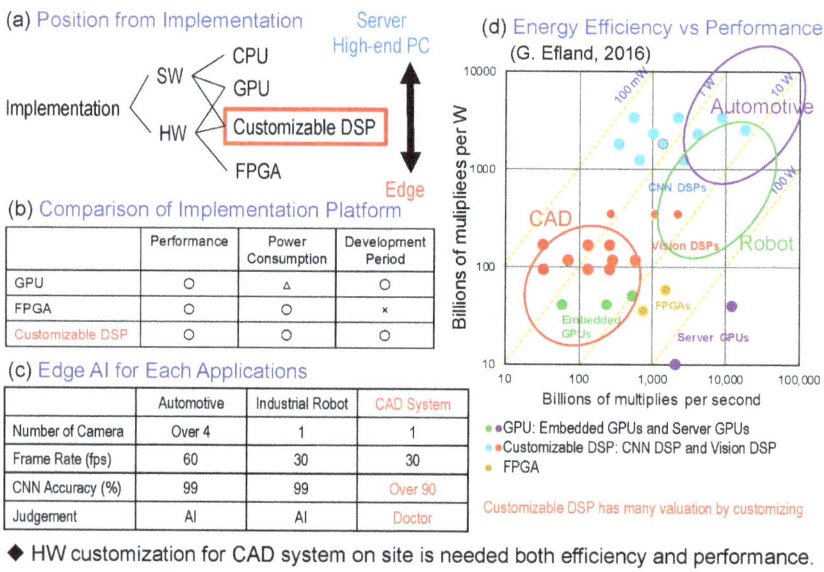

Figure 16.10 Positioning of CAD system from an implementation perspective.

16.3.2 Requirements for Hardware Platform of the CAD System Implementation

In general, there are some options for hardware implementation of CNN feature extraction and SVM classification (CNN-SVM) such as graphics processing unit (GPU), field programmable gate array (FPGA), and digital signal processor (DSP) (Figure 16.10). The processing speed is increased by applying several optimization methods. However, the power consumption is not reduced so much, and it also takes time for designing hardware (HW) in FPGA. The requirement for HW, which executes the CNN, is different for applications, automotive, industrial robots, and medical. It is necessary to change the HW configuration for each application to meet the requirements. Therefore, we selected a customizable embedded DSP for our target.

16.3.3 Overview of Customizable Embedded DSP Core

For efficient execution of CNN-SVM, the simultaneous execution of multiple instructions by multiple numbers of MAC (multiply-accumulate) and VLIW/SIMD execution units are required [20]. VLIW (very long instruction word) is one of the instruction set architectures designed to exploit instruction-level parallelism. SIMD (single instruction, multiple data) is a class of parallel computers with multiple processing elements that perform the same operation on multiple data simultaneously. Also, an efficient tiled image transfer by scatter-gather direct memory access (DMA) is required for video image processing.

We use the Cadence Tensilica® Vision P6 DSP core (VP6 core) [14], which is a customizable DSP core for embedded applications, as the target architecture to be implemented. Figure 16.11 shows the architecture of the VP6 core. The VP6 core has instruction sets specified for image processing and CNN processing, and it has a 256 parallel MAC operation unit of 8-bit × 8-bit for high-speed processing of convolution operation. It adopts a 5-slot VLIW for enabling the execution of instructions in 5 parallels. There are built-in 512-bit dual load/store data memories for high-performance video image processing. In the VP6 core, cache size, internal data memory size, internal instruction memory size, and vector floating point unit are customizable. It also allows designers to extend and add instructions.

We use the pre-trained AlexNet for the VP6 and optimized the bit width of the coefficient parameter to 8-bit [15]. As a result, the amount of memory is reduced, and the processing speed is improved. Table 16.3 shows comparison results of the memory usage and the recognition accuracy of the original 64-bit AlexNet and 8-bit optimized AlexNet, respectively. The recognition rate of 8-bit optimized AlexNet is within 1% of the error compared to the original 64-bit AlexNet [16]. We compared classification accuracy (***True-Positive***) by using these pre-trained AlexNet with the ImageNet database [12] of the general object recognition contest as the feature extraction to SVM endoscopic image classification. Figure 16.12 shows the accuracy comparison results. From these results, it is possible to construct the CAD system by reducing the memory size by 75% and keeping the average recognition accuracy of 90% using the SVM classifier relearning for the feature extractor with 8-bit optimized AlexNet.

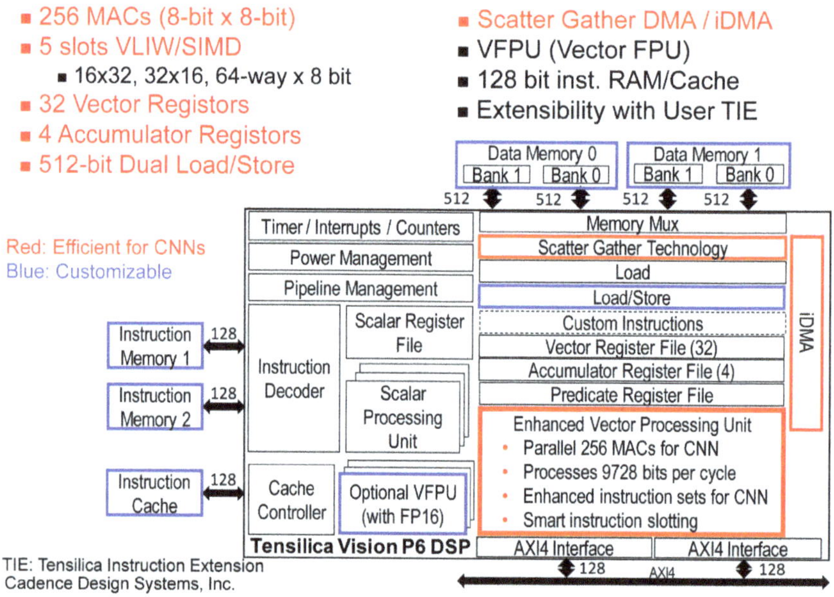

Figure 16.11 Overview of Vision P6 Core Architecture.

Table 16.3 Memory size and accuracy of the 8-bit optimized AlexNet with ImageNet

	Memory (Mb)	Top 1 accuracy (%)	Top 5 accuracy (%)
AlexNet (64-bit original)	243.9	57.10	80.20
AlexNet (8-bit optimized)	61.0	56.01	79.54

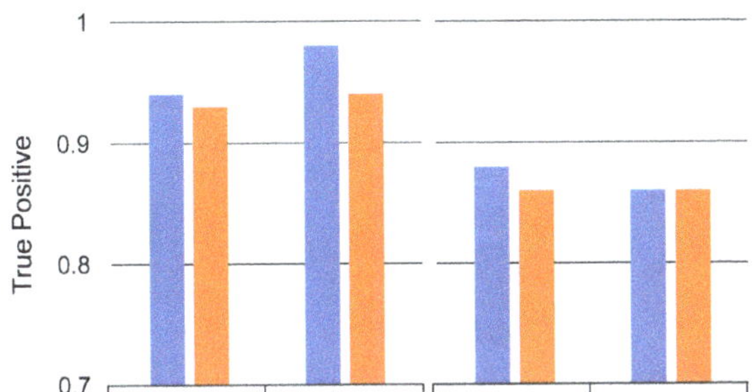

	Type 1	Type 2A/3	Type 2A	Type 3
64 bit pre-trained AlexNet + SVM	0.96	0.98	0.88	0.86
8 bit pre-trained AlexNet + SVM	0.93	0.94	0.86	0.86

Figure 16.12 SVM classification accuracy (true-positive) with feature extraction for 64-bit and 8-bit AlexNets which are pre-trained by the ImageNet database.

16.3.4 Hardware Design and Processing Flow

For developing the proposed CAD system, we decided to use an FPGA-based prototyping system for enabling rapid implementation of both HW and SW and real-time validation of the CAD system [17]. The prototyping system shown in Figure 16.13 is made up of two parts, a host computer that stores the endoscopic data and displays classification results and the Cadence rapid prototyping platform Protium® S1 in which the VP6 core and peripherals are installed. In the proposed CAD system, the main processing units such as the CNN feature extraction and the SVM classification are executed on the VP6 core. Protium S1 has good on-the-fly debugging functionality, and it is possible to observe the waveform of arbitrary signals in FPGA.

Figure 16.14 shows a block diagram of the developed system including the VP6 core and peripherals. In the developed system, two blocks of 1 Mb internal RAM for image buffering, 1 Mb internal ROM for system ROM, and 64 Mb work memory area for coefficients of CNN on external DRAM are implemented. We customized VP6's configuration as follows: (a) 48 kb instruction cache and (b) 256 kb × 2 blocks of built-in data memory are implemented, and (c) optional vector floating point unit (VFPU) is not implemented due to the area limitation of FPGA.

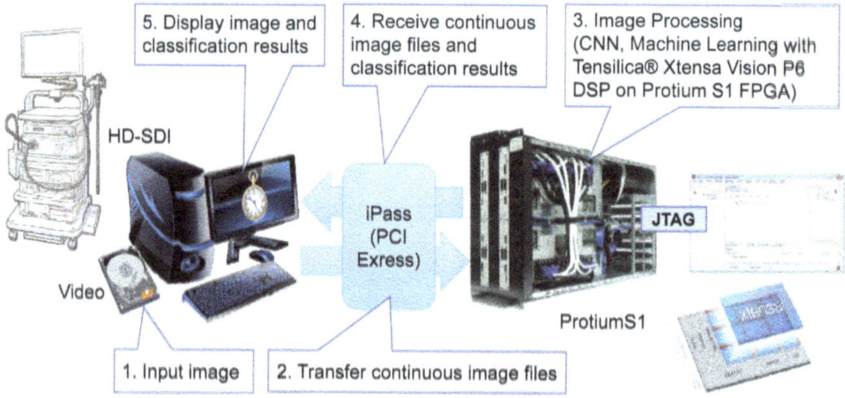

Figure 16.13 The developed prototyping CAD system overview.

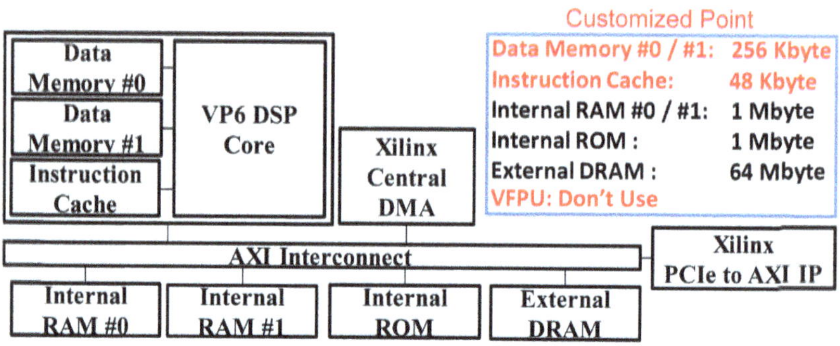

Figure 16.14 Block diagram of the implemented system.

Figure 16.15 shows the flowchart of the developed prototype system. When the system starts the image processing, the frame data is read as image data from the endoscopic video sequence. Next, as the input data to the CNN, an arbitrary region of 227 × 227 pixels is cut out from one frame of the endoscopic video as a staging region. A size other than 227 × 227 pixels can be also used as the staging region, and in that case, the staging region is resized to 227 × 227 pixels. Then the image data of the staging region is stored in the image buffering memory (Internal RAM # 0) shared between the host and the DSP. In the DSP, CNN feature extraction and SVM classification are performed to obtain the classification result for the staging region. The classification result is stored in the image buffering memory (Internal

RAM # 1) shared between the host and the DSP. Finally, the host reads the classification result and displays the staging region and the result together with the input frame image. The above process is repeated until the endoscopic video ends.

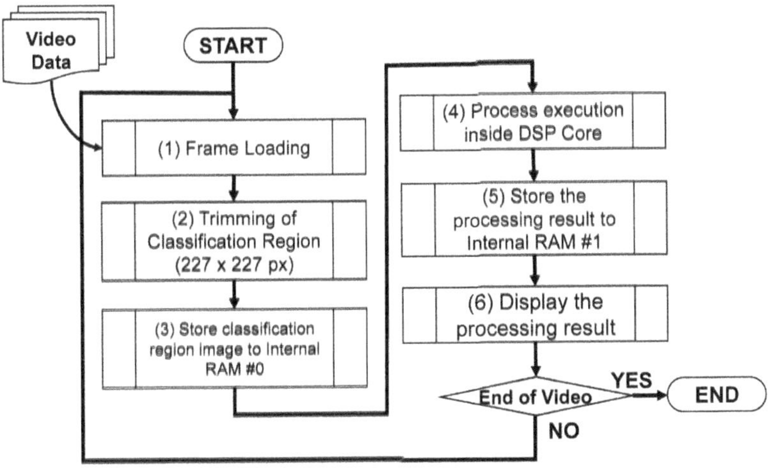

Figure 16.15 Flowchart of the developed CAD prototype system.

16.3.5 Processing Cycle Reduction and Implementation

Figure 16.16 shows the result of the processing cycle reduction. In endoscopic image diagnosis, the clinical doctor does not take care of the color information of the lesion and focuses on vessel pattern structure and surface structure of the lesion, therefore, the image can be gray-scaled to reduce the amount of processing data of AlexNet. This reduces the convolution layer processing cycle by approximately 8 M cycles, almost 47%.

For reducing the waiting time of DMA transfer for reading the weight coefficients of the fully connected (*fc*) layer from the external memory to the internal data RAM, we will use the intermediate data as the extracted feature before the fully connected layer in AlexNet. The process of AlexNet itself will be quitted at that stage. For implementing the CNN-SVM system to an embedded system, the number of dimensions of the intermediate data to be used is equivalent to the number of dimensions of the input data to the SVM classifier. Therefore, we have to consider the trade-off between the classification accuracy and the number of dimensions of the intermediate data from a hidden layer of AlexNet.

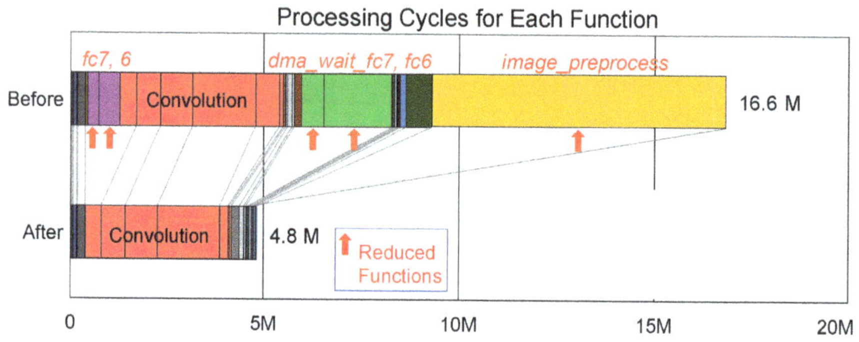

Figure 16.16 Result of optimization for processing cycles per one still image.

Figure 16.17 shows the number of dimensions on intermediate data as feature quantity from each hidden layer of AlexNet. The ***prob*** layer output at the final stage is the probability of 1,000 categories (dimensions) as AlexNet's outputs value. We use ***pool5***, ***fc6***, ***fc7***, ***fc8***, and ***prob*** as candidates for intermediate data as feature extraction. Thus, we evaluated the classification accuracy when these intermediate data are used as input data to the SVM classifier for comparison.

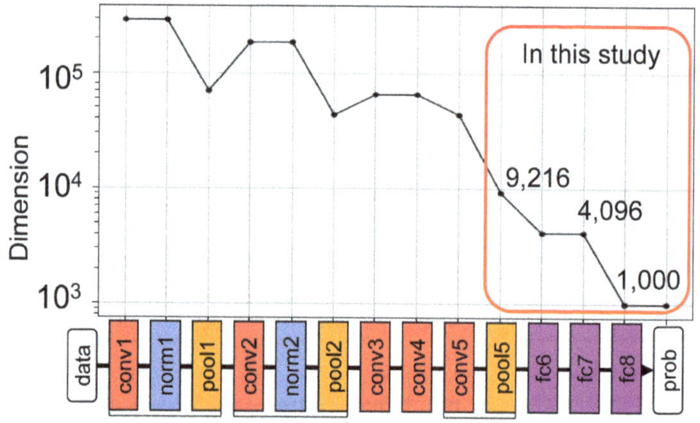

Figure 16.17 Feature dimensions of pre-trained AlexNet and the architecture.

Figure 16.18 shows the evaluation results. The classification accuracy was evaluated by F-measure performing 10-fold cross-validation (CV) to compare the classification accuracy of the proposed method. For comparison, we use a prior work on endoscopic image recognition have used D-SIFT [1]. The value of the F-measure shows over 97% classification of Type 1 and Type not 1 (Type 2A and Type 3). Compare to prior systems based on D-SIFT, accuracies for CNN feature extraction are higher for Type 2A and Type 3 classifications. From these results, it is possible to improve the CNN-SVM system speed with keeping high classification accuracy.

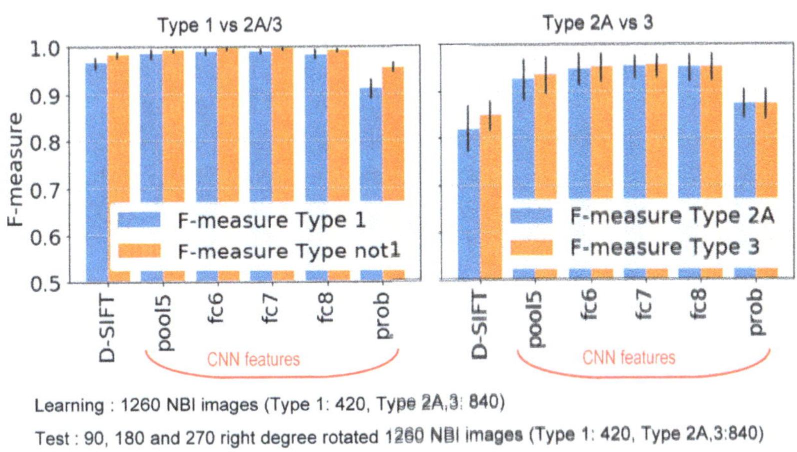

Figure 16.18 F-measure for each hidden layer of AlexNet.

The number of dimensions of the extracted feature from ***pool5*** increases by 9,216, about 9 times the number of dimensions from ***prob***. The number of processing cycles in SVM is approximately 0.06 M cycles when the output of ***prob*** is used as input and approximately 0.56 M cycles when the output of ***pool5*** is used as input. However, the number of processing cycles reduced by deleting the processing of ***dma_wait_fc6*** and ***dma_wait_fc7***, which are the cycles of DMA transfers, and ***fc6*** and ***fc7***, which are the cycles of fully connected layers, is 4 M cycles as shown in Figure 16.16. Using the 9,216-dimensional intermediate data as extracted feature from ***pool5*** is much more effective. The data transfer size by DMA is reduced to 56 Mb by using the output from ***pool5*** compared to using the output from ***prob***, which is the last layer in AlexNet. From these results, it is effective to use the output of ***pool5*** with dimension number 9,126 as the extracted feature of the input to SVM of the latter stage.

16.4 Evaluation of the Developed Prototype System

Figure 16.16 summarizes the comparison of the numbers of processing cycles before and after cycle reduction of the above-mentioned optimization. This result shows that the number of total processing cycles can be reduced by approximately 70%. The reason for the reduction of about 70% is the reduction of load/store of related data processing cycles, while a reduction of 61% is also expected. When the clock frequency is 200 MHz, the frame rate is 44.6 fps, which exceeds the input video frame rate of 30 fps, and also it is achieved the research target of 30 fps. We estimated power consumption is 66.6 mW under a 16 nm CMOS process by Xtensa Xplorer [14]. For example, Nvidia's Jetson AGX, an embedded GPU and LSI manufactured in the 12 nm CMOS process of TSMC, executes AlexNet 299 fps at 14 W by 15 W mode [18]. It is equivalent to 2.08 W when reducing the performance to the same frame rate of 44.6 fps as Vison P6. We compared it to other platforms and Table 16.4 shows the comparison results [18, 19]. The power consumption of our system is lower compared to the latest embedded GPUs. The latency of our system is about 22 ms, from Step 2 to Step 4 in Figure 16.15. The latency of the endoscopic camera transfer can be assumed to be almost equivalent, which corresponds to a delay of less than one frame when the frame rate of the input video image is 30 fps. There is no difference between the frame taken by the endoscope and the frame displaying the classification result. Thus, it is possible to provide information about the classification result that is also easier for the doctor to understand.

Table 16.4 Performance for AlexNet and power compared to other platforms

	Vision P6	Jetson AGX	Jetson Nano	Raspberry Pi 3B
Performance (fps)	44.6	299	21.7	0.35
Power (W)	0.0666	14	4.58	2.73
Power (W) per 1 fps	0.000149	0.0468	0.211	7.80
Clock frequency (MHz)	200 (DSP)	670 (GPU)	640 (GPU)	1200 (ARM A53)

We constructed the proposed CAD system on the hardware prototyping platform in Figure 16.13, Protium S1, and validated using the endoscopic video images. Since Protium S1 has a function of observing waveform data from each signal for debugging, there is a limitation to improving the operating clock frequency [17]. Therefore, the operating clock frequency is 22.97 MHz, which is equivalent to 4 fps in processing performance. Figure 16.19 shows the output display image of the developed system. The yellow and red rectangle areas are the staging regions. The classification results are displayed at the top of the endoscopic image.

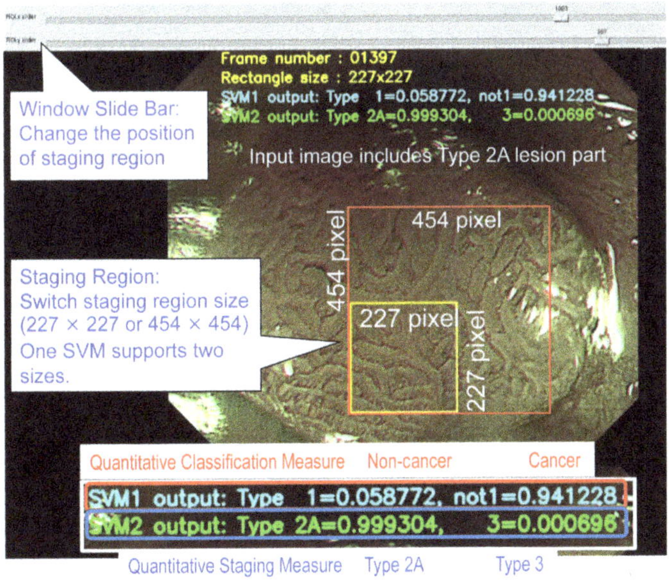

Figure 16.19 The classification result of the endoscopic video image on the real-time prototyping system (Type 2A).

The clinical doctors can switch the size of the staging region to 227 × 227 pixels (green rectangle) or 454 × 454 pixels (red rectangle), as shown in Figure 16.20 (a). The clinical doctors can set the staging region position or move the clear part of an endoscopic image into the staging region during observation (yellow rectangle), as shown in Figure 16.20 (b). Figure 16.21 shows output results from our CAD system, which provides the probability of each pathological type. After avoiding unclear regions, the probability of Type 3, as shown in Figure 16.21 (b), is improved from about 0.49 to 0.99 [22].

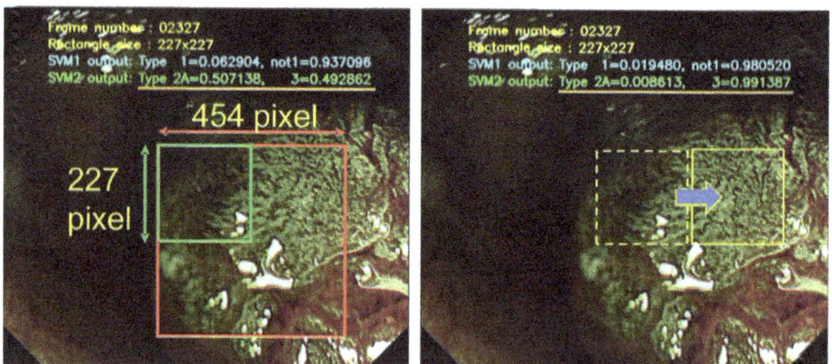

(a) Switch the classification region sizes (227 × 227 or 454 × 454)

(b) Move the classification region

Figure 16.20 Staging region setting.

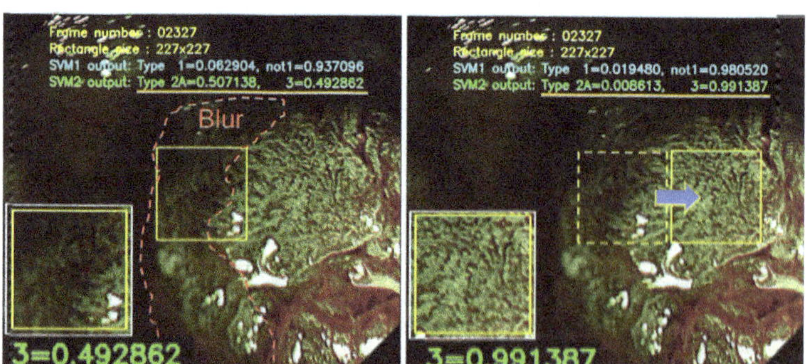

(a) Classification results at the boundary of the lesion including blur region.

(b) Classification results in the center of the lesion.

Figure 16.21 Real-time classification results from the boundary (blur region) to the center of the lesion of Type 3.

16.5 Conclusion

In this chapter, we presented the real-time CAD system with quantitative staging on customizable embedded DSP [20]. The proposed CAD system provides a quantitative and objective index of cancer stage to doctors based on the standard JNET classification [2], not only classifying cancer or not-cancer and implemented on a customizable embedded DSP. The developed CAD system achieved real-time quantitative staging classification for the endoscopic video image (44.6 fps throughput/22 ms latency at 200 MHz clock frequency, 66.6 mW power consumption), and sufficient classification accuracy (> 90%). From the above study, a quantitative and objective staging index is provided to the doctor more accurately in magnified NBI endoscopic observation, which is independent of the experience of doctors, and the diagnostic support method is established such as a "second opinion" at magnified NBI endoscopic observation on site. Future works include the automatic detection of the optimal classification region of the lesion, the consideration of the unclear video frame including blurring, color shift, or reflection of light, and the development of custom instructions of DSP core for more effective execution considering the trade-off between the performance and implementation cost.

Acknowledgments

Part of this work was supported by Grant-in-Aid for Scientific Researches (B) JSPS KAKENHI, Grant Number 20H04157, and collaborative research of the Research Center for Biomedical Engineering, respectively.

References

1. T. Tamaki, J. Yoshimuta, M. Kawakami, B. Raytchev, K. Kaneda, S. Yoshida, Y. Takemura, K. Onji, R. Miyaki, and S. Tanaka, "Computer-aided colorectal tumor classification in NBI endoscopy using local features," *Med. Image Anal.*, vol. 17, no. 1, pp. 78–100, Jan. 2013.

2. Y. Sano, S. Tanaka, S. Kudo, S. Saito, T. Matsuda, Y.Wada, T. Fujii, H. Ikematsu, T. Uraoka, N. Kobayashi, H. Nakamura, K. Hotta, T. Horimatsu, N. Sakamoto, K.-I Fu, O. Tsuruta, H. Kawano, H. Kashida, Y. Takeuchi, H. Machida, T. Kusaka, N. Yoshida, I. Hirata, T. Terai, H. Yamano, K. Kaneko, T. Nakajima, T. Sakamoto, Y. Yamaguchi, N. Tamai, N. Nakano, N. Hayashi, S. Oka, M. Iwatate, H. Ishikawa, Y. Murakami, S. Yoshida, and Y. Saito, "Narrow-band imaging (NBI) magnifying endoscopic classification of colorectal tumors proposed by the Japan NBI expert team," *Dig. Endosc.*, vol. 28, no. 5, pp. 526–533, 2016.
3. Y. Kominami, S. Yoshida, S. Tanaka, Y, Sanomura, T. Hirakawa, B. Raytchev, T. Tamaki, T. Koide, K. Kaneda, and K. Chayama, "Computer-aided diagnosis of colorectal polyp histology by using a real-time image recognition system and narrow-band imaging magnifying colonoscopy," *Gastrointest. Endosc.*, vol. 83, no. 3, pp. 643–649, 2016.
4. PJ. Chen, MC. Lin, MJ. Lai, JC. Lin, HH. Lu, and VS. Tseng, "Accurate classification of diminutive colorectal polyps using computer-aided analysis," *Gastroenterology*, vol. 154, pp. 568–575, 2018.
5. P. Wang, X. Xiao, JR. Brown, TM. Berzin, M. Tu, F. Xiong, X. Hu, P. Liu, Y. Song, D. Zhang, X. Yang, L. Li, J. He, X. Yi, J. Liu, and X. Liu, "Development and validation of a deep-learning algorithm for the detection of polyps during colonoscopy," *Nature Biomedical Engineering*, vol. 2, pp. 741–748, 2018; MF. Byrne, N. Chapados, F. Soudan, C. Oertel, M. Linares Pérez, R. Kelly, N. Iqbal, F. Chandelier, and DK. Rex, "Real-time differentiation of adenomatous and hyperplastic diminutive colorectal polyps during analysis of unaltered videos of standard colonoscopy using a deep learning model," *Gut*, vol. 68, pp. 94–100, 2019.
6. M. Min, S. Su, W. He, Y. Bi, Z. Ma, and Y. Liu, "Computer-aided diagnosis of colorectal polyps using linked color imaging colonoscopy to predict histology," *Scientific Reports*, vol. 9, Article number: 2881 (2019).
7. SE. Kudo, M. Misawa, Y. Mori, K. Hotta, K. Ohtsuka, H. Ikematsu, Y. Saito, K. Takeda, H. Nakamura, K. Ichimasa, T. Ishigaki, N. Toyoshima, T. Kudo, T. Hayashi, K. Wakamura, T. Baba, F. Ishida, H. Inoue, H. Itoh, M. Oda, and K. Mori, "Artificial intelligence-assisted system improves endoscopic identification of colorectal neoplasms," *Clinical Gastroenterology and Hepatology*, vol. 18, pp. 1874–1881, 2020.
8. JY. Lee, J. Jeong, EM. Song, C. Ha, HJ. Lee, JE. Koo, DH. Yang, N. Kim, and JS. Byeon, "Real-time detection of colon polyps during colonoscopy

using deep learning: Systematic validation with four independent datasets," *Scientific Reports*, vol. 10, pp. 8379, 2020.

9. T. Ozawa, S. Ishihara, M. Fujishiro, Y. Kumagai, S. Shichijo, and T. Tada. "Automated endoscopic detection and classification of colorectal polyps using convolutional neural networks," *Therapeutic Advances in Gastroenterology*, vol. 13, January 2020. doi:10.1177/1756284820910659.
10. Y. LeCun, B. Boser, J.S. Denker, D. Henderson, R.E. Howard, W. Hubbard, and L.D. Jackel, "Backpropagation applied to handwritten zip code recognition," *Neural Comput.*, vol. 1, no. 4, pp. 541–551, Dec. 1989.
11. K. Alex, I. Sutskever, and G.E. Hinton, "ImageNet classification with deep convolutional neural networks," *Proc. 25th International Conference on Neural Information Processing Systems*, vol. 1, pp. 1097–1105, 2012.
12. O. Russakovsky, J. Deng, H. Su, J. Krause, S. Satheesh, S. Ma, Z. Huang, A. Karpathy, A. Khosla, M. Bernstein, A.C. Berg, and L. Fei-Fei, "Image Net large scale visual recognition challenge," *International Journal of Computer Vision*, vol. 115, pp. 211–252, 2015.
13. V. Sze, Y. Chen, T. Yang, and J. S. Emer, "Efficient processing of deep neural networks: A tutorial and survey," *Proceedings of the IEEE*, vol. 105, no. 12, pp. 2295–2329, 2017.
14. Cadence Design Systems, Inc., "Vision DSPs for imaging and neural networks." https://ip.cadence.com/vision
15. G. Efland, S. Parikh, H. Sanghavi, and A. Farooqui, "High performance DSP for vision, imaging and neural networks," *IEEE Hot Chips 2016*, 2016.
16. G. Phillip, "Ristretto: Hardware-oriented approximation of convolutional neural networks," *arXiv preprint arXiv:1605.060402*, 2016.
17. Cadence Design Systems, "Protium S1 FPGA-based prototyping platform." https://www.cadence.com/news/protium.
18. Nvidia, "Jetson AGX Xavier: Deep learning inference benchmarks." https://developer.nvidia.com/embedded/jetson-agx-xavierdl-inference-benchmarks.
19. R. Hadidi, J. Cao, Y. Xie, B. Asgari, T. Krishna, and H. Kim, "Characterizing the deployment of deep neural networks on commercial edge devices," *Proc. 2019 IEEE International Symposium on Workload Characterization*, pp. 35–48, 2019.

20. Masayuki Odagawa, Takumi Okamoto, Tetsuhi Koide, Toru Tamaki, Bisser Raytchev, Kazufumi Kaneda, Shigeto Yoshida, Hiroshi Mieno, Shinji Tanaka, Takayuki Sugawara, Hiroshi Toishi, Masayuki Tsuji, and Nobuo Tamba, "A hardware implementation on customizable embedded DSP core for colorectal tumor classification with endoscopic video toward real-time computer-aided diagnosis system," *IEICE TRANSACTIONS on Fundamentals of Electronics, Communications and Computer Sciences*, vol. E104-A, no. 4, pp. 691–701, 2021.

21. Masayuki Odagawa, Takumi Okamoto, Tetsushi Koide, Toru Tamaki, Shigeto Yoshida, Hiroshi Mieno, and Shinji Tanaka, "Classification with CNN features and SVM on embedded DSP core for colorectal magnified NBI endoscopic video image," *IEICE TRANSACTIONS on Fundamentals of Electronics, Communications and Computer Sciences*, vol. E105-A, no. 1, pp. 58–62, 2022.

22. Masayuki Odagawa, Tetsushi Koide, Toru Tamaki, Shigeto Yoshida, Hiroshi Mieno, and Shinji Tanaka, "Feasibility study for computer-aided diagnosis system with navigation function of clear region for real-time endoscopic video image on customizable embedded DSP cores," *IEICE TRANSACTIONS on Fundamentals of Electronics, Communications and Computer Sciences*, vol. E105-A, no. 1, pp. 25–34, 2022.

Chapter 17

Medical Image Analysis

Yoshikazu Nakajima, Shinya Onogi, Takaaki Sugino, and Dongbo Zhou

Department of Biomedical Informatics,
Institute of Biomaterials and Bioengineering,
Tokyo Medical and Dental University, Japan

nakajima.bmi@tmd.ac.jp

Data-driven analysis is revolutionizing a wide range of research and business areas, including computational medicine, material informatics, and computational design of medical system development. Its potential is rapidly expanding and bringing fruitful results to our life. Deep neural networks (DNNs) and their learning technique, deep learning (DL), are presently becoming more common, but are even not perfect. Some problems are suitable for DNN solutions, while others are not. It is important to select and apply the appropriate computation algorithm for each process. This session will cover computational technologies using legacy and advanced methods, including DNNs.

Biomedical Engineering: Imaging Systems, Electric Devices, and Medical Materials
Edited by Akihiro Miyauchi and Hiroyuki Kagechika

ISBN 978-981-5129-16-8 (Hardcover), 978-1-003-46404-4 (eBook)
www.jennystanford.com

17.1 Image Processing

17.1.1 Correlation

Similarity assessment is one of the fundamental methodologies to divide incidents into two categories, for example, accepted or rejected cases. It can be given by their inner product, which is also expressed as "correlation" or "convolution." Let two functions be $f(x)$ and $g(x)$ with respect to a variable x, the inner product of them is given by

$$\langle f(x), g(x) \rangle = \int f(x)\bar{g}(x)dx, \tag{17.1}$$

where, $\bar{\cdot}$ notes the complex conjugate, i.e., $\bar{g}(x)$ notes the complex conjugate of $g(x)$. In particular, if $f(x)$ and $g(x)$ are a signal function and an orthonormal basis, this operation is called orthonormal transformation. For example, the Fourier transform is given by

$$\mathcal{F}(f) = \int f(x)e^{-i\omega x}dx, \tag{17.2}$$

where, if the functional variable is time, x can be expressed with time t. f and $\omega = 2\pi f$ are frequency and angular frequency, respectively. As well, Laplace transform is given by

$$\mathcal{L}\{f\}(s) = \int f(t)e^{-st}dt, \tag{17.3}$$

where, $s = \sigma + i\omega$ is a complex frequency-domain parameter with real numbers of σ and ω. In the description, the function $f(t)$ is expressed as a parameter of Laplace transform as $\mathcal{L}\{f\}$.

17.1.2 Filtering

For image processing, let vector $(\mathbf{x}, \mathbf{y})$ be the point geometry on an image, and $f(x, y)$ and $g(x, y)$ be the intensity functions of two images. Their correlation can be given with their inner product:

$$f * g = \langle f(x,y), g(x,y) \rangle = \iint f(x,y), g(x,y)dxdy \tag{17.4}$$

Pattern similarity of them can be given by the normalized correlation as

$$f * g = \left\langle \hat{f}(x,y), \hat{g}(x,y) \right\rangle, \tag{17.5}$$

where, $\wedge$ is normalization, for example,

$$\hat{f}(x,y) = \frac{f(x,y) - \overline{f(x,y)}}{\iint_{x,y} \left(f(x,y) - \overline{f(x,y)} \right)^2} \tag{17.6}$$

is normalization of $f(x)$. Where, $\overline{\cdot}$ is the average operation. The denominator term shows the variance of pixel intensities. For three-dimensional image volumes, it can be extended straightforwardly as

$$f * g = \left\langle \hat{f}(x,y,z), \hat{g}(x,y,z) \right\rangle, \tag{17.7}$$

where, (x, y, z) is the point geometry in the image volume. For filtering applications including pattern detection or diagnosis, signal images are assigned to a function f and each pattern to be detected is assigned to a function g. Correlation $f * g$ provides similarity of the signal image and required pattern. Introducing some evaluation computing, for example, threshold binarization, cross-entropy, or Bayesian estimation, the signal images can be divided into two or more classes.

17.2 Machine Learning

Machine learning is a technique for automatically finding latent patterns that frequently appear in data, which enables various data analyses such as regression, classification, clustering, dimensionality reduction, and recommendation. It assumes that latent patterns exist in data, and it is very effective in analyzing the data including frequently appeared patterns. Although machine learning includes supervised learning, unsupervised learning, and reinforcement learning, this section focuses on supervised learning, which is mostly used in medical image analysis.

Supervised learning is an algorithm that allows a machine to learn relationships and dependencies between inputs and target outputs. Supervised machine learning models for medical image analysis are trained using the known dataset of medical image data and the corresponding annotated data (i.e., ground-truth data), and subsequently, the trained models can be used to make predictions for image analysis tasks, such as classification and regression, on unknown medical image data. In this section, we will describe two supervised machine learning algorithms: support vector machine and convolutional neural network, although many machine learning algorithms have been proposed by researchers.

17.2.1 Support Vector Machine

Support vector machine (SVM) [1, 2] is a supervised machine learning model for classification tasks based on two key concepts of "kernel trick" and "margin maximization." The kernel trick is a technique of mapping linearly inseparable data into a higher dimensional space where the data can be linearly separable with less computational costs, while margin maximization is a strategy for maximizing "margin", the distance between the classification boundary and the data closest to it. These concepts allow SVMs to train classification models with better generalization performance that can address not only linearly separable problems but also linearly inseparable problems.

We here consider training an SVM classifier for binary classification based on N training data samples that belong to two classes c_1 and c_2. Suppose the training data samples consist of d-dimensional image feature vectors $\boldsymbol{x}_n$ (n = 1, ..., N) and the corresponding ground truth labels t_n defined as

$$t_n = \begin{cases} 1 & (\boldsymbol{x}_n \in c_1) \\ -1 & (\boldsymbol{x}_n \in c_2) \end{cases}. \tag{17.8}$$

The binary classification is equivalent to finding a boundary separating the classes by using a discriminant function. As shown in Figure 17.1(a), in the case of linearly separable problems, the linear discriminant function can be used for binary classification, defined as

$$f(\boldsymbol{x}_n) = \boldsymbol{w}^{\mathrm{T}}\boldsymbol{x}_n + b, \tag{17.9}$$

where $\boldsymbol{w}$ is a d-dimensional weight vector and b is a scalar constant, this is called the bias. The binary classification for all feature vectors $\boldsymbol{x}_{\mathrm{n}}$ is achieved by finding the weight vector $\boldsymbol{w}$ and the bias b that satisfy the following inequality:

$$f(\boldsymbol{x}_n) = \boldsymbol{w}^{\mathrm{T}}\boldsymbol{x}_n + b \begin{cases} \geq 0 & (\boldsymbol{x}_n \in c_1) \\ < 0 & (\boldsymbol{x}_n \in c_2) \end{cases}. \tag{17.10}$$

When $f(\boldsymbol{x}) = 0$, it corresponds to the decision boundary that separates the classes, which is called a hyperplane. In simple linearly separable problems, the hyperplane for separating the classes can be easily obtained by using classical linear discriminant analysis methods (e.g., least squares, Fisher's linear discriminant, and perceptron) based on data distribution patterns in a training dataset.

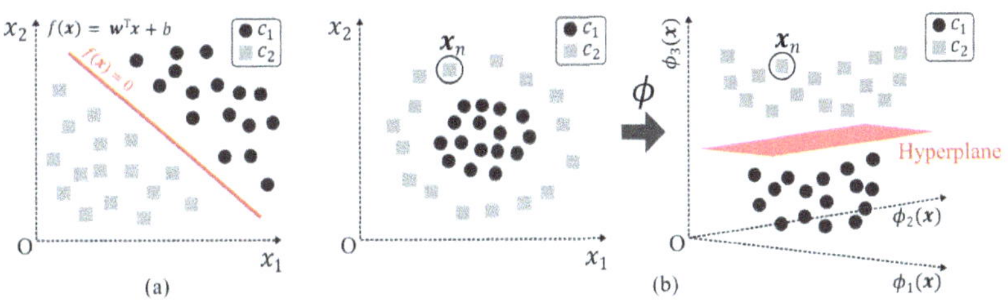

Figure 17.1 Examples of binary classification problems: (a) linearly separable case and (b) linearly inseparable case.

However, since the feature vectors in real-world image classification problems often have complex distributions, we have difficulty finding the hyperplane that linearly separates the classes in most cases. Thus, as shown in Figure 17.1(b), SVM introduces a kernel method, which uses a non-linear kernel function to map the feature vectors from a d-dimensional feature space to a higher D-dimensional feature space, so that it can deal with linearly inseparable problems as linearly separable problems. Theoretically, the feature vectors mapped to D-dimensional feature space can be always linearly separable when $N \leq D$. The non-linear transformation $\boldsymbol{\phi}$ is defined as

$$\boldsymbol{\phi}:\boldsymbol{x}=(x_1,x_2,\cdots,x_d)^{\mathrm{T}} \mapsto (\phi_1(\boldsymbol{x}),\phi_2(\boldsymbol{x}),\cdots,\phi_D(\boldsymbol{x}))^{\mathrm{T}}. \tag{17.11}$$

In the kernel method, the function $\boldsymbol{\phi}$ for non-linear transformation is defined through a kernel function instead of explicitly defining it. The kernel function k is defined as a function satisfying the following equation for the data samples $\boldsymbol{x}_{\mathrm{n}}$ and $\boldsymbol{x}_{\mathrm{m}}$ in the d-dimensional image feature space ($\boldsymbol{x}_n, \boldsymbol{x}_m \in \mathbb{R}^d$):

$$k(\boldsymbol{x}_n,\boldsymbol{x}_m)=\boldsymbol{\phi}(\boldsymbol{x}_n)^{\mathrm{T}}\boldsymbol{\phi}(\boldsymbol{x}_m). \tag{17.12}$$

Commonly used kernel functions include polynomial kernel and Gaussian kernel. Equation (17.12) means that the kernel function can replace calculations that use the dot product of the transformed image feature vectors $\boldsymbol{\phi}(\boldsymbol{x}_n)$ and $\boldsymbol{\phi}(\boldsymbol{x}_m)$ although the dot product operation is used to solve the optimization problem in Eq. (17.12) as described below. In other words, by using the kernel function, the computationally expensive dot product $\boldsymbol{\phi}(\boldsymbol{x}_n)^{\mathrm{T}}\boldsymbol{\phi}(\boldsymbol{x}_m)$ on high dimensional non-linear space can be computed as $k(\boldsymbol{x}_n, \boldsymbol{x}_m)$ on low dimensional linear space without giving a specific definition of $\boldsymbol{\phi}$; this is called the kernel trick. Therefore, the kernel method enables us to compute the operations using a non-linear transformation to higher dimensional space, which is necessary to obtain a non-linear SVM classifier, with lower computational cost.

Suppose the distribution of feature vectors transformed by the transformation $\boldsymbol{\phi}$ is obtained as shown in Figure 17.2(a). Then, the linear discriminant function on the D-dimensional feature space can be represented using the transformed vectors $\boldsymbol{\phi}(\boldsymbol{x})$ as

$$f(\boldsymbol{x}_n)=\boldsymbol{w}^{\mathrm{T}}\boldsymbol{\phi}(\boldsymbol{x}_n)+b\begin{cases}\geq 0 & (\boldsymbol{x}_n \in c_1)\\ <0 & (\boldsymbol{x}_n \in c_2)\end{cases}. \tag{17.13}$$

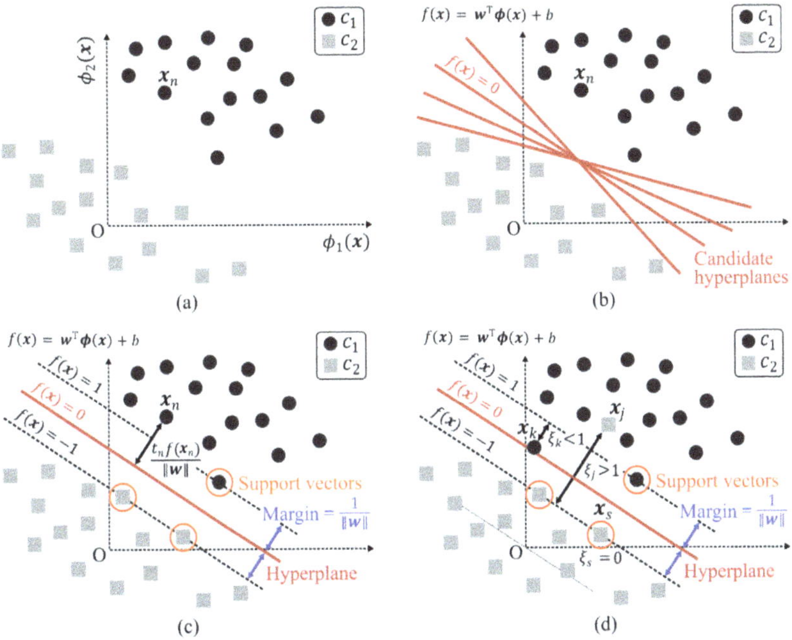

Figure 17.2 Examples of margin maximization by SVM: (a) data distribution in the feature space, (b) candidate hyperplanes, (c) hard margin, and (d) soft margin.

However, as shown in Figure 17.2(b), there can be an infinite number of candidate hyperplanes that separate the classes c_1 and c_2. To obtain an optimal hyperplane, SVM is trained to find the hyperplane with the largest as shown in Figure 17.2(c). In other words, the optimal hyperplane can be obtained by finding $\boldsymbol{w}$ and b that maximize the margin M under the constraint that all image feature vectors $\boldsymbol{x}_n (n = 1, ..., N)$ are far more than or equal to M from the hyperplane. As the distance d_n between the hyperplane and the vector $\boldsymbol{x}_n$ is $|f(\boldsymbol{x}_n)|/||\boldsymbol{w}||$, this can be given from Eqs. (17.8) and (17.13) by

$$\max_{\boldsymbol{w},b} M(\boldsymbol{w},b) \text{ subject to } d_n = \frac{\left|\boldsymbol{w}^{\mathrm{T}}\boldsymbol{\phi}(\boldsymbol{x}_n)+b\right|}{\|\boldsymbol{w}\|}$$

$$= \frac{t_n(\boldsymbol{w}^{\mathrm{T}}\boldsymbol{\phi}(\boldsymbol{x}_n)+b)}{\|\boldsymbol{w}\|} \geq M(n=1,\ldots,N) \quad (17.14)$$

The term $t_n(\boldsymbol{w}^{\mathrm{T}}\boldsymbol{\phi}(\boldsymbol{x}_n) + b)/||\boldsymbol{w}||$ is invariant to any constant scaling for $\boldsymbol{w}$ and b (i.e., even if $\boldsymbol{w}$ and b are multiplied by arbitrary scalar constants, the constants are canceled in the numerator and denominator). Given the scale satisfying $t_s(\boldsymbol{w}^{\mathrm{T}}\boldsymbol{\phi}(\boldsymbol{x}_s) + b) = 1$ for the support vector $\boldsymbol{x}_s$ as in Figure 17.2(c), Eq. (17.14) can be represented as follows:

$$\max_{w,\,b} \frac{1}{||\boldsymbol{w}||} \text{subject to } t_n(\boldsymbol{w}^{\mathrm{T}}\boldsymbol{\phi}(\boldsymbol{x}_n)+b) \geq 1 \; (n=1,2,\ldots,N)$$

$$\Rightarrow \min_{w,\,b} \frac{1}{2}||\boldsymbol{w}||^2 \text{ subject to } t_n(\boldsymbol{w}^{\mathrm{T}}\boldsymbol{\phi}(\boldsymbol{x}_n)+b) \geq 1 \; (n=1,2,\ldots,N). \quad (17.15)$$

Although the target classifier can be obtained by solving the minimization problem given by Eq. (17.15), it assumes maximizing the margin when the data samples are linearly separable in the feature space, which is called the hard-margin SVM classifier. However, since the data distributions in real-world image classification problems are complex as mentioned above, the overfitting occurs in most cases when we use the hard-margin SVM to train the separating hyperplane that satisfies the inequalities in Eq. (17.13) for all feature vectors of data samples in a training dataset. To solve this problem, we can introduce a slack variable ξ_n for each feature vector $\boldsymbol{x}_n$ and use the constraints modified from Eq. (17.10) to

$$f(\boldsymbol{x}_n) = \boldsymbol{w}^{\mathrm{T}}\boldsymbol{\phi}(\boldsymbol{x}_n) + b \begin{cases} \geq 1-\xi_n & (\boldsymbol{x}_n \in c_1) \\ < -1+\xi_n & (\boldsymbol{x}_n \in c_2) \end{cases}. \quad (17.16)$$

The slack variable $\xi_n \geq 0$ means the penalty for misclassification. As shown in Figure 17.2(d), the feature vector $\boldsymbol{x}_n$ with $\xi_n = 0$ is correctly classified, $\boldsymbol{x}_n$ with $0 < \xi_n \leq 1$ is in the margin but correctly classified, and $\boldsymbol{x}_n$ with $\xi_n > 1$ is misclassified. To obtain the optimal hyperplane in linearly inseparable problems, we need to find $\boldsymbol{w}$, b, and $\boldsymbol{\xi}$ that maximize the margin as well as minimize the sum of slack variables while satisfying Eq. (17.15). Therefore, Eq. (17.14) can be modified as follows:

$$\min_{w,b,\xi} \left(\frac{1}{2}||\boldsymbol{w}||^2 + C\sum_{n=1}^{N}\xi_n \right)$$

$$\text{subject to } t_n(\boldsymbol{w}^{\mathrm{T}}\boldsymbol{\phi}(\boldsymbol{x}_n)+b) \geq 1-\xi_n \text{ and } \xi_n \geq 0 \, (n=1,2,\ldots,N), \quad (17.17)$$

where $C > 0$ is a hyperparameter that controls the trade-off between the margin and the penalty of slack variables. A larger C imposes more severe penalties for misclassifications, which results in the hyperplane with a narrower margin. Although the margin obtained from Eq. (17.17) is called the soft margin, it is equivalent to the hard margin when $C \to \infty$. On the other hand, a smaller C means the allowance of more misclassifications and leads to the hyperplane with a wider margin. The constrained minimization problem in Eq. (17.17) can be solved using the Lagrange multiplier method. The Lagrange function L for the minimization problem is given as

$$
\begin{aligned}
&L(\boldsymbol{w},\boldsymbol{b},\xi,\boldsymbol{\alpha},\boldsymbol{\beta}) \\
&=\frac{1}{2}\|\boldsymbol{w}\|^2+C\sum_{n=1}^{N}\xi_n-\sum_{n=1}^{N}\alpha_n\left\{t_n(\boldsymbol{w}^{\mathrm{T}}\boldsymbol{\phi}(\boldsymbol{x}_n)+b)-1+\xi_n\right\}-\sum_{n=1}^{N}\beta_n\xi_n \\
&\qquad \text{subject to}\, \alpha_n\left\{t_n(\boldsymbol{w}^{\mathrm{T}}\boldsymbol{\phi}(\boldsymbol{x}_n)+b)-1+\xi_n\right\}=0 \\
&\qquad \text{with}\, \alpha_n \geq 0 \,\text{and}\, \beta_n\xi_n=0 \,\text{with}\, \beta_n \geq 0,
\end{aligned} \tag{17.18}
$$

where α_n and β_n are Lagrange multipliers. From the partial derivatives of $L(\boldsymbol{w}, \boldsymbol{b}, \xi, \boldsymbol{\alpha}, \boldsymbol{\beta})$ with respect to $\boldsymbol{w}$, b, and ξ_n, we can obtain the following results:

$$\frac{\partial L}{\partial \boldsymbol{w}}=0 \Rightarrow \boldsymbol{w}=\sum_{n=1}^{N}a_n t_n\boldsymbol{\phi}(\boldsymbol{x}_n) \tag{17.19}$$

$$\frac{\partial L}{\partial b}=0 \Rightarrow \sum_{n=1}^{N}a_n t_n=0 \tag{17.20}$$

$$\frac{\partial L}{\partial \xi_n}=0 \Rightarrow C=a_n+\beta_n. \tag{17.21}$$

Hence, we can plug these partial derivative results of Eqs. (17.19), (17.20), and (17.21) to obtain the dual Lagrange function $\tilde{L}$ and represent the optimization problem in Eq. (17.17) with one variable $\boldsymbol{\alpha}$ and the kernel function in Eq. (17.12) as

$$\max_{\boldsymbol{\alpha}}\left(\tilde{L}(\boldsymbol{\alpha})=\sum_{n=1}^{N}\alpha_n-\frac{1}{2}\sum_{n=1}^{N}\sum_{m=1}^{N}\alpha_n\alpha_m t_n t_m \boldsymbol{\phi}(\boldsymbol{x}_n)^{\mathrm{T}}\boldsymbol{\phi}(\boldsymbol{x}_m)\right)$$
$$\Rightarrow \max_{\boldsymbol{\alpha}}\left(\tilde{L}(\boldsymbol{\alpha})=\sum_{n=1}^{N}\alpha_n-\frac{1}{2}\sum_{n=1}^{N}\sum_{m=1}^{N}\alpha_n\alpha_m t_n t_m k(\boldsymbol{x}_n,\boldsymbol{x}_m)\right)$$
$$\text{subject to } 0\le\alpha_n\le C \text{ and} \sum_{n=1}^{N}\alpha_n t_n=0. \quad (17.22)$$

Therefore, the optimal hyperplane can be found by using optimization methods such as sequential minimal optimization [3] to solve for $\boldsymbol{\alpha}$ based on Eq. (17.22).

SVMs are a powerful machine learning model, which has high classification performance even when the data dimension is large and can always find a global optimal solution. However, there are some limitations to SVM-based medical image analysis. First, SVMs are difficult to train on large datasets because the computational costs for training increase exponentially with increasing training data samples. Second, SVMs are an algorithm for mainly applying to binary classification tasks although they can also be applied to regression and multi-class classification tasks. Third, SVMs often require preprocessing to extract and select effective image feature vectors for classification tasks. Additionally, SVMs require an appropriate selection of the kernel functions and their hyperparameters to enhance the classification performance.

17.2.2 Convolutional Neural Network

Convolutional neural network (CNN), which is a type of neural network that is mainly used for image analysis, has a hierarchical structure that mimics the mechanism of the human visual cortex. It originated from Neocognitron [4] and LeNet [5]. As with neural networks, every CNN has input, hidden, and output layers, and especially a CNN with two or more hidden layers is known as a deep convolutional neural network (DCNN), which is one of the deep learning-based image analysis methods. CNNs usually consist of convolution layers, pooling layers, and fully connected layers. The convolution layers extract features from input images, pooling layers aggregate the salient information from the extracted features, and fully connected layers are used in typical neural networks and provide output prediction results based on the aggregated features.

As in Section 17.2.1, we here consider training a CNN for binary classification based on N training data samples that belong to two classes c_1 and c_2. Suppose the training data samples are grayscale images $\boldsymbol{x}_n (n = 1, ..., N)$ with the size of H × W × 1 (height × width × channel) and the CNN architecture consists of one convolution layer, one pooling layer, and one fully connected layer. Figure 17.3 shows an overview of the CNN architecture. The CNN model can be trained with feedforward and backpropagation processes.

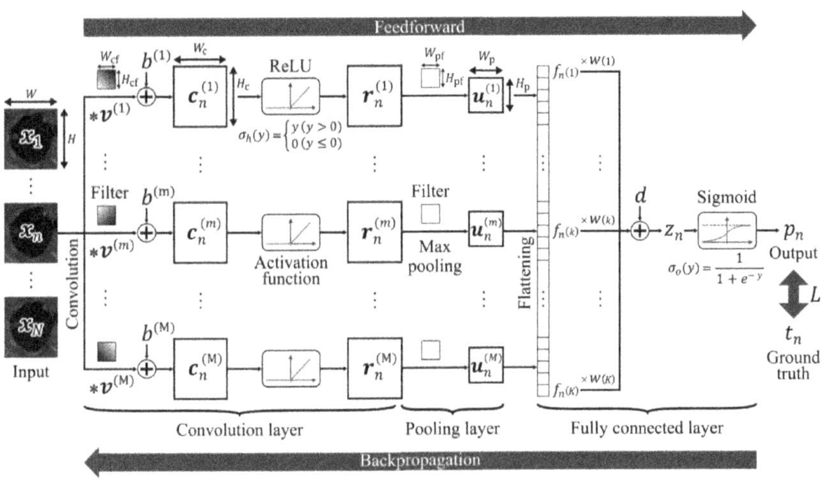

Figure 17.3 Overview of CNN architecture.

In the feedforward process, the CNN output prediction results $p_n (n = 1, ..., N)$ through convolution, pooling, and fully connected layers. It first uses a convolution layer to extract feature maps $\boldsymbol{r}_n$ from input images $\boldsymbol{x}_n$. The convolution layer uses M convolution filters with the size of H_{cf} × W_{cf} to perform convolution operations, which are a dot product operation between the convolution filter sliding over the input image and the overlapped local region as shown in Figure 17.4(a), adds a bias to the convolution output, and subsequently applies an activation function σ_h to the convolution result $\boldsymbol{c}_n$. The outputs

$\boldsymbol{c}_n^{(m)}$ and $\boldsymbol{r}_n^{(m)}$ resulting from m-th convolution filter are represented as

$$c_n^{(m)}(i_c, j_c) = \sum_{i_{cf}=1}^{H_{cf}} \sum_{j_{cf}=1}^{W_{cf}} (v^{(m)}(i_{cf}, j_{cf}) x_n(i, j)) + b^{(m)}, \tag{17.23}$$

$$r_n^{(m)}(i_c, j_c) = \sigma_h(c_n^{(m)}(i_c, j_c)),$$
$$\begin{pmatrix} i = 1, \ldots, H, j = 1, \ldots, W, i_{cf} = 1, \ldots, H_{cf}, j_{cf} = 1, \ldots, \\ W_{cf}, i_c = 1, \ldots, H_c, \text{and } j_c = 1, \ldots, W_c \end{pmatrix} \tag{17.24}$$

$$i_c = \frac{i - i_{cf} + P_c}{S_c} + 1 \text{ and } j_c = \frac{j - j_{cf} + P_c}{S_c} + 1. \tag{17.25}$$

$$H_c = \left\lfloor \frac{H - H_{cf} + 2P_c}{S_c} \right\rfloor + 1 \text{ and } W_c = \left\lfloor \frac{W - W_{cf} + 2P_c}{S_c} \right\rfloor + 1, \tag{17.26}$$

where $v^{(\mathrm{m})}$ is a set of values (i.e., weights) in m-th convolution filter. (i, j), (i_{cf}, j_{cf}), and (i_c, j_c) denote the indices of (row, column) of the input image $\boldsymbol{x}_n$, the convolution filter $v^{(\mathrm{m})}$, and the output $\boldsymbol{c}_n^{(m)}$, respectively. $b^{(m)}$ denotes the bias adding to the convolution result from m-th filter. P_c and S_c mean the amount of zero padding (adding zero values around images for size adjustment) and stride (shift for filter sliding), respectively. The convolution operation has two important characteristics of "local receptive field" and "weight sharing". The local receptive field means the restriction of the receptive field, which is defined as the input region to a particular layer, to a local region based on the concept that the closer pixels in an image have stronger connections to each other. While weight sharing means applying a single filter, instead of different filters, to different regions on an image because similar image features may exist in the different image regions. These characteristics allow CNNs to acquire position invariance, i.e., to capture image features regardless of position, while significantly reducing the computational cost. The activation function plays a crucial role in defining how the inputs are transformed into the outputs in convolution and fully connected layers. CNNs typically use non-linear activation functions that help the model acquire the non-linearity for learning complex data patterns, although a linear activation function (i.e., identity function) is exceptionally used in the output layer for regression models.

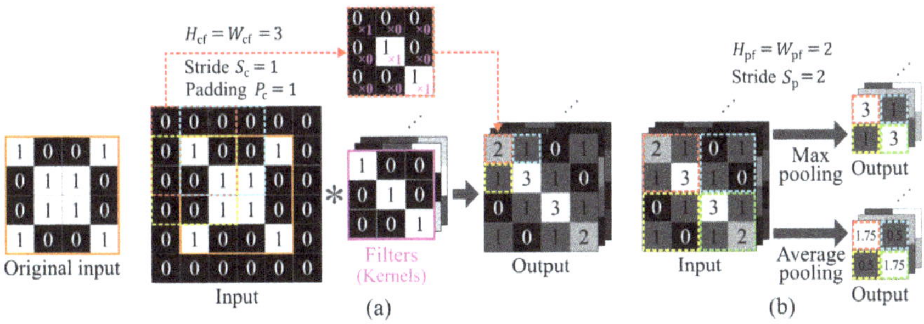

Figure 17.4 Key operations for CNNs: (a) convolution and (b) pooling.

After the convolution layer, the CNN uses a pooling layer to downsample the feature maps extracted by the convolution layer. The pooling operation, which takes a salient feature from the local region overlapped with the pooling filter sliding over the input feature map, as shown in Figure 17.4(b), is performed for each of M feature maps. There are two types of pooling operations: max pooling and average pooling. The max pooling takes the max value from the local image region overlapped with the pooling filter, while the average pooling computes the average value in the overlapped local image region. The output $u_n^{(m)}$ of pooling operation for m-th feature map is defined as

$$u_n^{(m)}(i_p, j_p) = \text{pooling}(r_n^{(m)}(i_c, j_c)),$$
$$(i_c = 1,\cdots,H_c, j_c = 1,\cdots,W_c, i_p = 1,\cdots,H_p, \text{and } j_p = 1,\cdots,W_p) \quad (17.27)$$

$$i_p = \frac{i_c - i_{pf}}{S_p} + 1 \text{ and } j_p = \frac{j_c - j_{pf}}{S_p} + 1, \quad (17.28)$$

$$H_p = \left\lfloor \frac{H_c - H_{pf}}{S_p} \right\rfloor + 1 \text{ and } W_p = \left\lfloor \frac{W_c - W_{pf}}{S_p} \right\rfloor + 1, \quad (17.29)$$

where, pooling $(\cdot)$means the pooling operation. (i_p, j_p) denotes the index of (row, column) of the output $\boldsymbol{u}_n$ from the pooling operation. The pooling operation contributes to improving the robustness of position gaps of objects in images.

Finally, the CNN converts the two-dimensional feature maps $\boldsymbol{u}_n$ into a one-dimensional array by flatten operations and uses a fully connected layer to perform a linear transformation to the flattened features $\boldsymbol{f}_n$ and output the prediction result p_n via the activation function σ_o. The flatten operation is represented as

$$f_n(k) = \text{flatten}(u_n^{(m)}(i_p, j_p)), \quad (k = 1, \ldots, K) \tag{17.30}$$

where

$$k = H_p W_p(m-1) + W_p(i_p - 1) + j_p, \tag{17.31}$$

$$k = H_p W_p M. \tag{17.32}$$

k is the index of the flattened features. And then, the output p_n from the fully connected layer is represented by the following equations:

$$z_n = \sum_{k=1}^{K} w(k) f_n(k) + d, \tag{17.33}$$

$$p_n = \sigma_o(z_n). \tag{17.34}$$

where $\boldsymbol{w}$ and d denote the weight and the bias for linear transformation, respectively. z_n is the linear transformation result in the fully connected layer. σ_o denotes the activation function in the fully connected layer (i.e., output layer).

In the backpropagation process [6], the CNN uses a loss function to evaluate the error between the prediction results p_n and their corresponding ground truths t_n, called "loss", subsequently optimizes the weights (i.e., $\boldsymbol{v}$ and $\boldsymbol{w}$) and the biases (i.e., b and d) in convolution and fully connected layers based on the error with the gradient descent method. In the gradient descent method, the weights and the biases are updated by computing the partial derivatives of the loss function $L(\boldsymbol{w}, d, \boldsymbol{v}, \boldsymbol{b})$ with respect to $\boldsymbol{w}$, d, $\boldsymbol{v}$, and $\boldsymbol{b}$ from backward as follows:

$$w \leftarrow w - \eta \frac{\partial L}{\partial w}, \tag{17.35}$$

$$d \leftarrow d - \eta \frac{\partial L}{\partial d}, \tag{17.36}$$

$$v \leftarrow v - \eta \frac{\partial L}{\partial v}, \tag{17.37}$$

$$\boldsymbol{b} \leftarrow \boldsymbol{b} - \eta \frac{\partial L}{\partial \boldsymbol{b}}, \tag{17.38}$$

where η, called a learning rate, is an important hyper-parameter that controls the number of updates for weights and biases, namely gradient. The partial derivatives of L with respect to $\boldsymbol{w}$ and d in the fully connected layer can be computed as follows:

$$\frac{\partial L}{\partial w(k)} = \frac{\partial L}{\partial p_n} \frac{\partial p_n}{\partial z_n} \frac{\partial z_n}{\partial w(k)} = \frac{\partial L}{\partial p_n} \frac{d\sigma_o(z_n)}{dz_n} f_n(k), \tag{17.39}$$

$$\frac{\partial L}{\partial d} = \frac{\partial L}{\partial p_n} \frac{\partial p_n}{\partial z_n} \frac{\partial z_n}{\partial d} = \frac{\partial L}{\partial p_n} \frac{d\sigma_o(z_n)}{dz_n}. \tag{17.40}$$

These equations include the partial derivatives of activation and loss functions. Table 17.1 summarizes the typical combination of activation and loss functions for CNNs. In the case of binary classification tasks, we can usually use the sigmoid activation function in the output layer and the binary cross-entropy loss function with the ground truth t_n = {0, 1}. By using the combination of activation function σ_o and loss function L indicated in Table 17.1, Eqs. (17.39) and (17.40) can be represented in the following simple equations:

Table 17.1 Typical combination of activation and loss functions for CNNs

Tasks	Functions: Activation function: Hidden layers	Output layer	Loss function
Regression	ReLU function $\sigma_h(y)=\begin{cases} y\,(y>0) \\ 0\,(y\le 0)\end{cases}$	Identity function $\sigma_o(y)=y$	Mean squared error function $L=\frac{1}{2N}\sum_{n=1}^{N}(p_n-t_n)^2$
Binary classification		Sigmoid function $\sigma_o(y)=\frac{1}{1+e^{-y}}$	Binary cross-entropy loss function $L=-\frac{1}{N}\sum_{n=1}^{N}\{t_n\log(p_n)+(1-t_n)\log(1-p_n)\}$
Multi-class classification		Softmax function $\sigma_o(y_c)=\frac{e^{y_c}}{\sum_{c=1}^{C}e^{y_c}}$	Categorical cross-entropy loss function $L=-\frac{1}{N}\sum_{c=1}^{C}\sum_{n=1}^{N}(t_{nc}\log(p_{nc}))$

$$\frac{\partial L}{\partial w(k)}=\frac{1}{N}\sum_{n=1}^{N}(p_n-t_n)f_n(k), \tag{17.41}$$

$$\frac{\partial L}{\partial d}=\frac{1}{N}\sum_{n=1}^{N}(p_n-t_n). \tag{17.42}$$

These equations mean the weights $\boldsymbol{w}$ and the bias d are updated when there are prediction errors. In addition, the partial derivatives of L with respect to $\boldsymbol{v}$ and $\boldsymbol{b}$ in the convolution layer (i.e., hidden layer) can be computed as follows:

$$\begin{aligned}\frac{\partial L}{\partial v^{(m)}(i_{\mathrm{cf}},j_{\mathrm{cf}})}&=\frac{\partial L}{\partial r_n^{(m)}(i_c,j_c)}\frac{\partial r_n^{(m)}(i_c,j_c)}{\partial c_n^{(m)}(i_c,j_c)}\frac{\partial c_n^{(m)}(i_c,j_c)}{\partial v^{(m)}(i_{\mathrm{cf}},j_{\mathrm{cf}})}\\&=\sum_{i_c=1}^{H_c}\sum_{j_c=1}^{W_c}\frac{\partial L}{\partial r_n^{(m)}(i_c,j_c)}\frac{d\sigma_h(c_n^{(m)}(i_c,j_c))}{dc_n^{(m)}(i_c,j_c)}x_n(i,j),\end{aligned} \tag{17.43}$$

$$\frac{\partial L}{\partial b^{(m)}} = \frac{\partial L}{\partial r_n^{(m)}(i_c, j_c)} \frac{\partial r_n^{(m)}(i_c, j_c)}{\partial c_n^{(m)}(i_c, j_c)} \frac{\partial c_n^{(m)}(i_c, j_c)}{\partial b^{(m)}}$$
$$= \sum_{i_c=1}^{H_c} \sum_{j_c=1}^{W_c} \frac{\partial L}{\partial r_n^{(m)}(i_c, j_c)} \frac{d\sigma_h(c_n^{(m)}(i_c, j_c))}{dc_n^{(m)}(i_c, j_c)}. \tag{17.44}$$

The partial derivative of L with respect to $\boldsymbol{r}_n$ in Eqs. (17.43) and (17.44) is obtained by performing the reverse of the flatten and pooling operations on the partial derivative of L with respect to $\boldsymbol{f}_n$ as

$$\frac{\partial L}{\partial f_n(k)} = \frac{\partial L}{\partial p_n} \frac{\partial p_n}{\partial z_n} \frac{\partial z_n}{\partial f_n(k)} = \frac{1}{N} \sum_{n=1}^{N} (p_n - t_n) w(k). \tag{17.45}$$

From Eqs. (17.43) to (17.45), the weights and the biases in the hidden layer are updated with the gradient obtained by multiplying the error propagated from one previous layer by the derivative of activation function σ_h, which means that as the number of hidden layers increases, the number of derivatives of activation function σ_h to be multiplied increases. Thus, in the case of DCNNs with more hidden layers, we encounter the problem of model training and convergence failure because the gradient becomes vanishingly small when the activation function with small derivative values, such as the sigmoid function, is used in hidden layers. This problem is known as the vanishing gradient problem. To overcome this problem, the rectified linear unit (ReLU) function [7] is often used as activation functions σ_h in the hidden layers, which has the derivative as

$$\frac{d\sigma_h(y)}{dy} = \begin{cases} 1 & (y > 0) \\ 0 & (y \leq 0) \end{cases}. \tag{17.46}$$

The ReLU function is mathematically indifferentiable at $y = 0$, but can be used by defining the derivative at $y = 0$ as zero.

DCNNs, which can automatically perform image processing from appropriate feature extraction to classification or regression, have attracted much attention as an image analysis method with higher performance compared to other machine learning-based image analysis methods. In fact, computer-aided diagnosis systems equipped with DCNN-based image analysis techniques have been put into practical use. However, there are some limitations in utilizing DCNNs for image analyses. First, DCNNs need to manually design their architectures including the number of layers and filters, and tune the hyperparameters for training, such as the number of epochs, learning rate, and batch size, according to target tasks and datasets. Second, DCNNs generally require powerful computing resources of graphics processing units and long computing time for training.

17.3 Applications

17.3.1 Applications for Image Diagnosis

Diagnostic assistance using medical image analysis, known as computer-aided diagnosis (CAD), is one of the most popular applications. Since the concept of CAD was established in the 1980s, CAD schemes have been developed widely [8]. Medical image analysis techniques underlying CAD devices include classification, detection, segmentation, denoising, and super-resolution. Figure 17.5 shows an example of the image analysis techniques.

Classification is a technique that classifies images into pre-defined classes and can be applied to support differential diagnosis, including the identification of conditions such as presence/absence, type, malignancy, and grade of lesions from medical images. Detection is a technique that provides the bounding boxes (or ellipses) circumscribed around target objects in medical images and their classes. It can help reduce false negatives (i.e., overlooking of lesions) and false positives (i.e., over-detection of lesions) for image diagnosis. Segmentation is a technique that extracts the shape of target objects in medical images by pixel-wise (or voxel-wise) image classification. It allows doctors to not only localize lesion areas but also quantitatively evaluate the size, volume, and shape of lesions for diagnosis. Denoising is a technique that reduces some noises (e.g., Gaussian, salt-and-pepper, speckle, Poisson, and blurred noises) in medical images, while super-resolution is a technique that enhances the resolution of medical images from low resolution to high resolution. Both denoising and super-resolution can lead to improvement in the visual quality of medical images. These medical image analysis techniques are indispensable for CAD devices and are still being actively studied for further advancement and expanded applications. Especially in the past decade, with the development of deep learning, AI-based medical image analysis techniques using DCNNs have been increasingly developed for CAD applications [9].

As described in Section 17.2, DCNNs consist of the components such as convolution layers, pooling layers, fully connected layers (or upsampling/deconvolution layers), and activation functions, and can be trained using loss functions based on the stochastic gradient descent algorithm. DCNNs for medical image analyses (i.e., classification, detection, segmentation, and denoising/super-resolution) in diagnostic applications have been proposed by changing the combination of these components and loss functions for training according to the desired outputs. Figure 17.6 shows examples of basic DCNN architectures for classification, detection, segmentation, and denoising/super-resolution. The cuboids in this figure mean the outputs (e.g., feature maps) from convolution blocks and deconvolution, pooling, and fully connected layers. The width and height of each cuboid denote the dimension of each output, while the length of it denotes the number of channels.

DCNNs for classification (Figure 17.6(a)), which output the probability of pre-defined classes based on medical image information, have been utilized to assist in the differential diagnosis (e.g., the diagnosis of lesion type, malignancy, and grade) or triage. Representative DCNNs for classification include VGG16 [10], ResNet [11], DenseNet [12], and so on. Moreover, DCNNs with attention mechanisms, which allow the network to focus on more relevant image features, have been proposed for better classification performance [13, 14].

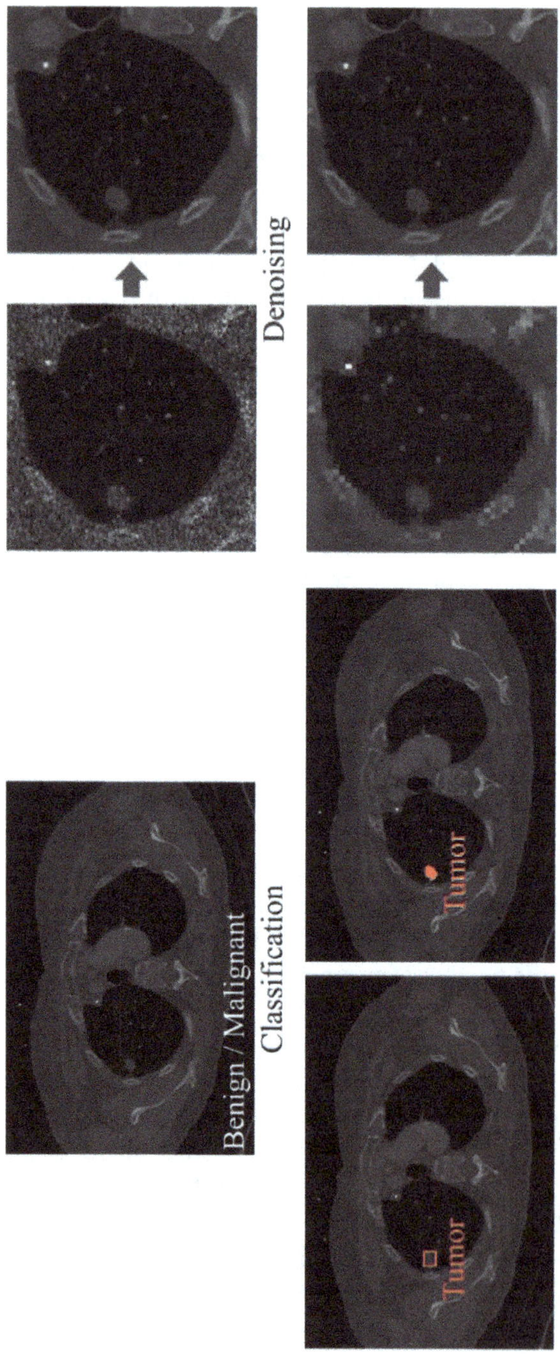

Figure 17.5 Example of medical image analysis for diagnosis.

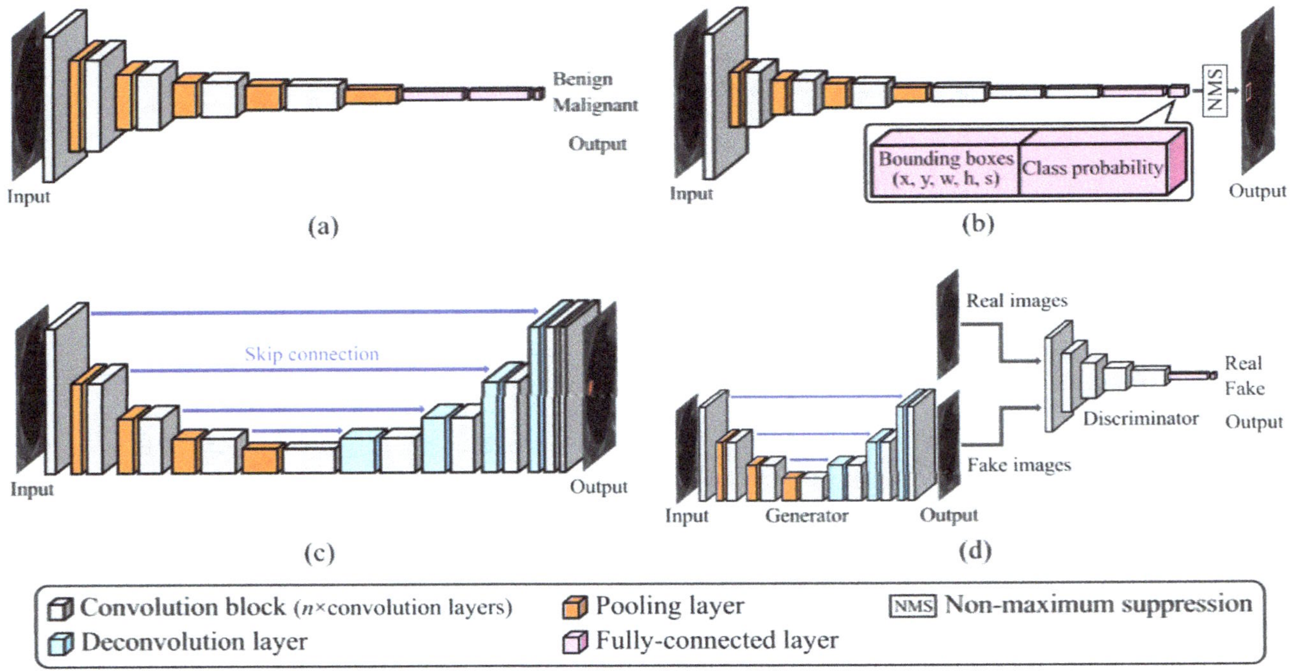

Figure 17.6 Examples of DCNN architectures for medical image analysis: (a) DCNN for classification (e.g., VGG16 [10]), (b) DCNN for detection (e.g., YOLO [16]), (c) DCNN for segmentation (e.g., U-Net [19]), and (d) DCNN for denoising/super-resolution (e.g., DCGAN [21]).

DCNNs for detection (Figure 17.6(b)), which can automatically localize target objects in medical images, are particularly effective to detect lesions in real-time and avoid overlooking lesions and thus have been popularly applied to computer-aided detection for endoscopy. They output the center coordinates (x, y), width w, height h, and confidence score s of bounding boxes and their class probability to predict both positions and classes of target objects in medical images. Subsequently, they provide the final output through non-maximum suppression (NMS), a post-processing algorithm for reducing redundant candidate bounding boxes. They include two types of detectors: two-stage and one-stage detectors. The two-stage detectors (e.g., Faster R-CNN [15]) first generate region proposals (bounding boxes) and then classify the boxes; and one-stage detectors (e.g., YOLO [16] and SSD [17]) predict the bounding boxes and their classes at once. The former tends to have better detection accuracy, while the latter achieves faster detection speed. For the trade-off between accuracy and speed, they are used differently depending on the application and its requirements.

DCNNs for segmentation (Figure 17.6(c)), which can create a pixel-wise (or voxel-wise) mask of each target object in medical images, have been used for not only lesion localization but also differential diagnosis through quantitative analysis of the shape and volume of anatomical structures and lesions. They are called "fully convolutional networks (FCNs)" [18] since they replace all fully connected layers with convolution layers to prevent the loss of spatial information in images. As shown in Figure 17.6(c), FCNs consist of the encoder part for extracting meaningful features from input images by convolution and pooling layers and the decoder part for restoring the downsized features to the input image size by upsampling/deconvolution layers. The most famous FCN architecture is U-Net [19, 20], a symmetrical encoder-decoder architecture that uses skip connections to combine multi-scale image features of the encoder path and the corresponding decoder path for performance improvement, and many of FCNs for medical image segmentation are designed based on U-Net.

DCNNs for denoising/super-resolution (Figure 17.6(d)) include deep convolutional generative adversarial networks (DCGANs) [21], which can generate sophisticated synthetic images. As shown in Figure 17.6(d), they consist of two network models: generator and discriminator. A generator model is trained to create images that look real, while a discriminator model is trained to distinguish between real images and fake images created by the generator model. The generator models in DCGANs trained using noisy and clear images or low-resolution and high-resolution images can be used to image data augmentation and image quality improvement (i.e., denoising and super-resolution) [22].

Traditionally, CAD devices had mainly meant computer-aided detection (CADe) that can help physicians detect lesions on medical images; in fact, all CAD devices commercialized from 1998 (when the first commercial CAD device was launched) until 2016 were only CADe [23]. However, with the development of CAD, especially AI-based CAD (AI-CAD), CAD devices have been recently commercialized not only for detection but also for a wide variety of applications such as the acquisition of high-quality medical images, screening, differential diagnosis, and triage. According to the classification of medical device products by the U.S. Food and Drug Administration (FDA), AI-CAD devices are currently classified into the following types: computer-aided detection (CADe), computer-aided diagnosis (CADx), computer-aided detection/diagnosis (CADe/x), computer-aided acquisition/optimization (CADa/o), and computer-aided triage and notification (CADt). Table 17.2 summarizes the classification of CAD device types defined by the FDA. Moreover, as shown in Figure 17.7, the usage patterns of AI-CAD devices in clinical practice can be categorized into the following three patterns [23, 24]:

(a) **Second reader:** A physician first reads medical images without AI-CAD (1st reading), subsequently, if necessary, he/she reviews the images based on the findings of AI-CAD (2nd reading) and then makes a diagnosis. In addition, interactive AI-CAD [25], which allows a physician to review the computer-estimated findings on the region of his/her interest in the images, is included in this usage pattern.

(b) **Concurrent reader:** A physician reads medical images and the computer-estimated findings from AI-CAD simultaneously and makes a diagnosis.

(c) **First reader:** A physician reads only the image slices with the computer-estimated findings from AI-CAD and makes a diagnosis. Hence, this usage pattern can significantly reduce the time required for reading and diagnosis.

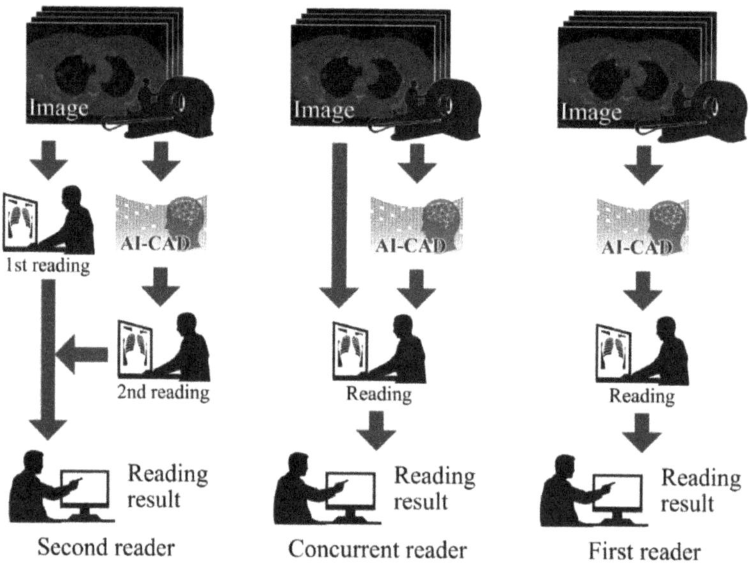

Figure 17.7 Usage patterns of AI-CAD systems (modified from [23, 24]).

Table 17.2 Classification of CAD device types

Type	Description
CADe	Aids in localizing/marking regions that may reveal specific abnormalities
CADx	Aids in characterizing/assessing disease, disease type, severity, stage, and progression
CADe/x	Aid in localizing and characterizing conditions
CADa/o	Aid in the acquisition/optimization of images/diagnostic signals
CADt	Aids in prioritizing/triaging time-sensitive patient detection and diagnosis

Compared to second- and concurrent-reader AI-CAD devices, first-reader AI-CAD devices can reduce the burden on physicians for diagnosis but have a greater impact on physicians' diagnoses and require higher accuracy. Therefore, it should be noted that at present, commercial AI-CAD products, approved by the FDA, include only second- and concurrent-reader AI-CAD devices; most of them are second-reader AI-CAD devices.

As described above, AI-CAD devices have been rapidly developed and commercialized in recent years. However, it should be noted that AI-CAD devices are intended not to make a diagnosis instead of physicians but to reduce the burden on physicians in reading images and to support the decision-making for diagnosis. Even if AI-CAD is used for diagnosis, physicians are basically responsible for diagnosis and making a final diagnostic decision. Therefore, AI-CAD devices do not replace physicians in diagnostic tasks but work collaboratively with physicians to further improve diagnostic accuracy. As medical big data are being accumulated and utilized for AI-CAD worldwide, more and more AI-CAD products will be developed in the future. It is expected that an AI-CAD product that acts as an avatar of experienced physicians will be developed so that the physicians can interactively discuss their diagnosis when they are unsure of it.

17.3.2 Applications for Surgical Navigation

Surgical navigation technology enables surgeons to precisely provide instrument positions and project the instrument onto the pre- or intra-operative imaging data. The goal of surgical navigation is to maximize the effect of surgery and minimize complications to patients by avoiding damage. Especially, navigation systems have been clinically employed in orthopedic surgery and brain surgery and their overcomes have been reported [26–29].

Figure 17.8 shows a typical surgical navigation, which consists of a computer workstation with pre-operative images, a position sensor, and a tracked tool. The tool is visualized in the navigation view, then surgeons can intuitively understand the relative position of the tool and the anatomical structure.

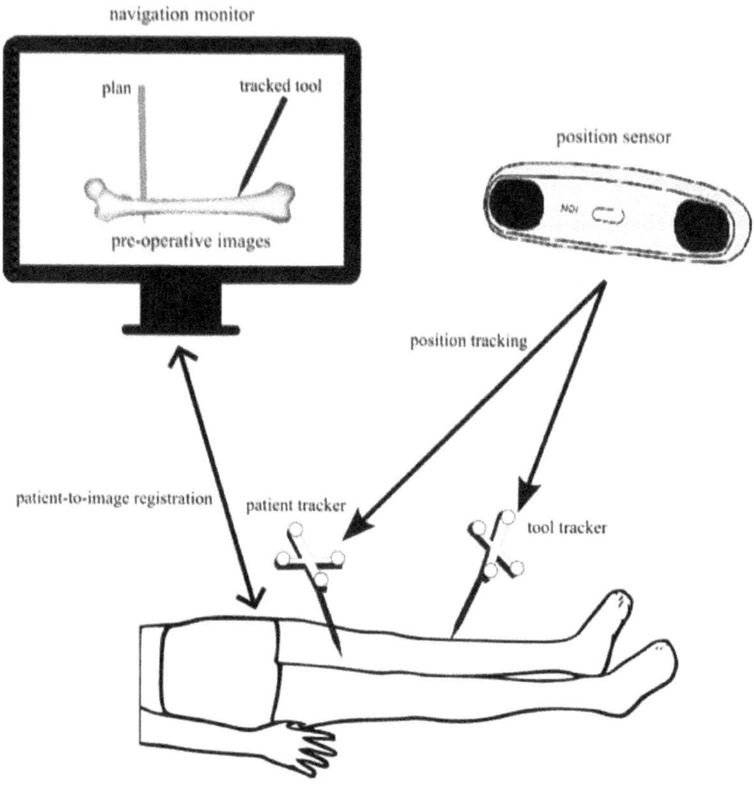

Figure 17.8 Surgical navigation system.

17.3.2.1 Positional sensor

A position sensor is indispensable to measure the relative positions between a patient and instruments. The important specifications of a position sensor are accuracy, sampling rate, latency, working volume, and size of markers and sensors. Two types of tracking technologies, as shown in Table 17.3, have been applied in clinical settings.

Optical tracking

Optical tracking measures a full 6-DOF position of fiducial markers by triangulation using two or more cameras. Near-infrared (IR) optical tracking system is widely used in surgical navigation. Passive markers reflect infrared light, emitted by IR LEDs on the position sensor, meanwhile, active markers actively emit infrared light. The limitation of optical tracking is that the line of sight between the tracked marker and the cameras must be clear.

Electromagnetic tracking

Electromagnetic tracking measures a 5-DOF position of a sensor coil from induced current by the magnetic field generated by a transmitter. A full 6-DOF position can be measured by the combination of two sensor coils. The magnetic field is unobstructed by a human body and some materials such as plastics; therefore, no line-of-sight is needed. Thus, EM tracking supports the tracking of instruments inserted into a patient body. Meanwhile, the working volume is limited rather than optical tracking, and ferromagnetic instruments are not useful due to magnetic field disturbance.

Table 17.3 Features of an optical and electromagnetic tracking

	Optical tracking	Electromagnetic tracking
Features	Wireless	Usable inside a body
Limitation	Camera occlusion	Magnetic field disturbance

17.3.2.2 Intra-operative registration

Registration estimates the transformation between medical images and a patient body to integrate both the coordinate system. Typical approaches are landmark-based registration, surface-based registration, and image-based registration.

Landmark-based registration

Landmark-based registration computes the best match transformation between two sets of points (landmarks) in different coordinate systems, as shown in Figure 17.9. In surgical navigation, external fiducial markers or anatomical landmarks are used. The problem is summarized as follows: Let $\{P_1, P_2\}$ be two pointsets in the patient and preoperative image coordinate systems. These must contain at least three points, respectively. The problem is to find the best transformation T to minimize the sum of square error as

$$T^* = \arg\min_T \sum_i^N || p_1 - Tp_2 ||^2, \tag{17.47}$$

where N is the number of points, T is all possible transformations. The best translation can be determined as the centroids of the two pointsets, and the best rotation is obtained by solving the energy function using singular value decomposition (SVD)[30].

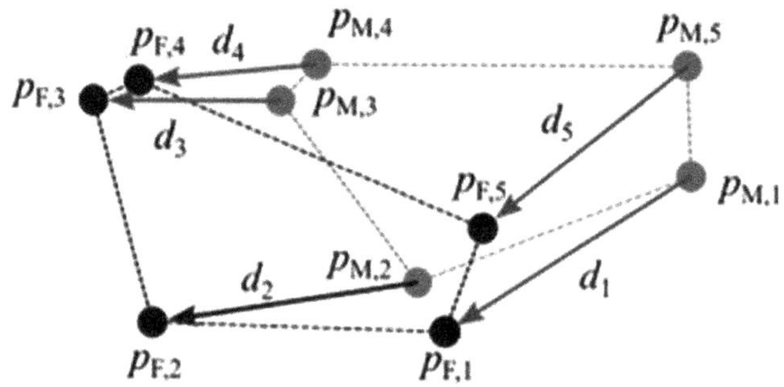

Figure 17.9 Landmark-based registration. The transformation from the moving coordinate system to the fixed coordinate system is estimated by a least square method.

Surface-based registration

The accuracy of the landmark-based registration highly depends on the measurement accuracy of the landmarks. On the other hand, surface-based registration, known as iterative closest point (ICP) registration, is more robust registration than landmark-based registration [31]. In surface-based registration, the best transformation as well as the corresponding points are found between two point clouds on the surfaces, as shown in Figure 17.10. In ICP registration, the best transform is estimated to minimize the sum of square differences $\sum||d_i||^2$ between the closest point pairs. Firstly, the points are chosen from the moving points, then the best transform is computed in the point pair. The computation is repeated until the sum of residual errors becomes sufficiently small. The performance of the surface-based registration depends on the initial transformation, which is generally provided by landmark-based registration.

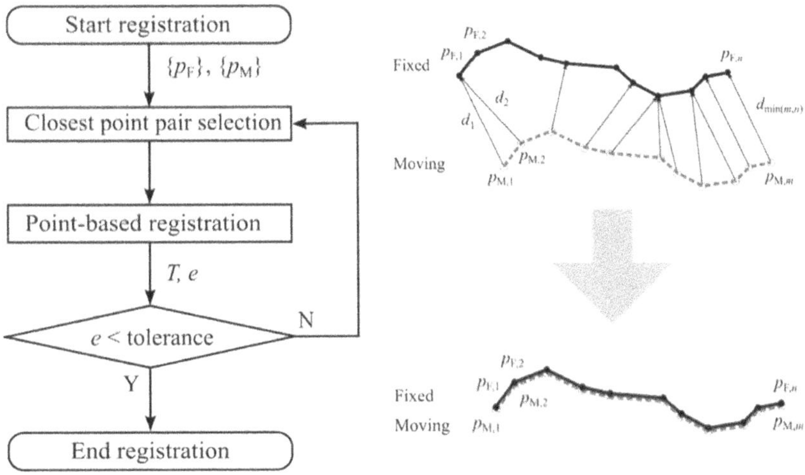

Figure 17.10 Flowchart of ICP registration, which iterates point-based registration if the error is less than tolerance.

Image-based registration

Image-based registration is another registration algorithm between pre- and intra-operative images such as pre-operative CT and intra-operative X-ray fluoroscopy. The algorithm estimates the best transform, which maximizes the similarity or minimizes the difference between two images. Especially, the registration between pre-operative CT and intra-operative X-ray is known as 2D/3D registration. The following metrics are generally used as the energy function.

Mean square difference: The mean squared pixel-wise difference computes the difference in image intensity between two images.

Correlation: Pixel-wise cross-correlation measures the similarity of two images. To reduce the effect of the contrast difference, cross-correlation is normalized by the square root of auto-correlation of the images.

Mutual information: Mutual information derived from entropy is a robust energy function, and is available for multi-modality registration [32, 33].

Figure 17.11 shows the typical algorithm of 2D/3D registration, which determines the posture of the X-ray fluoroscope in the CT coordinate system and evaluates the tentative fluoroscope posture, virtual X-ray.

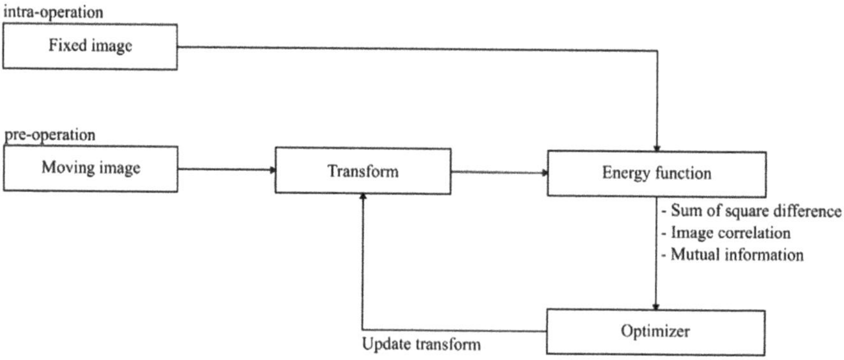

Figure 17.11 Block diagram of image registration.

17.3.2.3 Visualization

Two visualization methods, virtual reality (VR) and augmented reality (AR), are used in surgical navigation. Respective methods are selected for medical procedures such as percutaneous, endoscopic, etc.

Virtual Reality

A VR approach is very similar to a car navigation system. In place of a road map, pre- or intra-operative images are used as an anatomical map. Raw medical images or 2D slices are used as well as 3D models generated by segmentation of 3D volume. On the 'map', surgical plans and intra-operative tracked tools are visualized for surgeons to intuitively understand the relative positions. Figure 17.12 shows an example of VR visualization in the surgical navigation system. Surgeons can intuitively understand the relative position between the vertebra and the surgical tool.

Augmented Reality

AR superimposes the information to surgical views. For example, there is a system that superimposes important tissues such as blood vessels, nerves, and lesions in organs obtained from pre-operative images onto the endoscopic view. A surgeon can see the internal structure intuitively. Figure 17.13 shows an example of AR visualization for brain surgery. You can see the brain structure with the tumor superimposed onto the real scene.

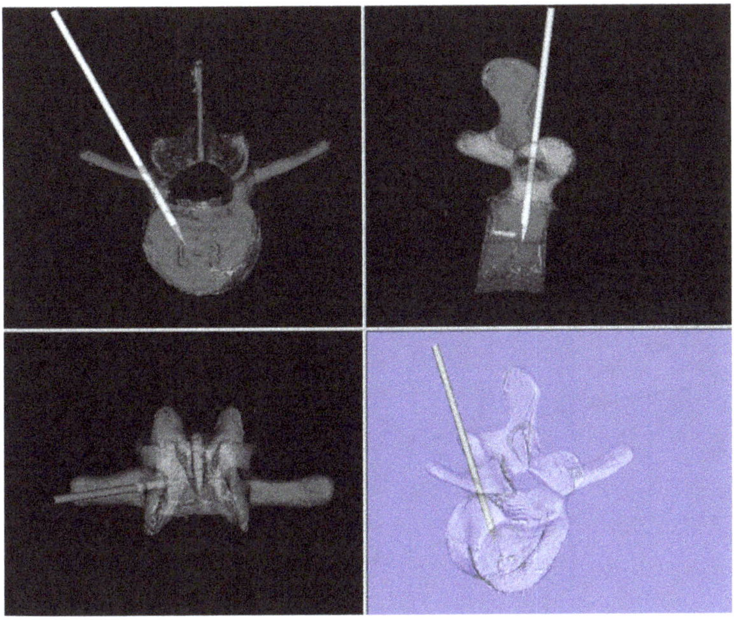

Figure 17.12 An example of VR visualization.

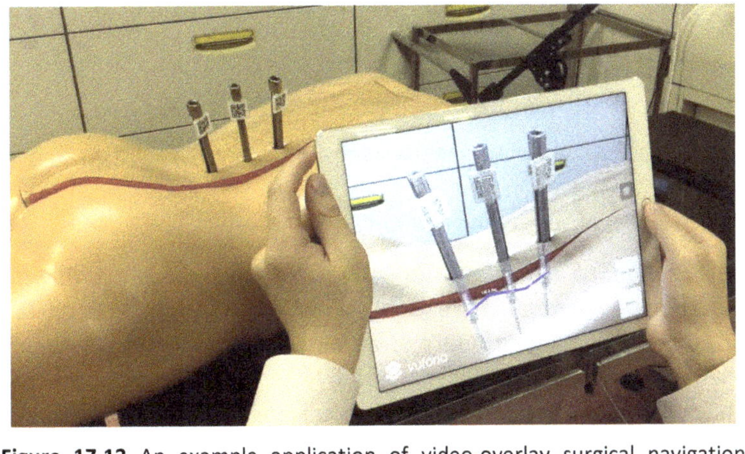

Figure 17.13 An example application of video-overlay surgical navigation systems.

To superimpose virtual data onto video frames, a virtual 3D point $p(x,y,z)$ in the world coordinate system is transformed to a pixel position $p'(u,v)$ in the image coordinate system, shown in Figure 17.14. The transformation is expressed as

$$\begin{pmatrix} u \\ v \end{pmatrix} = C_I C_E \begin{pmatrix} x \\ y \\ z \\ 1 \end{pmatrix} = \begin{pmatrix} f_x & 0 & c_x \\ 0 & f_y & c_y \\ 0 & 0 & 1 \end{pmatrix} \begin{pmatrix} r_{11} & r_{12} & r_{13} & t_1 \\ r_{21} & r_{22} & r_{23} & t_2 \\ r_{31} & r_{32} & r_{33} & t_3 \end{pmatrix} \begin{pmatrix} x \\ y \\ z \\ 1 \end{pmatrix}, \quad (17.48)$$

where C_I and C_E are respectively the intrinsic and extrinsic matrices of a camera. The camera properties are determined by camera calibration [34].

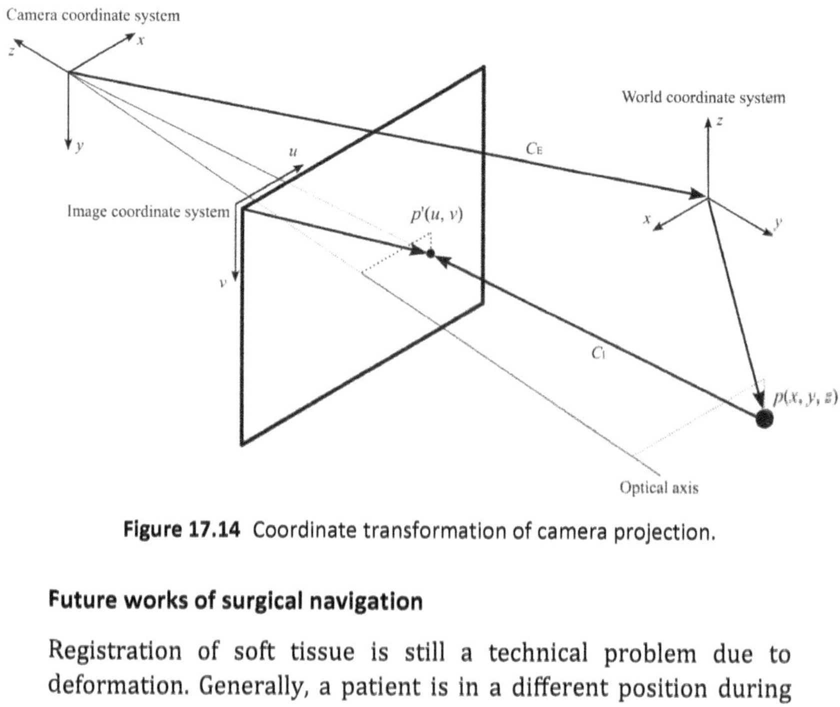

Figure 17.14 Coordinate transformation of camera projection.

Future works of surgical navigation

Registration of soft tissue is still a technical problem due to deformation. Generally, a patient is in a different position during pre-operative imaging and operation. Organ shape and its inner structure are significantly changed by the operative position of a patient. Therefore, accurate navigation is very difficult in a surgery targeting soft organs such as abdominal surgery.

17.3.3 Applications for Medical Robotics

17.3.3.1 Visual feedback

The word "visual feedback" in this context means giving visual information to users of the medical robot. Nearly every medical robot in the market now works with visual aids like RGB views, stereo laparoscopic images, CT pictures, OCT imaging, etc. However, these are basic visual feedback directly received from visual apparatuses like endoscopic cameras. In this section, we will discuss two types of sophisticated visual feedback: AR and 3D reconstruction, which process the users' fundamental visual data and present them with additional information.

AR is a popular research field over the past decades. According to the definition [35], AR is used in 3D virtual items that are blended into a 3D real environment in real-time.

Examples of typical AR applications in medical robotics include improving the recognition of key vascular, pinpointing the location of the affected parts using image segmentation, drawing the safe operation area, etc. The fundamental challenge with AR is correctly positioning the user and the object in the 3D space. The most common method for 3D positioning in medical robotics is simultaneous localization and mapping (SLAM) because of the robot's great positioning precision.

Besides the inside information of the surgery space, understanding the external geometry of the operational target organ is also important. One technique is 3D reconstruction, which mimics the shape and appearance of real objects. This process can be accomplished either by active or passive methods.

The active method uses the depth map to reconstruct the 3D shape by numerical approximation approach. This method mechanically interferes with the objective organ. Figure 17.15 shows a schematic approach to reconstructing the shape of eyeball for the robotic-assisted eye surgery using an ophthalmic endoscope inserted into the patient's eye. For each pixel in the endoscopic image ($(u, v)^T$ is the position of the pixel in the image coordinate $\sum_i$), first calculate the position of the corresponding fundus point (x_c, y_c, z_c) in the camera coordinate $\sum_c$ by methods of distance estimation such as neural network, second, and transfer (x_c, y_c, z_c) to that in the world coordinate (x_W, y_W, z_W) by using the kinematics of the robot, then use the point cloud (x_W, y_W, z_W) to reconstruct the fundus shape. The passive methods follow a similar pattern but do not interfere with the objective organ. They employ sensors such as OCT, X-ray, MRI, etc. to measure the radiance reflected from the objective organ to deduce its 3D structure through methods of image processing.

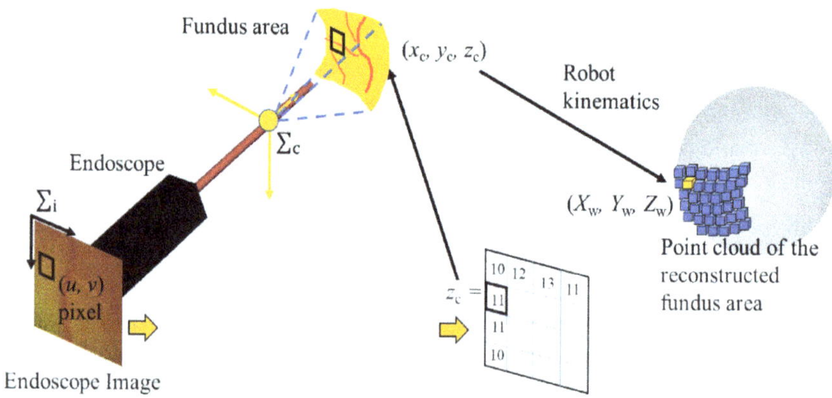

Figure 17.15 Schematic of active 3D reconstruction using an ophthalmic endoscope inserted into the patient's eye.

17.3.3.2 Force feedback

Adding force feedback to the medical robotic system has advantages such as improving operational safety and efficiency. Force measurement and force presentation are the two key components of realizing force feedback.

Force measurement is about the instrument side. The conventional method of using force sensors is inapplicable to medical robots. In comparison to disposable surgical equipment, the cost of a compact force sensor is significant (more than 5,000 dollars). Moreover, the precision of the force sensor is compromised by the moist in-vivo environment. These reasons account for the absence of the force feedback function in the current commercialized surgery assistant robot systems like Da Vinci (Intuitive Surgical, USA), and Hinotori (Medicaroid Corp., Japan).

One alternative method is using strain gauges. The low cost and the layout flexibility of the strain gauges allow the system designers to locate them at the robot components outside the human body. Then, the interaction force with the organ that appeared at the tip of the robot instrument can be calculated from the measured value of the strain gauges and the position/gesture of the robot instrument. Another method is designing a disturbance observer in the control system, which considers the interaction force as an external disturbance. For a medical robot system, measuring the tiny forces during the surgery is necessary. Hence, the key point of realizing disturbance observer in a medical robot system is the backdrivability of the actuator and the accurate dynamic model of the robot. The bi-lateral drive gear [36] is a potential option for developing a conventional motor-gear-actuated medical robot with an external force observer. Some studies use novel actuators with high back-drivability such as pneumatical cylinders to realize sensor-less external force measurement [37].

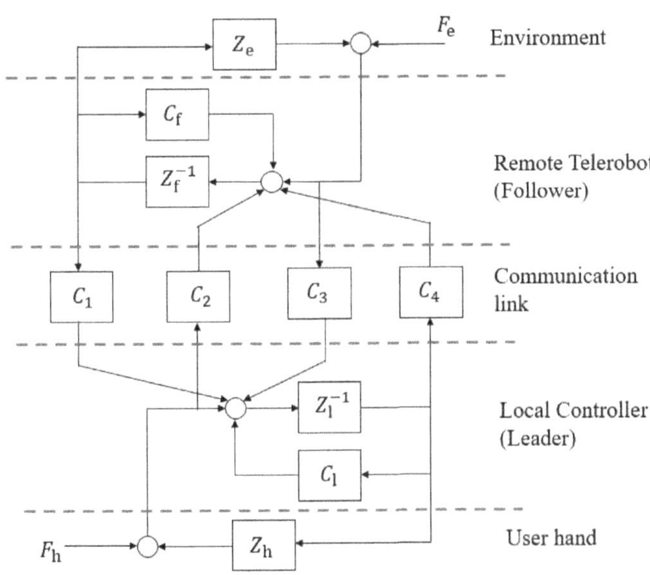

Figure 17.16 General diagram of teleoperation system.

Force presentation is about the user side. "Transparency" is an indicator of the force presentation. When using a transparent system, because the force fed back to the user is the same as what occurred at the instrument side, users feel that they are directly operating the organ by hand.

In medical robots, teleoperation is typically utilized to realize force feedback. Figure 17.16 is the general diagram of the teleoperation system. The blocks are the system factors including the mechanical impedance, the organ stiffness, the time lag, etc. Because of these factors, an absolutely transparent teleoperation system does not exist. However, the system designer can adjust the system factors to make the force fed back to the user's hand (F_h) close to that of the environment (F_e). When doing this, multiple theories like system stability, modern control theory, control theory, etc. should be used.

17.3.3.3 Material informatics

In general, the performance of the instruments used in the medical robot is determined by the property of the material. For example, robotic forceps with a wrist joint made of PEEK plastic can provide high bending flexibility in a small space and durability after being bent more than 10 thousand times [38]. An organ-grasping device consisting of two overlapping beams that are elastic in the bending direction and rigid in the axial direction, and can realize the tunable stiffness. This organ-grasping device can mimic the shape of the organ in the low stiffness condition, and efficiently transfer the force from the surgical instruments to the objective organ in the high stiffness condition [39].

Material informatics (MI) is used to increase the efficiency of materials development by applying the information science technologies such as artificial intelligence (AI). Currently, the approach of MI is used to search for the optimal materials with desired properties from many options.

In the past, researchers developed materials by thoroughly cataloging all potential elements and formations through countless experiments. By using MI, researchers can find the target materials more quickly than before. For example, using machine learning to analyze the data in past experiments, papers, and simulations, several guesses are made about the molecular structure of the material, element combinations, and manufacturing methods.

Researchers can implement verification experiments based on the advised results.

One of the open MI tools is Matlantis, a general-purpose simulator developed by ENEOS. Co and Preferred Networks, Inc. By using deep learning, this simulator can reproduce materials at the atomic level and search for new materials, and it can perform simulations in a few seconds.

In addition to the software technologies such as machine learning, improvements in hardware technologies such as computing power are also essential for the development of MI. Expectations are also high for the use of quantum computers in the future.

References

1. Boser B. E., Guyon I. M., Vapnik V. (1992). A training algorithm for optimal margin classifiers. *Proc. the Fifth Annual Workshop on Computational Learning Theory*, pp. 144–152.
2. Cortes C., Vapnik V. (1995). Support-vector networks. *Machine Learning*, **20(3)**, pp. 273–297.
3. Platt J. C. (1998). Sequential minimal optimization: A fast algorithm for training support vector machines. *Microsoft Research Technical Report*, MSR-TR-98-14.
4. Fukushima K., Miyake S. (1982). Neocognitron: A new algorithm for pattern recognition tolerant of deformations and shift in position. *Pattern Recognit.*, **15(6)**, pp. 455–469.
5. LeCun Y., Bottou L., Bengio Y., Haffner P. (1998). Gradient-based learning applied to document recognition. *Proc. IEEE*, **86(11)**, pp. 2278–2324.
6. Rumelhart D. E., Mcclelland, J. (1986). Parallel distributed processing: explorations in the microstructure of cognition. *MIT Press*.
7. Nair V., Hinton G. E. (2010). Rectified linear units improve restricted Boltzmann machines. *Proc. Int. Conf. Mach. Learn.*
8. Doi K. (2007). Computer-aided diagnosis in medical imaging: historical review, current status and future potential. *Comput. Med. Imaging Graph.*, **31(4–5)**, pp. 198–211.
9. Litjens G., Kooi T., Bejnordi B. E., Setio A. A. A., Ciompi F., Ghafoorian M., Van Der Laak J. A., Van Ginneken B., Sánchez C. I. (2017). A survey on deep learning in medical image analysis. *Med. Image Anal.*, **42**, pp. 60–88.

10. Simonyan K., Zisserman A. (2014). Very deep convolutional networks for large-scale image recognition. *arXiv preprint arXiv:1409.1556*.
11. He K., Zhang X., Ren S., Sun J. (2016). Deep residual learning for image recognition. *Proc. IEEE Comput. Soc. Conf. Comput. Vis. Pattern Recognit.*, pp. 770–778.
12. Huang G., Liu Z., Van Der Maaten L., Weinberger K. Q. (2017). Densely connected convolutional networks. *Proc. IEEE Comput. Soc. Conf. Comput. Vis. Pattern Recognit.*, pp. 4700–4708.
13. Wang F., Jiang M., Qian C., Yang S., Li C., Zhang H., Wang X., Tang X. (2017). Residual attention network for image classification. *Proc. IEEE Comput. Soc. Conf. Comput. Vis. Pattern Recognit.*, pp. 3156–3164.
14. Hu J., Shen L., Sun G. (2018). Squeeze-and-excitation networks. *Proc. IEEE Comput. Soc. Conf. Comput. Vis. Pattern Recognit.*, pp. 7132–7141.
15. Ren S., He K., Girshick R., Sun J. (2015). Faster R-CNN: Towards real-time object detection with region proposal networks. *Adv. Neural. Inf. Process. Syst.*, **28**.
16. Redmon J., Divvala S., Girshick R., Farhadi A. (2016). You only look once: Unified, real-time object detection.
17. Liu W., Anguelov D., Erhan D., Szegedy C., Reed S., Fu C. Y., Berg A. C. (2016). SSD: Single shot multibox detector. *European Conference on Computer Vision*, pp. 21–37. *Proc. IEEE Comput. Soc. Conf. Comput. Vis. Pattern Recognit.*, pp. 779–788.
18. Long J., Shelhamer E., Darrell T. (2015). Fully convolutional networks for semantic segmentation. *Proc. IEEE Comput. Soc. Conf. Comput. Vis. Pattern Recognit.*, pp. 3431–3440.
19. Ronneberger O., Fischer P., Brox T. (2015). U-Net: Convolutional networks for biomedical image segmentation. *Med. Image Comput. Comput. Assist. Interv.*, pp. 234–241.
20. Çiçek Ö., Abdulkadir A., Lienkamp S. S., Brox T., Ronneberger O. (2016). 3D U-Net: learning dense volumetric segmentation from sparse annotation. *Med. Image Comput. Comput. Assist. Interv.*, pp. 424–432.
21. Radford A., Metz L., Chintala S. (2015). Unsupervised representation learning with deep convolutional generative adversarial networks. *arXiv preprint arXiv:1511.06434*.
22. Yi X., Walia E., Babyn P. (2019). Generative adversarial network in medical imaging: A review. *Med. Image Anal.*, **58**, 101552.

23. Fujita H. (2020). AI-based computer aided diagnosis (AI-CAD): The latest review to read first. *Radiol. Phys. Technol.*, **13(1)**, pp. 6–19.

24. Beyer F., Zierott L., Fallenberg F. M., Juergens K. U., Stoeckel J., Heindel W., Wormanns D. (2007). Comparison of sensitivity and reading time for the use of computer-aided detection (CAD) of pulmonary nodules at MDCT as concurrent or second reader. *Eur. Radiol.*, **17(11)**, pp. 2941–2947.

25. Rodríguez-Ruiz A., Krupinski E., Mordang J. J., Schilling K., Heywang-Köbrunner S. H., Sechopoulos I., Mann R. M. (2019). Detection of breast cancer with mammography: Effect of an artificial intelligence support system. *Radiology*, **290(2)**, pp. 305–314.

26. Wirtz C. R., Knauth M., Staubert A., Bonsanto M. M., Sartor K., Kunze S., Tronnier V. M. (2000). Clinical evaluation and follow-up results for intraoperative magnetic resonance imaging in neurosurgery. *Neurosurgery*, **46(5)**, pp. 1112–1122.

27. Foley K. T., Simon D. A., Rampersaud Y. R. (2001). Virtual fluoroscopy: Computer-assisted fluoroscopic navigation. *Spine*, **26(4)**, pp. 347–351.

28. Kosmopoulos V., Schizas C. (2007). Pedicle screw placement accuracy: A meta-analysis. *Spine*, **32(3)**, pp. E111–E120. DOI: 10.1097/01.brs.0000254048.79024.8b

29. Parratte S., Argenson J.-N. A. (2007). Validation and usefulness of a computer-assisted cup-positioning system in total hip arthroplasty: A prospective, randomized, controlled study. *The Journal of Bone & Joint Surgery*, **89(3)**, pp. 494–499. DOI: 10.2106/JBJS.F.00529

30. Berthold K. P. H. (1987). Closed-form solution of absolute orientation using unit quaternions. *J. Opt. Soc. Am. A.*, **4**, pp. 629–642.

31. Besl P. J., McKay N. D. (1992). A method for registration of 3-D shapes. *IEEE Transactions on Pattern Analysis and Machine Intelligence*, **14(2)**, pp. 239–256. DOI: 10.1109/34.121791.

32. Wells W. M., Viola P., Atsumi H., Nakajima S., Kikinis R. (1996). Multi-modal volume registration by maximization of mutual information. *Medical Image Analysis*, **1(1)**, pp. 35–51. https://doi.org/10.1016/S1361-8415(01)80004-9.

33. Pluim J. P., Maintz J. B. A., Viergever M. A. (2003). Mutual-information-based registration of medical images: A survey. *IEEE Transactions on Medical Imaging*, **22(8)**, pp. 986–1004.

34. Zhang Z. (2000). A flexible new technique for camera calibration. *IEEE Transactions on Pattern Analysis and Machine Intelligence,* **22(11)**, pp. 1330–1334. DOI: 10.1109/34.888718.
35. Azuma R.T. (1997). A survey of augmented reality. *Presence: Teleoperators Virtual Env.,* **6**, pp. 355–385.
36. Matsuki H., Nagano L., Fujimoto Y. (2009). Bilateral drive gear: A highly backdrivable reduction gearbox for robotic actuators. *IEEE/ASME Transactions on Mechatronics,* **24(6)**, pp. 2661–2673.
37. Zhou D., Haraguchi D. (2022). Design and evaluation of a robotic forceps with flexible wrist joint made of PEEK Plastic. *IEEE Robotics and Automation Letters,* **7(3)**.
38. Zhou D., Sanada K., and Haraguchi D. (2020). Robotic forceps with a flexible wrist joint made of super engineering plastic. *Sensors and Materials,* **32(3)**, pp. 1027–1039.
39. Kim J., Nakajima Y., Kobayashi K. (2018). A suction-fixing, stiffness-tunable liver manipulator for laparoscopic surgeries. *IEEE/ASME Trans. on Mechatronics,* **23(1)**, pp. 262–273.

Index

For Product Safety Concerns and Information please contact our EU
representative GPSR@taylorandfrancis.com
Taylor & Francis Verlag GmbH, Kaufingerstraße 24, 80331 München, Germany

www.ingramcontent.com/pod-product-compliance
Lightning Source LLC
LaVergne TN
LVHW020627300926
849161LV00004B/632
* 9 7 8 9 8 1 5 1 2 9 1 6 8 *